THE HUMAN BRAIN AND NEUROPLASTICITY

The HUMAN BRAIN and NEUROPLASTICITY

edited by
Jordan Grafman
Paolo Nichelli

THE GUILFORD PRESS
New York London

A Division of Guilford Publications, Inc.
www.guilford.com

Printed in the United States of America

This book is printed on acid-free paper.

For product and safety concerns within the EU, please contact *GPSR@taylorandfrancis.com,* Taylor & Francis Verlag GmbH, Kaufingerstraße 24, 80331 München, Germany.

Last digit is print number: 9 8 7 6 5 4 3 2 1

This publication is intended to provide helpful and informative material. It is not intended to diagnose, treat, cure, or prevent any health problem or condition, nor is it intended to replace the advice of a health professional. No action should be taken based solely on the contents of this book. Always consult your physician or qualified health care professional on any matters regarding your health and before adopting any suggestions in this book or drawing inferences from it.

The authors and publisher specifically disclaim all responsibility for any liability, loss, or risk, personal or otherwise, which is incurred as a consequence, directly or indirectly, from the use or application of any contents of this book.

Any and all product names referenced within this book are the trademarks of their respective owners. Always read all information provided by the manufacturers' product labels before using their products. The authors and publisher are not responsible for claims made by manufacturers.

Library of Congress Cataloging-in-Publication Data

Names: Grafman, Jordan editor | Nichelli, Paolo F., editor
Title: Human brain and neuroplasticity / edited by Jordan Grafman, Paolo F. Nichelli.
Description: New York : The Guilford Press, [2026] | Includes bibliographical references and index. |
Identifiers: LCCN 2025038855 | ISBN 9781462562435 cloth
Subjects: LCSH: Neuroplasticity | Brain--Physiology | Neural networks (Neurobiology) | BISAC: PSYCHOLOGY / Neuropsychology | PSYCHOLOGY / Cognitive Neuroscience & Cognitive Neuropsychology
Classification: LCC QP363.3 .H86 2026
LC record available at ***https://lccn.loc.gov/2025038855***

About the Editors

Jordan Grafman, PhD, is Director of Brain Injury Research and Chief of the Cognitive Neuroscience Laboratory at the Shirley Ryan AbilityLab and Professor in the Department of Physical Medicine and Rehabilitation at Northwestern University. He served as Chief of the Cognitive Neuroscience Laboratory at the National Institute of Neurological Disorders and Stroke for several decades. With more than 600 publications, Dr. Grafman currently focuses his research on the brain bases of belief and the brain networks supporting reward and reinforcement. He also leads the Vietnam Head Injury Study. Dr. Grafman is a recipient of the U.S. Department of Defense Meritorious Service Award, the National Institutes of Health Award of Merit, the National Institutes of Health Director's Award, and the Research Award from the Alexander von Humboldt Foundation in Germany.

Paolo Nichelli, MD, is a retired Full Professor of Neurology at the University of Modena and Reggio Emilia in Modena, Italy, and former Clinical Director of the Neuroscience Department at the Sant'Agostino-Estense Modena Hospital. Since the beginning of his career, his research has focused on clinical and experimental neuropsychology. As a Visiting Scientist in the Cognitive Neuroscience Laboratory at the National Institute of Neurological Disorders and Stroke in the early 1990s, Dr. Nichelli became interested in using functional neuroimaging methods, which he later helped implement in Modena. A founding member and past president of the Italian Society of Neuropsychology, Dr. Nichelli has published over 280 scientific articles and book chapters.

About the Editors

Contributors

Georgette Argiris, PhD, Division of Cognitive Neuroscience, Columbia University, New York, New York

Valentina Azzollini, MD, Department of Translational Research and New Technologies in Medicine and Surgery, University of Pisa, Pisa, Italy

Amitabh Bhattacharya, PhD, Krembil Research Institute, Toronto, Ontario, Canada

Louis Bherer, PhD, Montreal Heart Institute and Department of Medicine, University of Montreal, Montreal, Quebec, Canada

Maxime Bleau, PhD candidate, School of Optometry, University of Montreal, Montreal, Quebec, Canada

Luca Bonfanti, DVM, PhD, Department of Veterinary Sciences and Neuroscience Institute Cavalieri Ottolenghi, University of Turin, Grugliasco, Italy

Davide Bottari, PhD, IMT School for Advanced Studies, Lucca, Italy

Davide B. Cappon, PhD, Hinda and Arthur Marcus Institute for Aging Research, Harvard Medical School, Boston, Massachusetts

Rachel Chang, BMSc, Krembil Research Institute, Toronto, Ontario, Canada

Christine J. Charvet, PhD, Department of Anatomy, Physiology, and Pharmacology, College of Veterinary Medicine, Auburn University, Auburn, Alabama

Robert Chen, MA, MSc, Department of Neurology, University of Toronto, Toronto, Ontario, Canada

Leonardo G. Cohen, MD, PhD, National Institute of Neurological Disorders and Stroke, National Institutes of Health, Bethesda, Maryland

Manuela Costa, PhD, Center for Biomedical Technology, Universidad Politécnica de Madrid, Madrid, Spain

Naaz Desai, PhD, Krembil Research Institute, Toronto, Ontario, Canada

Dario Farina, PhD, Department of Bioengineering, Imperial College, London, United Kingdom

Dustin Fetterhoff, PhD, Center for Biomedical Technology, Universidad Politécnica de Madrid, Madrid, Spain

Joyce Gomes-Osman, PhD, Department of Neurology, Miller School of Medicine, University of Miami, Miami, Florida

Jordan Grafman, PhD, Shirley Ryan Ability Lab and Department of Physical Medicine and Rehabilitation, Northwestern University, Chicago, Illinois

Christian Habeck, PhD, Department of Neurology, Vagelos College of Physicians and Surgeons, Columbia University, New York, New York

Ali Jannati, MD, PhD, Linus Health, Boston, Massachusetts

Tara Keck, PhD, Division of Biosciences, University College London, London, United Kingdom

Martin Korte, PhD, Department of Cellular Neurobiology, TU Braunschweig Zoological Institute, Braunschweig, Germany

Natalie Mrachacz-Kersting, PhD, BrainLinks BrainTools and Department of Sport and Sport Science, Albert Ludwigs University of Freiburg, Freiburg, Germany

Negar Nasrkhani, BMSc, Krembil Research Institute, Toronto, Ontario, Canada

Elena Nava, PhD, Department of Psychology, University of Milan–Bicocca, Milan, Italy

Paolo Nichelli, MD, Department of Biomedical, Metabolic, and Neural Sciences, University of Modena and Reggio Emilia, Modena, Italy

Alvaro Pascual-Leone, MD, PhD, Deanna and Sidney Wolk Center for Memory Health, Harvard Medical School, Boston, Massachusetts

Maurice Ptito, MD, PhD, School of Optometry, University of Montreal, Montreal, Quebec, Canada

Nasem Raies, MSc, Krembil Research Institute, Toronto, Ontario, Canada

Nishaad Sheth, BHSc, Faculty of Medicine, University of Toronto, Toronto, Ontario, Canada

Bryan Strange, PhD, Center for Biomedical Technology, Universidad Politécnica de Madrid, Madrid, Spain

Yaakov Stern, PhD, Division of Cognitive Neuroscience, Columbia University, New York, New York

Tudor Vrinceanu, PhD, Department of Medicine, University of Montreal, Montreal, Quebec, Canada

Preface

The human brain has long been regarded as one of nature's most complex and fascinating structures—a dynamic, living network capable of remarkable feats of adaptation. In recent years, few areas in neuroscience have captured the imagination of researchers and the broader public as vividly as *neuroplasticity*: the brain's ability to reorganize its structure, function, and connections in response to experience, learning, injury, or environmental changes.

Although the notion that the brain is malleable is not new—early observations of functional recovery after brain injury date back centuries—it is only in the last few decades that the tools of modern neuroscience have allowed us to observe, measure, and even harness plasticity in rigorous and transformative ways. Advances in neuroimaging, molecular biology, noninvasive brain stimulation, and computational modeling have opened new avenues for exploring how the brain changes throughout life. This burgeoning field now spans everything from basic cellular studies in animal models to clinically relevant interventions to promote recovery from stroke or enhance cognitive function in aging populations.

We conceived this book with the idea that *neuroplasticity has become too important, too expansive, and intertwined with multiple disciplines for anyone to track easily.* Our goal was to create a clear, accessible primer for students, postdoctoral trainees, and academic professionals who might be approaching this topic for the first time, or who find themselves overwhelmed by the rapid pace of discovery and the sheer breadth of approaches being used.

Instead of pursuing an encyclopedic review, we chose to create a focused, *multi-authored volume* that guides the reader through the conceptual foundations, research methods, and clinical implications of neuroplasticity. Each chapter is authored by experts actively engaged in the field, providing a synthesis of current knowledge and a glimpse into where future investigations might lead.

What You'll Find in This Book

The book begins with a foundational chapter introducing the core concept of brain plasticity—its story, what it is, how it works, and why it matters. We then progress into a series of chapters devoted to the *methods used to study plasticity* in animal models and human participants, ranging from invasive electrophysiology to functional magnetic resonance imaging and noninvasive neurophysiological techniques. This section aims to familiarize readers with the tools that have enabled the modern study of neuroplasticity.

Understanding plasticity requires appreciating its various forms and levels, as well as how these differ across brain regions, developmental stages, and species. To that end, the next set of chapters discusses the *diverse expressions of plasticity*—from the basic mechanisms underlying learning and memory to specialized changes in the developing visual system, and how these processes evolve with age.

A particularly vital section addresses *adaptive plasticity*: the capacity of the nervous system to reorganize itself after damage, as seen in stroke recovery, sensory deprivation, or early-life brain lesions. Here, we explore the factors that constrain or promote recovery, including the remarkable abilities of children's brains to compensate for injury.

The book then explores the *clinical implications of modulating brain plasticity*. Several chapters examine therapeutic interventions aimed at altering brain excitability and network connectivity—from invasive techniques like deep brain stimulation to noninvasive approaches such as transcranial magnetic and electrical stimulation. These chapters not only survey current clinical applications, but also discuss the challenges of translating neuroplasticity research into effective, individualized treatments for neurological and psychiatric disorders.

One of the most rapidly advancing frontiers of applied neuroplasticity is the integration of *brain–computer interfaces* (BCIs), which leverage the brain's learning capacity to restore communication and movement in individuals with severe disabilities. The book highlights both classic applications and the more recent, innovative uses of BCIs to enhance sensory feedback.

Finally, no exploration of human brain plasticity would be complete without considering the profound ways our *digital environment* is reshaping cognition, attention, and brain organization. The book's penultimate chapter reflects on how the pervasive presence of internet-connected devices and artificial intelligence influences the structure and function of our brains in ways we are only beginning to understand.

The volume concludes with a set of final thoughts that summarize key themes and point toward future challenges: Which forms of plasticity are truly adaptive? How can we leverage them to support health and well-being across the lifespan? And what ethical considerations arise as we increasingly learn to intervene in the brain's natural capacity for change?

Why This Book, and Why Now?

If you are new to this field or seeking a concise yet comprehensive guide to the landscape of neuroplasticity research, we hope this book serves as a valuable starting point. It brings together diverse perspectives—from molecular neurobiology to cognitive neuroscience and clinical rehabilitation—and presents them in a format designed to be approachable, informative, and forward-looking.

We believe that understanding the principles and possibilities of brain plasticity is not merely of academic interest, but essential for anyone concerned with how the brain adapts, learns, recovers, and sometimes falters in the face of challenges. As neuroscience continues to advance in mapping and manipulating plasticity, the insights gained will have more direct implications for education, medicine, and society as a whole.

We invite you to explore this book as a window into one of the most vibrant and consequential areas of neuroscience today.

Contents

THE HUMAN BRAIN AND NEUROPLASTICITY

CHAPTER 1

Introduction

WHAT IS BRAIN PLASTICITY?

Paolo Nichelli and Jordan Grafman

Introduction

Brain plasticity is critical for behavioral development, normal learning and memory, and recovery/maintenance of function in the context of brain disorders. The concept of "plasticity" of the nervous system encompasses a broad variety of phenomena, including changes in neural structure or function throughout the lifespan. Not surprisingly, it is difficult to ascribe the primacy of the term *plasticity* in the field of neuroscience.

William James addressed the problem of plasticity in his *Principles of Psychology* (James, 1890). He linked the property of plasticity with behavioral habits and with the habilitation of specific brain paths with repeated use. He also proposed that brain components happening to be active at the same time could drain into each other, thus forming new association paths (Berlucchi & Buchtel, 2009).

However, since neuronal plasticity is strongly related to the synapses' functioning, an essential contribution to its definition should be credited to the work of the Spanish neuroanatomist Santiago Ramón y Cajal. He was the proponent of the neuron theory that, between the 19th and 20th centuries, defined the neuron, though not using this name, as the key anatomical, physiological, and metabolic unit of the nervous system (Ramón y Cajal, 1899–1904). He took advantage of the silver staining technique discovered by the Italian anatomist Camillo Golgi. This method, by staining a limited number of cells at random in their entirety, allowed him, with unprecedented clarity, to visualize not only the cell soma, but also the axon and the branching dendrites in their entire length. Golgi published the first picture made by his technique in 1873 (Golgi, 1873). He was convinced that neurons formed a continuous network that he called the "diffuse nervous network." He stubbornly fought against the neuron theory throughout his life.

In this introductory chapter, we provide a brief overview of the concept of brain plasticity that emerged from a better understanding of synapse functioning and its role in learning and memory. Then, we provide a definition of neuronal plasticity and take a stab at identifying the different forms of brain plasticity.

The Synapse

Among the proponents of neuronal plasticity, some authors began to ask themselves what caused one neuron to seek the connection to another neighboring neuron. They compared neuronal dendrites and axons to the pseudopods of amoebae and leucocytes and suggested that neuronal endings could have limited movements of extension and retraction, which would alter interneuron conduction. Such alteration in conduction caused mental association and memory and corresponded to different conscious states. This theory, called "neuronal amoeboidism" (Demoor, 1896), attracted much attention between 1895 and 1900. Lacking empirical support after 1900, the concept of amoeboidism faded into oblivion (Black, 1981). Later, Cajal's view of mental activity as a product of cortical interneuronal association became widely accepted both in neurological and psychological thinking. Then, it was up to the scientists who claimed that the existing evidence pointed to the nervous system as an *aggregate* of neurons separated by tiny distances to introduce the concept of synaptic plasticity.

The term *synapse* was introduced by Sherrington in 1897 (Tansey, 1997) to convey the idea of an instrument of contact, rather than something that enables contact. Even before the term *synapse* was coined by Sherrington, Eugenio Tanzi, a professor of psychiatry at the University of Palermo, proposed that the distance between neurons was reduced by the small growth of associate neurons, allowing the facilitation of waves of neuronal excitation and hence learning (Tanzi, 1893). Ernesto Lugaro, a disciple of Tanzi and professor of Psychiatry at the University of Florence, linked the notion of synaptic plasticity to neural plasticity as early as 1906 (Berlucchi & Buchtel, 2009). He was also the first to foresee the chemical nature of synaptic transmission in the central nervous system, to note that the nervous elements can grow, and to propose that their plasticity, which allows the internal relations to be molded by external stimuli, decreases as the years go by.

After Sherrington named the synapse, in the first two decades of the 19th century, the concept of synaptic plasticity, the basis of cognitive functioning, obtained significant support but also provoked critical reactions. One argument revolved around the putative causal role of psychological forces (e.g., the will) in directing the growth of new associations between neurons. Karl Lashley proposed other critiques (Lashley, 1924). Lashley was a strong and influential proponent of the theory that large parts of the cerebral cortex have similar potential to perform complex memory and cognitive functions (equipotentiality) and of the hypothesis that the size of the brain damage is proportional to the decreased ability of memory functions (mass action). His views belittled the role of dedicated neural circuits as substrates for cognitive functions. He noted that learned responses could be attained using neural paths that had never been used before, an example of equipotentiality. Lashley based this claim on the demonstration that, in rats, transferring brightness discrimination from one eye to the other is not affected by bilateral removal of the visual cortex. Later split-brain experiments (Sperry, 1961) demonstrated that this can happen due to the convergence of information through the corpus callosum or other interhemispheric connections. Lashley also argued against the role of synapses in learning, noting that there are many instances of learning that do not require the repetition of stimuli and responses. However, later studies have proven that this can occur due to synaptic transmission changes produced by expectation, motivation, or instructions, facilitating some responses and inhibiting the competing ones (Berlucchi & Buchtel, 2009).

The Role of Synapses in Learning

Due to the enormous influence of Lashley's ideas of mass action and functional equipotentiality of the cortex, the issue of brain plasticity remained limited to the analyses of functional recovery after brain damage without including studies examining the neuronal and synaptic levels.

The scientific landscape changed in the late 1940s with Jerzy Konorski and Donald O. Hebb. Jerzy Konorski, a Polish neurophysiologist studying classical Pavlovian conditioning, observed that conditioned responses can occur after as little as two trials. He argued that it was inconceivable that newborn connections could arise with that speed between spatially distant brain centers (Bijoch et al., 2020). He claimed that neural plasticity results from a remodeling of existing synapses created during ontogenesis (Konorski, 1948). At the same time, Donald Hebb described a theory of the cellular mechanism of learning as a change in connection quality between neurons (Hebb, 1949). He developed an associative learning theory to explain how the perceptual system can recognize an object, even if it sees it from a different angle than it had previously seen. His theory, later known as "Hebbian learning," is based on a simple assumption: *When an axon of cell A is near enough to excite cell B and repeatedly or persistently takes part in firing it, some growth process or metabolic change takes place in one or both cells such that A's efficiency, as one of the cells firing B, is increased.* This is often referred to as "Hebb's law": *Neurons that fire together wire together.* Hebb favored the hypothesis of an increase in the efficiency of existing synapses, as opposed to the formation of new ones, but made a point that this was not a new idea, but an old one he revived in a new physiological context (Berlucchi & Buchtel, 2009).

Many decades after observations and theories by Konorski and Hebb, experimental neuroscience provided evidence that synaptic plasticity was indeed the process underlying learning. An essential step in experimentally demonstrating that synapses are plastic in the mammalian brain was the discovery of long-term potentiation (LTP). The first observation of this phenomenon was due to Terje Lomo. In 1966, Lomo was a PhD student in Per Andersen's lab of the Department of Physiology in Oslo when he observed that brief trains of stimuli affecting the perforant path to dentate granule cells in the hippocampus of anesthetized rabbits resulted in increased efficiency of transmission at the cell synapses that could last for hours. In 1968, Tim Bliss came to Andersen's lab and joined Lomo to follow up his preliminary results. Together, they did experiments and published a paper that was considered the basic reference for discovering LTP (Bliss & Lomo, 1973). These findings were made possible using hippocampal slice preparation, a technical development also obtained in Andersen's lab (Skrede & Westgaard, 1971). Since then, research using the LTP paradigm has continued to improve our understanding of synaptic plasticity. In 1977, Lynch and colleagues (1977) described long-term depression (LTD), a postsynaptic correlate of LTP. Experimental studies have clarified what occurs during the brief stimulation that induces LTP, in what way the LTP can change the synapses both at the presynaptic and postsynaptic sites, the role and the interplay of glutamate with *N*-methyl-D-aspartate and alpha-amino-3-hydroxy-5-methyl-4-isoxazolepropionic acid receptors, and the relationship of LTP with memory (Nicoll, 2017).

The Synapse and the Biology of Memory

Further steps toward understanding the biology of memory and its linkage with synapse plasticity were possible by studying simple forms of learning in the context of implicit memory. The most influential experiments were those based on the gill-withdrawal defensive reflex of the sea slug *Aplysia* (Kandel, 2012). This molecular research indicated the mechanisms underlying short-term and long-term learning-related synaptic plasticity and the conservation of molecular memory mechanisms across different brain regions within a species and across species widely separated by evolution. Short-term memory, as studied by sensitizing, with a single noxious stimulus, the tail of *Aplysia*, leads to the activation of modulatory neurons using serotonin as a neurotransmitter, which determines the increase of synaptic strength. Long-term memory differs from short-term memory in that it involves the growth of new synaptic connections, which in *Aplysia* occurs not only in the connections between sensory and motor neurons, but also in the connections between sensory neurons and interneurons. The growth of new synapses represents the most stable phase of long-term memory storage. This process requires the synthesis of new proteins and is mediated by the activation of specific patterns of gene expression (Kandel, 2001). This is true for memory storage of a defensive reflex of a slug, but further studies have demonstrated that this type of plasticity and the exact molecular strategies are conserved in mammals and can also explain more complex cases of implicit and explicit memory storage (Asok et al., 2019).

Today, we have converging evidence from electrophysiological recordings, optogenetics, and other techniques supporting that synapses are plastic preexisting connections. More recent studies (Magee & Grienberger, 2020) have elucidated how different plasticity rules, by combining neuromodulation and eligibility traces, can represent more powerful directed types of synaptic plasticity, which can account for different aspects of brain plasticity.

Defining Brain Plasticity

Neuroplasticity does not refer only to learning and synaptic functioning. The term is currently used for a wide range of phenomena (e.g., plasticity of phenotypic expressions, morphologic plasticity, sensory–motor coordination plasticity, behavioral plasticity, etc.). Yet, according to Paillard (Will et al., 2008b), the word *plasticity* is only appropriate when related to the ability of a system to achieve *novel* functions, either by transforming its internal connectivity or by changing the elements of which it is made. So, not every change in the nervous system can be attributed to novel plasticity. Functional adaptation based on preprogrammed or expected environmental changes should be considered examples of neural network flexibility rather than plasticity. Living systems show plasticity through the self-governing reorganization of their inner wiring that impacts their functional assignment (Will et al., 2008a).

Tools for Investigating Brain Plasticity

The last three decades have seen rapid advances in noninvasive techniques to examine the human brain and its functional networks both in adults and in young children, at rest and during learning, in health, and during diseases or brain lesions. These techniques have increased and deeply modified our view of brain plasticity. They include event-related potentials, magnetoencephalography, structural and functional magnetic resonance imaging, near-infrared spectroscopy, and noninvasive brain stimulation.

Event-Related Potentials

Event-related potentials (ERPs) have been widely used to study cognitive processes. They reflect scalp-recorded voltage fluctuations time-locked to a particular event. ERPs can follow the onset of a specific sensory stimulus or indicate a cognitive process, such as recognizing a grammatical violation in a sentence. ERPs can also precede a cue signaling motor preparation, motor execution, or covert mental operations (e.g., imagery). ERPs provide very accurate time resolution (in the range of milliseconds). However, the spatial resolution of the source of the recorded brain activation is limited.

Magnetoencephalography

Magnetoencephalography (MEG) is a neuroimaging technique that records the magnetic fields produced by the electrical currents occurring in the brain. MEG signals were first recorded by David Cohen in 1968, but it was only in the 1980s, after the development of magnetometers based on superconducting quantum interference devices and their arrangement in multiple arrays to cover a larger area of the head, that this technique began to be used to explore brain activity. Typically, MEG arrays contain 300 sensors set in a helmet-shaped vacuum flask that covers most of the head. Spatial resolution is better compared to that attainable by ERPs. To increase the portability of the MEG apparatus, spin exchange relaxation-free (SERF) magnetometers, which are relatively small and would not require a cooling system to operate, are being considered. The first experiment using SERF has already been validated (Koshev et al., 2021).

Structural Magnetic Resonance Imaging

Structural magnetic resonance imaging (sMRI) was developed in the 1970s and 1980s and can produce remarkably precise images of human brain structure. It is often combined with physiological activity acquired with ERP or MEG to increase the spatial resolution of these methods. Using diffusion tensor imaging, a technique based on analyzing the movement of water molecules in brain tissue, sMRI allows white matter bundles to be mapped in three dimensions. The method, also called tractography, allows the reconstruction of connections between brain areas.

Functional Magnetic Resonance Imaging

Functional magnetic resonance imaging (fMRI) was developed in the early 1990s and soon became the most used tool in brain mapping research due to its wide availability and because it does not involve exposure to ionizing radiation like computed assisted tomography. Instead, fMRI uses the magnetic properties of oxygen-rich blood captured by the blood-oxygen-level–dependent sequence of radiofrequency pulses. Unlike ERP and MEG, fMRI does not directly measure the neural activity but rather the increase of blood oxygenation occurring during neural activation. fMRI signals need to be processed to remove unwanted artifacts and transform the data into a standard format. Statistical analysis can determine the voxels in the image that show a response to the stimulus and allow the displaying of activation images with probability values associated with statistical confidence. fMRI is an indirect correlational tool to assess the functional specialization of the brain areas and the network subserving specific cognitive processes. It provides a rather good spatial resolution but a somewhat coarse temporal resolution. For this reason, researchers may combine fMRI with ERPs or, even better, with MEG.

Near-Infrared Spectroscopy

Near-infrared spectroscopy (NIRS) uses the absorption of light, which is sensitive to the concentration of hemoglobin, to assess oxygenation and microvascular function of the brain and how they vary with neural activity. It can be used as a partial replacement for fMRI techniques. However, it can only be used to scan cortical tissue, whereas fMRI can be used to measure activation throughout the brain. NIRS is much more portable than fMRI machines and can also be used on infants (Bortfeld et al., 2007) and, using wireless instrumentation, on freely moving subjects.

Noninvasive Brain Stimulation

Repetitive transcranial magnetic stimulation (rTMS) causes brain stimulation of a specific brain area through a magnetic coil applied to the scalp. The coil, by electromagnetic induction, determines an electric stimulation that, depending on the stimulated region and the characteristics of the stimulation, can show diagnostic or therapeutic effects. Low-frequency rTMS, with a stimulus frequency less than 1 Hz, is believed to inhibit cortical firing, while a stimulus frequency greater than 1 Hz can provoke cortical firing. It has been suggested that its influence on brain tissue is due to a change in synaptic efficacy related to LTP- and LTD-like plasticity (Fitzgerald et al., 2006). Similar noninvasive brain stimulation techniques, such as transcranial direct current stimulation or vagal nerve stimulation, are also widely used.

Different Kinds of Brain Plasticity

The late Giorgio Innocenti (Innocenti, 2022) recently summarized the many facets of brain plasticity in development and adulthood. We list here some critical historical milestones in this effort.

Developmental Plasticity

Synaptic plasticity, as well as learning and memory, peaks soon after birth and declines at a variable rate with increasing age. During development, there are phases (critical periods) of significantly increased plasticity for specific sensory or sensorimotor interactions. This is true for the filial imprinting of birds, who, during a few hours after hatching, learn to follow around their mother, but also in human infants who learn language following a stereotypical pattern (Kuhl, 2010). Developmental plasticity depends on neurogenesis, neuronal death, neuronal migration, neuronal differentiation, cytoarchitectonic specialization, and the formation of new connections.

The birth of experimental neurobiology can be traced back to the first half of the 19th century. Marian Lidia Shorey, a biology student at Frank R. Lillie's laboratory in Chicago, demonstrated that removing the primordia of some muscles of chick embryos before nerve fibers penetrated them determined well-defined defects in the nervous system due to the failure of neuroblasts to develop (Shorey, 1909). Twenty-five years later, Viktor Hamburger, working in the same laboratory, confirmed the results obtained by Marian Shorey, adding a semiquantitative method to correlate hypoplasia of the motor column to muscle loss. These experiments and similar observations led to the concept that innervation of the peripheral territory (skin or muscle) is necessary for neuronal survival and eventually to the discovery of neurotrophins, as described by Hamburger (Hamburger, 1988). In 1986, Rita Levi Montalcini and Stanley Cohen received the Nobel prize for the discovery of neural growth factor, the first and the best known of the neurotrophins, but regrettably, the early contribution of Marian Shorey was forgotten (Strata & Pareti, 2019). The brain's cell number is determined by neuronal production and neuronal death. Some developmental diseases are associated with microcephaly, but it is still debated whether they are due to arrested neurogenesis or excessive apoptosis.

Neuronal Migration

An important feature of neural cells in the developing brain is their ability to migrate from their germinal zone to their final position in cell assemblies. Frederick Tilney,

Professor of Neurology at Columbia University in New York, was the first to describe the different stages of neuronal migration (Tilney, 1933) during brain development. However, the pattern of migration he described was erroneous. Studying the development of the cerebral cortex between the 16th day of fetal life and the day of birth using autoradiographs, Berry and Rogers (1965) demonstrated that neuroblasts formed by cell division in the ependymal layer populated different layers of the cerebral cortex at different times.

Further investigations (Nadarajah & Parnavelas, 2002) have demonstrated that different types of neurons adopt three distinct modes of migration: (1) Somal translocation is adopted by early generated neurons; (2) glial-guided locomotion is used predominantly by pyramidal cells; and (3) cortical interneurons, which originate in the ventral telencephalon, migrate tangentially into the cortex and then seek the ventricular zone before moving radially to take up their position in the cortical anlage. A significant number of patients affected by drug-resistant epilepsy have cortical malformations caused by disorders of neuronal migration. These disorders include polymicrogyria, where the brain presents multiple small gyri; schizencephaly, where the brain is split by a cleft connecting the surface of the cerebral hemisphere to the lateral ventricle; lissencephaly, where the brain appears smooth, as it lacks the normal folding; and focal cortical dysplasia, where the neurons failed to migrate to their proper destination.

Neuronal Differentiation and Formation of Connections

Acquiring the final neuronal phenotype is a complex process that requires both progressive and regressive events involving the dendritic system and the axon. Progressive events include elongation, radial growth, branching, and formation of spines or synaptic branches. Regressive events involve eliminating part of the dendritic arbor, also called pruning. The term *pruning* was introduced by Irving Feinberg in 1982. However, Peter Huttenlocher (1979) described the first demonstration of pruning in humans as being in the frontal cortex. Huttenlocher was a pediatric neurologist at the University of Chicago. Counting synapses with an electron microscope, he showed that in the frontal cortex synaptic density increased during infancy, reaching a maximum at ages 1–2 years, which was about 50% above the adult mean. The decline in synaptic density observed between ages 2 and 16 years was accompanied by a slight decrease in neuronal density. He demonstrated that while synaptic density was relatively low in neonates, the brain grew new synapses very quickly, reaching levels *far above* those of adults. The density peaked at different brain centers over time—in some areas at about 3 months, in others at 3 years of age. Then synapse numbers in the declined to adult levels by age 12. Interestingly, Anna Huttenlocher, his daughter, a pediatric rheumatologist, recently published a book about her father and his discovery (Huttenlocher, 2023). Further studies have targeted the mechanisms underlying these changes. From a clinical standpoint, there is some evidence supporting the view of schizophrenia as a disconnection syndrome caused by failed stabilization of connections in development and that disordered pruning in the frontal lobe might underlie those cases of schizophrenia that emerge in adolescence.

Adult Plasticity

Neurogenesis

Adult neurogenesis had been considered impossible in mammals until the first observations by Joseph Altman (1962). He traumatized the lateral geniculate body of adult rats and injected tritiated thymidine, a cell proliferation marker, into the lesions. The autoradiograms obtained from rats sacrificed 1 day to several months after the lesion demonstrated the labeling of some neurons and neuroblasts in the thalamus and cortex. This indicates that neurons can come into existence in the brains of adult mammals. In the following year, using a similar experimental model, he observed newly labeled neurons in the dentate gyrus of the hippocampus and the cortex of rats and cats. However, even though Altman had respected academic credentials in the neuroscientific community, his findings were subjected to wide criticism, and it took nearly three decades to be accepted with qualifications. Adult neurogenesis in humans is still a debated issue (Kempermann et al., 2018). The prevailing view is that it is restricted to the hippocampus, but even in this case, knowledge about this process might change our ideas about the structural substrates of human cognition, cognitive aging, and disorders affecting the hippocampus, such as Alzheimer's disease, stress-related disorders, and depression.

Neural Network Functional Plasticity

From a clinical standpoint, brain plasticity has been investigated mainly as the reorganization of neural networks following brain lesions or deprivation of regular peripheral input to the brain. One of us (Grafman, 2000) has suggested that at least four forms of neuroplasticity can be studied in humans: homologous area adaptation, cross-modal reassignment, map expansion, and compensatory masquerade.

Homologous Area Adaptation

Homologous area adaptation is the possibility that, after a brain lesion, a particular cognitive process is taken care of by the homologous area in the opposite hemisphere. This kind of plasticity is more active during the early stages of human development and is especially relevant after large brain lesions, as following a hemispherectomy, a radical surgical procedure where the diseased half of the brain is wholly removed, partially removed and entirely disconnected or just disconnected from the normal hemisphere. Walter Dandy introduced this procedure in 1928 to treat five patients with glioblastoma, the most aggressive brain tumor. At that time, the median survival rate for glioblastoma was just 3 months. The procedure never panned out for brain tumors but found a space in functional neurosurgery, especially for the treatment of severe forms of childhood drug-resistant epilepsy. In a recent small series of three young patients with Rasmussen encephalitis treated with left functional hemispherectomy on the dominant hemisphere for severe epilepsy associated with the disease, all benefited from a favorable cognitive outcome (Borne et al., 2022). Their ages at the operation were 5.5, 8.5, and 14.0. They were followed up for more than 8 years. All of them showed recovery of cognitive function, including language. The more rapid and complete recovery was in the patient who was 5.5 years old, thus demonstrating a shift of language abilities to the intact hemisphere. The patient, 8.5 years of age at the operation, presented a reorganization of language and memory function that seemed to have been at the expense of nonverbal ones, a result that has led to the idea that the brain area accepting a cognitive operation previously assigned to the diseased hemisphere becomes more crowded with distinct cognitive representation.

Cross-Modal Reassignment

Cross-modal reassignment occurs when new inputs are introduced to a brain region that is deprived of its original input. A positron emission tomography study is the first example of this form of neuroplasticity (Sadato et al., 1996), which demonstrated the activation of the visual areas of the occipital cortex in early blind subjects involved in tactile discrimination of geometric forms (e.g., Braille letters). Similar cross-modal reassignment has been reported in other instances of sensory loss (e.g., deafness).

Map Expansion

Map expansion can occur whenever a given function is performed by a brain region more extensive than that previously associated with that task or adjacent to that previously associated with it. The first experimental evidence of this mechanism can be traced to studies of Sherrington and coworkers at the beginning of the 20th century. In different experiments on monkeys, as reported by Wiesendanger (2011), Sherrington observed functional recovery after large or small lesions of the motor cortex, particularly for arm-hand representation. He noticed that 6 months after an almost complete lesion of the arm area of the right motor cortex, the movements of the left arm gradually improved and became stronger and demonstrated that "recovery is not due to taking over by the corresponding area of the other cortex of the movements of both arms" and that "it is not due to the taking over postcentral cortex of the function of the motor cortex." Similar observations were reported after a small cortical lesion of the same motor area, demonstrating that after a focal injury to the thumb cortical representation of the thumb, the recovery was associated with remapping in the adjacent cortical territory. Map expansion has also been reported in normal subjects when they are learning a new skill. In the early stages of skill acquisition, map expansion might be associated with brain volume expansion in task-relevant areas. Then, volume expansion is followed by a selection process operating on this new tissue, leading to a complete or partial return to the baseline of the overall volume after selection has ended (Wenger et al., 2017). In 1930, Karl Spencer Lashley formulated the principle of motor equivalence by which when some motor organs are rendered nonfunctional by removal or paralysis, there is a spontaneous use of other systems that had not been previously associated with or used in the performance of that activity. As an example, he proposed shifting the writing with fine fingering to movements of the whole arm. In a broader context, this is called *compensatory masquerade*, a form of reorganization that, at a cognitive level, includes the novel use of intact components to perform a task previously dependent on impaired processes.

Conclusion

The concept of brain plasticity has its roots in the discovery of neurons, their shape and location, and their interaction with other neural elements, including glial cells, and hence on the foundation of modern neuroscience. In the last 30 years, the development of functional neuroimaging and neurophysiological techniques allowed not only the recording of brain activity, but also the stimulation of the brain, allowing significant progress in our knowledge about neuronal plasticity, its possibilities, its limits, and our chances to influence them. The chapters that follow this one will introduce different aspects of neuroplasticity in more detail, building upon the research conducted over the last 150 years. The concept of brain plasticity is evolving before our eyes!

REFERENCES

Altman, J. (1962). Are new neurons formed in the brains of adult mammals? *Science, 135*, 1127–1128.

Asok, A., Leroy, F., Rayman, J. B., & Kandel, E. R. (2019). Molecular mechanisms of the memory trace. *Trends in Neurosciences, 42*(1), 14–22.

Berlucchi, G., & Buchtel, H. A. (2009). Neuronal plasticity: Historical roots and evolution of meaning. *Experimental Brain Research, 192*(3), 307–319.

Berry, M., & Rogers, A. W. (1965). The migration of neuroblasts in the developing cerebral cortex. *Journal of Anatomy, 99*(Pt. 4), 691–709.

Bijoch, L., Borczyk, M., & Czajkowski, R. (2020). Bases of Jerzy Konorski's theory of synaptic plasticity. *European Journal of Neuroscience, 51*(9), 1857–1866.

Black, S. E. (1981). Pseudopods and synapses: The amoeboid theories of neuronal mobility and the early formulation of the synapse concept, 1894–1900. *Bulletin of the History of Medicine, 55*(1), 34–58.

Bliss, T. V., & Lomo, T. (1973). Long-lasting potentiation of synaptic transmission in the dentate area of the anaesthetized rabbit following stimulation of the perforant path. *Journal of Physiology, 232*(2), 331–356.

Borne, A., Perrone-Bertolotti, M., Jambaque, I., Castaignede, C., Dorfmuller, G., Ferrand-Sorbets, S., et al. (2022). Cognitive outcome after left functional hemispherectomy on dominant hemisphere in patients with Rasmussen encephalitis: Beyond the myth of aphasia. Patient series. *Journal of Neurosurgery Case Lessons, 4*(22), case 22410.

Bortfeld, H., Wruck, E., & Boas, D. A. (2007). Assessing infants' cortical response to speech using near-infrared spectroscopy. *Neuroimage, 34*(1), 407–415.

Demoor, J. (1896). La plasticité morphologique des neurones cérébraux. *Archives de Biologie (Bruxelles), 14*, 723–751.

Fitzgerald, P. B., Fountain, S., & Daskalakis, Z. J. (2006). A comprehensive review of the effects of rTMS on motor cortical excitability and inhibition. *Clinical Neurophysiology, 117*(12), 2584–2596.

Golgi, C. (1873). Sulla struttura della sostanza grigia del cervello. *Gazzetta Medica Italiana-Lombardia, 6*, 244–246.

Grafman, J. (2000). Conceptualizing functional neuroplasticity. *Journal of Communication Disorders, 33*(4), 345–355.

Hamburger, V. (1988). Ontogeny of neuroembryology. *Journal of Neuroscience, 8*(10), 3535–3540.

Hebb, D. O. (1949). *The organization of behavior: A neuropsychological theory.* Wiley.
Huttenlocher, A. (2023). *From loss to memory: Behind the discovery of synaptic pruning.* Cambridge University Press.
Huttenlocher, P. R. (1979). Synaptic density in human frontal cortex—developmental changes and effects of aging. *Brain Research Bulletin, 163*(2), 195–205.
Innocenti, G. M. (2022). Defining neuroplasticity. In A. Quartarone, M. F. Ghilardi, & F. Boller (Eds.), *Handbook of clinical neurology* (Vol. 184, pp. 3–18). Elsevier.
James, W. (1890). *The principles of psychology.* Macmillan.
Kandel, E. R. (2001). The molecular biology of memory storage: A dialogue between genes and synapses. *Science, 294*, 1030–1038.
Kandel, E. R. (2012). The molecular biology of memory: cAMP, PKA, CRE, CREB-1, CREB-2, and CPEB. *Molecular Brain, 5*, 14.
Kempermann, G., Gage, F. H., Aigner, L., Song, H., Curtis, M. A., Thuret, S., et al. (2018). Human adult neurogenesis: Evidence and remaining questions. *Cell Stem Cell, 23*(1), 25–30.
Konorski, J. (1948). *Conditioned reflexes and neuron organization.* Cambridge University Press.
Koshev, N., Butorina, A., Skidchenko, E., Kuzmichev, A., Ossadtchi, A., Ostras, M., et al. (2021). Evolution of MEG: A first MEG-feasible fluxgate magnetometer. *Human Brain Mapping, 42*(15), 4844–4856.
Kuhl, P. K. (2010). Brain mechanisms in early language acquisition. *Neuron, 67*(5), 713–727.
Lashley, K. S. (1924). Studies of cerebral function in learning (VI). *Psychological Review, 31*(5), 369–375.
Lynch, G. S., Dunwiddie, T., & Gribkoff, V. (1977). Heterosynaptic depression: A postsynaptic correlate of long-term potentiation. *Nature, 266*, 737–739.
Magee, J. C., & Grienberger, C. (2020). Synaptic plasticity forms and functions. *Annual Review of Neuroscience, 43*, 95–117.
Nadarajah, B., & Parnavelas, J. G. (2002). Modes of neuronal migration in the developing cerebral cortex. *Nature Review Neuroscience, 3*(6), 423–432.
Nicoll, R. A. (2017). A brief history of long-term potentiation. *Neuron, 93*(2), 281–290.
Ramón y Cajal, S. (1899–1904). *Textura del sistema nervioso del hombre y de los vertebrados.* Nicolás Moya.
Sadato, N., Pascual-Leone, A., Grafman, J., Ibanez, V., Deiber, M. P., Dold, G., & Hallett, M. (1996). Activation of the primary visual cortex by Braille reading in blind subjects. *Nature, 380*, 526–528.
Shorey, M. L. (1909). The effect of the destruction of peripheral areas on the differentiation of the neuroblasts. *Journal of Experimental Zoology, 7*(1), 25–63.
Skrede, K. K., & Westgaard, R. H. (1971). The transverse hippocampal slice: A well-defined cortical structure maintainedin vitro. *Brain Research, 35*(2), 589–293.
Sperry, R. W. (1961). Cerebral organization and behavior: The split brain behaves in many respects like two separate brains, providing new research possibilities. *Science, 133*, 1749–1757.
Strata, P., & Pareti, G. (2019). A new season for experimental neuroembryology: The mysterious history of Marian Lydia Shorey. *Endeavour, 43*(4), 100707.
Tansey, E. M. (1997). Not committing barbarisms: Sherrington and the synapse, 1897. *Brain Research Bulletin, 44*(3), 211–212.
Tanzi, E. (1893). I fatti e le induzioni dell'odierna istologia del sistema nervoso. *Rivista Sperimentale di Freniatria e Medicina Legale, 19*, 419–472.
Tilney, R. (1933). Behavior in its relation to the development of the brain. Part II. Correlation

between the development of the brain and behavior in the albino rat from embryonic states to maturity. *Bulletin of the Neurological Institute of New York, 2*, 252–358.

Wenger, E., Brozzoli, C., Lindenberger, U., & Lovden, M. (2017). Expansion and renormalization of human brain structure during skill acquisition. *Trends in Cognitive Sciences, 21*(12), 930–939.

Wiesendanger, M. (2011). Postlesion recovery of motor and sensory cortex in the early twentieth century. *Journal of the History of the Neurosciences, 20*(1), 42–57.

Will, B., Dalrymple-Alford, J., Wolff, M., & Cassel, J. C. (2008a). The concept of brain plasticity—Paillard's systemic analysis and emphasis on structure and function (followed by the translation of a seminal paper by Paillard on plasticity). *Behavioural Brain Research, 192*(1), 2–7.

Will, B., Dalrymple-Alford, J., Wolff, M., & Cassel, J. C. (2008b). Reflections on the use of the concept of plasticity in neurobiology. Translation and adaptation by Bruno Will, John Dalrymple-Alford, Mathieu Wolff, and Jean-Christophe Cassel from J. Paillard, J Psychol 1976;1:33-47. *Behavioural Brain Research, 192*(1), 7–11.

CHAPTER 2

Neurobiology Methods for Studying Neuronal Plasticity in Animal Models

Tara Keck

Introduction

Animal models have long been used to study the mechanisms of neuronal plasticity. Over the past decades, there have been many advances in tools and techniques that now allow for unprecedented measurements of neuronal plasticity and manipulation of neuronal circuits and activity to induce and disrupt plasticity. This chapter provides an overview of the commonly used methodologies for plasticity induction and measurement, and the frequently used animal models.

Plasticity Induction and Measurement

Plasticity Induction

Plasticity is ongoing in the brain through a combination of experience-dependent plasticity, which includes learning and memory formation encoding daily experiences, and homeostatic plasticity mechanisms, which help balance neuronal properties such as firing rate or calcium levels and are necessary for these properties to stay in a physiological range. These ongoing changes, however, can be challenging to measure, as they may be dispersed throughout the brain and cannot be easily time-matched to an experience or behavior. Thus, many studies will use a plasticity induction protocol and record the plasticity measurement before and after this timed induction. Plasticity induction generally falls into three categories: manipulation of sensory input, learning, and manipulation of activity. Each of these plasticity paradigms tends to be used in combination with different experimental approaches.

Manipulation of Sensory Input

The manipulation of sensory input can be done (1) through manipulation of the environment to which the animal is exposed, such as dark rearing, dark exposure, extended light exposure, odor exposure, or high levels of sound exposure or (2) through the manipulation of the sensory system itself, for example, through eyelid suture, focal retinal lesions, enucleation, removable plugging of the ear or nose, temporary binding of digits together, or whisker trimming (Fabian & Sachse, 2023; Holtmaat & Svoboda, 2009). These types of manipulation have been shown to result in a change in activity levels associated with the change in sensory input. These changes in activity and sensory input often trigger a combination of molecular, synaptic, cellular, and network plasticity in the brain (Barnes & Finnerty, 2010). One advantage of these approaches is that the highly specific timing of the paradigm induction can be correlated with the subsequent plasticity, as the paradigms result in the immediate change in feed-forward sensory stimulation. A challenge associated with these paradigms is that many of them result in a dramatic change in activity levels, which reflects the types of plasticity that the brain is capable of but may differ in some ways from more nuanced ongoing experience-dependent plasticity.

Learning

Learning paradigms have long been used to induce plasticity in different animal models and can include reward-based learning, fear conditioning, associative learning, and natural behavior learning, among others. Paradigms are often designed for animals to learn to associate sensory stimuli with outcomes (reward or fear conditioning aversive outcomes), which also helps in determining which brain areas to target to measure plasticity. One advantage of learning paradigms is that they can be designed to translate well to learning paradigms in humans, particularly paradigms that are used in nonhuman primates (Hubbard et al., 2009).

One challenge is that some forms of reward-based learning and associative learning can occur over several days, or in some instances even weeks or months, with performance improving gradually over time. It can therefore be difficult to correlate the timing of changes to molecules, synapses, cells, and networks of cells with the behavior, as many other changes are ongoing during this extended period.

Natural behaviors can result in quicker acquisition (Cisek & Green, 2024). These behaviors include escape behaviors in rodents, hunting behaviors in larval zebrafish, and auditory responses to pup calls in rodent mothers, among others. Fear conditioning also has a fast time course for learning, often occurring in a single trial. Use of these faster learning paradigms can help with temporally correlating neuronal plasticity and behavioral changes.

Manipulation of Activity

Studies of the mechanisms of plasticity, often conducted with *in vitro* preparations such as acute slices or cultured neurons, frequently use manipulation of activity. This manipulation can be achieved through electrical stimulation or optical stimulation, such as with optogenetic tools or caged neurotransmitters (see the "Methodologies and Tools for Measuring Plasticity" section). This type of stimulation can be temporally precise and has helped uncover many of the temporal rules of plasticity induction related to long-term potentiation, long-term depression, and short-term plasticity.

The use of these approaches in *in vitro* preparations also allows for concurrent manipulation with applications of agonists and/or antagonists for receptors, which has facilitated the characterization of the roles of specific receptors in neural plasticity (Hille, 2001). When combined with the manipulation of sensory input or learning *in vivo*, *ex vivo* preparations from animals that have undergone *in vivo* manipulations combined with these forms of stimulation have helped uncover the subcellular underpinnings of plasticity associated with behavioral changes.

Methodologies and Tools for Measuring Plasticity

A key challenge in studying neuronal plasticity is measuring it. Over the past decades, there have been numerous advances in technologies, tools, and methodologies that allow for measurements of forms of neuroplasticity in animal models. Whether the plasticity in question is occurring at the level of gene expression, molecules, synapses, single cells or networks of cells, or is being reflected in changes in the behavior of the animal, there is a myriad of ways to measure these changes and the interactions between plasticity at these different scales.

Recent methodologies have focused on approaches that chronically measure the same plasticity measurement in a single animal over time, which allow for more direct measures of the changes that occur after plasticity paradigms and reduce the effects of animal variability. Changes to a number of outcomes can be measured to infer plasticity. These include changes in neuronal activity (both sub- and suprathreshold activity), neuronal anatomy, functional synaptic release, gene/protein/receptor expression, and behavior. Below we highlight the commonly used methods and how these methods are often used in combination to study scientific questions addressing neuronal plasticity.

Optogenetic Tools

The use of optogenetic tools has dramatically increased since their introduction to neuroscience over 20 years ago. These optogenetic tools are ion channels, pumps, or enzymes that are engineered to be light-sensitive and are typically genetically or virally expressed in cells of interest (Emiliani et al., 2022; Fenno et al., 2011). They are activated when exposed to their designated wavelength of light. While early tools were engineered to cause a de- or hyperpolarization in cells, depending on the specifics of the channel, light-modulated tools have since been developed for a wide variety of uses, including targeting second messenger systems, G protein signaling, kinases, transcription, and translation (Emiliani et al., 2022; Kim et al., 2017; Rost et al., 2017).

Many optogenetic tools that de- or hyperpolarize cells have short onset and decay times, which allows for temporally and spatially precise control of neuronal activity in individual neurons or subsets of neurons (Shemesh et al., 2017). While titration of light intensity does influence the degree of activation, controlling the precise delivery of light in highly dense brain regions can be a challenge in using these tools, particularly for *in vivo* preparations (Kim et al., 2017). To date, these tools have been used to provide precise stimulation, such as with inductions of plasticity paradigms of long-term potentiation and long-term depression (Fenno et al., 2011), and to silence or activate brain regions to understand their role in particular behaviors (Kim et al., 2017).

The development of new tools to target second messenger systems and other subcellular signaling could be useful to help further elucidate their roles in plasticity induction (Rost et al., 2017). One challenge with optogenetic tools is that the time for which they can be effectively activated is limited, but broadly, optogenetic tools have been critical in helping establish causality in neuroscience experiments (Emiliani et al., 2022; Kim et al., 2017).

Chemogenetic Tools

Chemogenetic tools are a complement to optogenetic tools and can be used in combination with them (Jiang et al., 2017). The most commonly used chemogenetic receptors are designer receptors exclusively activated by designer drugs (DREADDs), which are genetically or virally expressed in specific genetically identifiable subsets of cells (Campbell & Marchant, 2018). These DREADDs are activated only when the designer ligand, often C21 (11-(1-piperazinyl)-5*H*-dibenzo[*b*,*e*][1,4]diazepine) or CNO (clozapine *N*-oxide) (Zhang et al., 2022), is systemically injected into the animal expressing the DREADDs.

DREADD activation can either increase or decrease neuronal activity (depending on the specific DREADD), most commonly through the action of G protein signaling pathways (Campbell & Marchant, 2018), and there continue to be more receptor–ligand pairs developed for use in experimental neuroscience. Having more than one designer drug–designer ligand pair allows for independent manipulation of multiple different subsets of cells, for example, excitatory and inhibitory cell types, in the same animal.

The effects of DREADDs can be long lasting, up to 9 hours (Alexander et al., 2009). DREADDs have the advantage of easy delivery of the activation method via systemic injections, but they do not have the same high temporal or spatial resolution of optogenetics (Jiang et al., 2017). Spatial resolution instead can be achieved to some degree by specific labeling of cell types or by intracranial injection of the designer ligand into a specific brain region (Campbell & Marchant, 2018).

Genetically Encoded Calcium Indicators

One of the most commonly utilized tools for measuring proxies of activity in neurons over the past decade are genetically encoded calcium indicators (GECIs; Day-Cooney et al., 2023; Kim & Schnitzer, 2022; Zhang & Looger, 2024). GECIs have been developed in several different excitation wavelengths, allowing for coexpression of and measurement from GECIs in different cell types in the same brain region. They have been used in both *in vivo* and *in vitro* plasticity experiments. GECIs exhibit a change in fluorescence when there is a calcium influx, which is typically associated with action potential firing. Deconvolution methods can facilitate distinguishing individual action potentials, but this can at times be challenging, particularly distinguishing single action potentials within bursts of action potentials. GECIs can be measured with high spatial resolution, allowing for calcium measurements in dendritic spines, dendrites, and cells.

GECIs have mixed temporal resolution. They have fast onset kinetics but traditionally have had slower offset kinetics, which limits their temporal resolution relative to electrophysiology measurements. However, newer iterations of GECIs have improved temporal kinetics (Zhang et al., 2023). Because they are genetically encoded, GECIs allow for repeated measures of the same spines, dendrites, cells, and network of cells over time, which is critical for plasticity experiments where activity can be measured both before and after a learning or plasticity intervention is induced (Huber et al., 2012; Keck et al., 2013; Rose et al., 2016).

The ability to measure activity in individual dendritic spines also allows for proxy measures of changes in synaptic strength, as well as the identification of the input properties (Barnes et al., 2022). These features allow for the design of plasticity experiments that determine which inputs to a cell are undergoing plasticity following induction paradigms and which inputs are more stable, adding a layer to our understanding of how plasticity is induced in circuits. Finally, GECIs allow for spatial interactions to be quantified, particularly which neurons are coactive through measuring the correlation of GECI activity between neighboring cells and their spatial relationships (Barnes et al., 2015).

Voltage-Sensitive Dyes

Voltage-sensitive dyes are less commonly used than GECIs in neuroscience research due to their higher levels of noise and the relative difficulty in measuring signals compared with GECIs (Bando et al., 2019; Day-Cooney et al., 2023; Kim & Schnitzer, 2022). Still, they do have several advantages over GECIs. These include (1) being able to measure subthreshold changes in neuronal voltage, (2) high temporal and spatial resolution (Grinvald et al., 2016), and (3) a direct measure of voltage instead of a proxy measurement of calcium with GECIs. As voltage-sensitive dyes continue to develop, they could be extremely beneficial for experiments measuring neuronal plasticity, providing a way to measure subthreshold changes in activity levels in cells, dendrites, and dendritic spines and temporally precise changes that are often associated with forms of long-term potentiation, such as spike-timing dependent plasticity. Understanding subthreshold changes *in vivo* would allow for a much more nuanced understanding of synaptic plasticity in response to learning and other plasticity paradigms.

Structural Markers

While there are many tools to measure and manipulate neuronal activity, plasticity can also take the form of structural or anatomical changes to neurons, including changes to axons, dendrites, boutons, and spines (Holtmaat & Svoboda, 2009).

Fluorescent proteins (FPs) have been developed in a wide spectrum of wavelength excitations, and they allow for co-labeling of different molecular, subcellular, synaptic, and cellular structures in the same brain regions. Repeated visualization of the same structures over time facilitates measuring structural plasticity, as a baseline for synaptic structure presence and size can be established prior to induction of plasticity or learning and probed again after for changes (Holtmaat & Svoboda, 2009). These changes include either changes in size or loss/gain of synaptic structures. Similarly, plasticity can occur in the growth and retraction of axons or dendrites, which can be visually tracked over time in FP-labeled cells (Lee et al., 2006). Because FPs are relatively stable over time, the same labeled structures can be monitored *in vivo* over many months (Keck et al., 2008; Trachtenberg et al., 2002), allowing for the investigation of the long-term consequences of plasticity induction and the effects of repeated plasticity paradigm induction—either the same paradigm repeated or differing paradigms interleaved. These types of experiments may be particularly useful in investigating learning, retrieval, and extinction of memory, which can happen over longer time scales.

One challenge of FP expression is the associated concerns of interfering with the normal physiology of the cells through overexpression. Gene-editing tools are now being used to fluorescently label receptors of interest in plasticity, such as alpha-amino-3-hydroxy-5-methyl-4-isoxazolepropionic acid (AMPA) receptors (Fang et al., 2021). These tools are relatively new, but they have great potential for use in plasticity studies, with a reduced risk of affecting the physiology of the cells.

Structural markers can also be used to map synaptic connections at a single time point. A commonly used approach for monosynaptic tracing of presynaptic partners is to use a rabies-based virus, which is adapted so that the FP expression is only in cells with monosynaptic connections with the neuron of interest (Wickersham et al., 2007). These viral tools for mapping monosynaptic connections cannot yet be used longitudinally, so they have to be used in experiments that compare groups that have undergone plasticity induction and control groups that have not. Still, these tools are extremely powerful for studying plasticity and determining how, for example, early life changes in the environment can result in a fundamental rewiring of circuits during development.

Identifying Cell Types

A key benefit of these tools is that the development of approaches to target cell types—for example, Cre-recombinase animal lines (Madisen et al., 2010) and the GAL4-UAS system (Brand & Perrimon, 1993)—means that they can be targeted to a genetically identifiable set of neurons, allowing the manipulation and measurement of activity from specific subsets of neurons. This includes targeting specific brain regions, cell layers, cell types (excitatory neurons, inhibitory neurons, glia, astrocytes), and cell subtypes (e.g., subsets of inhibitory neurons—neuropeptide Y, vasoactive intestinal polypeptide–expressing, calretinin, or parvalbumin; Gavériaux-Ruff & Kieffer, 2007). This specificity of activity manipulation and functional and structural measurement allows for the characterization of the role of specific cell types in plasticity.

Cell types undergoing plasticity can also be identified by optically measuring plasticity *in vivo* using imaging tools, followed by post hoc identification of these specific cell types using postexperimental reconstructions and labeling of cell types using either immunohistochemistry (Barnes et al., 2015; Kerlin et al., 2010) or transcriptomics (Bugeon et al., 2022). These reconstructions can either be done in tissue that has been sectioned or through the use of tissue-clearing techniques, which allows for three-dimensional imaging of the entire brain (Ueda et al., 2020) or large parts of it. Together, these approaches allow for measuring plasticity in specific cell types throughout the brain and considering how this cell-type plasticity may interact to facilitate network plasticity and behavioral changes.

Imaging Approaches

Over the past decades, multiphoton imaging has been used extensively in neuroscience research in animal models (Yang & Yuste, 2017). Multiphoton imaging, when combined with genetic tools for labeling cell structure or activity, allows for a clear spatial readout and concurrent recordings from multiple cells. When combined with genetic labeling techniques or reconstructions, it also allows for *in vivo* measures from specific cell types in the brain (Svoboda & Yasuda, 2006). Multiphoton imaging provides high spatial resolution, but somewhat limited depth penetration, making measurements from deep brain structures more challenging. Some studies have overcome this barrier through the use of GRIN (gradient-index) lenses (Reed et al., 2002), which allow for imaging of deeper structures. The ease of repeated measurements with multiphoton imaging techniques has made it a popular method for neuronal plasticity experiments, examining changes before and after plasticity induction of activity proxies in networks, cells, and synapses (Barnes et al., 2022; Huber et al., 2012; Rose et al., 2016), as well as in the structure of cells and synapses (Holtmaat & Svoboda, 2009). It also facilitates the identification of inactive and extremely sparsely active cells, which can be visually identified and characterized with low or no activity.

In vitro, multiphoton imaging can be used for high-resolution visualization of synapses and cells, combined with localized stimulation through uncaging of caged molecules, such as glutamate or GABA (gamma-aminobutyric acid; Matsuzaki & Kasai, 2011). These approaches have helped uncover dendritic and synaptic properties, as well as nonlinear interactions on dendrites (Branco et al., 2010), which may be changed by subcellular plasticity, for example, via changes in relative receptor density or activation. *In vitro* experiments also allow for the local application of receptor agonists or antagonists while imaging structural or functional plasticity following an induction protocol. These approaches have been valuable in identifying the role of specific receptors in plasticity induction (Hille, 2001), particularly in the dendrites and axons of the cell, which are harder to measure and isolate using other techniques. Imaging *in vitro* may also be combined with single-cell electrophysiology to link calcium and voltage measures within a cell, or to deliver agonists or antagonists intracellularly and co-measure structural or functional plasticity outcomes.

Imaging approaches can also be used in combination with optogenetics and chemogenetics to allow for concurrent manipulation of activity and measuring the outcomes of those manipulations (Emiliani et al., 2022; Simpson & Looger, 2018). More recently, single- or two-photon imaging has been used in head-attached implants, which allow for imaging in freely moving animals (Ghosh et al., 2011; Zong et al., 2022). While resolution in these experiments is limited, these approaches can be used to more directly link a wider range of behavioral changes to neuronal plasticity.

Super-resolution microscopy has been used to study subcellular plasticity (Tønnesen & Nägerl, 2013). These approaches include STED (stimulated emission depletion), SUSHI (super-resolution shadow imaging), PALM (photoactivated localization microscopy), STORM (stochastic optical reconstruction microscopy), SIM (structured illumination microscopy), and PAINT (point accumulation imaging in nanoscale topography) (Tønnesen & Nägerl, 2013). These approaches use either single molecule localization approaches or a depletion light beam to increase resolution, allowing for subcellular high-resolution imaging of synapses and molecules, although these techniques are also limited by depth penetration into live tissue. Electron microscopy is also frequently used in the study of synaptic plasticity, as it allows for high-resolution imaging of synapses, including synaptic vesicles and synaptic scaffolding proteins in fixed tissue (Bourne & Harris, 2012; Denk & Horstmann, 2004).

On the opposite end of the resolution spectrum, imaging approaches have also been used to examine wide-field activity in and across brain regions. These approaches include intrinsic optical imaging (Grinvald et al., 1986) and, more recently, wide-field imaging using GECIs (Scott et al., 2018). These approaches allow for measures of large-scale changes in activity, such as following loss of input in a stroke model or focal peripheral input deprivation paradigms. While these approaches have lower spatial resolution and reflect the activity of many neurons in a region, they can be used in combination with other tools to measure plasticity outcomes. By identifying the spatial location of affected areas where activity changes are ongoing in plasticity paradigms, more fine-tuned measures can be made in these regions, such as imaging of structural or functional changes in synapses and cells (Keck et al., 2008).

Electrophysiology

Electrophysiology has been used for many decades to measure neuronal activity. *In vivo* approaches span several key parameters, including (1) intracellular and extracellular recording approaches, (2) the number of recording sites, with recording electrodes spanning from one recording site to hundreds, and (3) acute experiments, made at a single point in time, and chronic experiments, which can last for days to weeks. The best method depends on the nature and spatial scale of the plasticity that is being measured, and we highlight a subset of these approaches below.

Tetrodes have been used for decades to measure neural activity over time in freely behaving animals, with multiple electrodes per experiment and four recording sites on each electrode (O'Keefe & Recce, 1993; Wilson & McNaughton, 1993). Recently developed large-scale silicon probe arrays, such as Neuropixels probes, have hundreds of recording sites along an extended vertical axis (Jun et al., 2017). These probes allow for the measurement of many cells across an extended spatial region of the brain, often including much of a single brain region or multiple brain regions. Both tetrodes and silicon probe arrays require spike sorting analyses to separate individual neurons that appear on multiple recording sites.

These *in vivo* electrophysiology approaches can be combined with manipulation of activity using optogenetics or chemogenetics, as well as learning paradigms. Electrophysiology has high temporal resolution and can directly measure action potentials, rather than the proxy of calcium that is commonly used in multiphoton imaging experiments. With the newer silicon probe arrays, activity correlations between neighboring neurons can be measured, allowing for the quantification of putative subnetworks of neurons (Jun et al., 2017). Both tetrodes and silicon probes can be used to measure from the same local region, but not necessarily the same cells, for weeks or more. Therefore, plasticity induction taking place over a shorter timeframe (within hours to days) can be well quantified at the level of cells and subnetworks of cells with high temporal resolution. In *in vivo* intracellular electrophysiology approaches, subthreshold activity and subsequent plastic changes can also be measured (Tao et al., 2015). One important consideration is that some electrophysiology measurements are biased toward active cells and identifying inactive cells or those with very low firing rates can be a challenge.

In vitro electrophysiology has been critical in the study of plasticity as well. *In vitro* electrophysiology experiments have characterized Hebbian plasticity, long-term potentiation, long-term depression, short-term plasticity, and homeostatic plasticity, which includes synaptic scaling, changes in the balance between excitation and inhibition, changes in the threshold for long-term potentiation and long-term depression induction, and changes in excitability (Bear & Abraham, 1996; Bliss & Lomo, 1973; Turrigiano & Nelson, 2000; Zucker & Regehr, 2002). *In vitro* preparations allow for the use of agonists and antagonists to quantify the roles of receptors and second messenger pathways in plasticity (Hille, 2001). The more recent use of *ex vivo* preparations, where animals undergo deprivation, stimulation, or learning paradigms *in vivo* and then are prepared for *in vitro* experiments, has allowed for in-depth characterizations of the subcellular mechanisms associated with these *in vivo* changes. *In vitro* preparations limit the ability to make comparisons within the same animal before and after plasticity induction, so sham plasticity controls are necessary for these instances. Imaging and optogenetics, both in specific cell types, can be combined with *in vitro* electrophysiology to measure voltage changes, sub- and suprathreshold, together with the manipulation of activity or measurements of structure and function (Emiliani et al., 2022).

Behavioral Readouts

Linking changes in behavior to neuronal plasticity has been ongoing for decades (Kupfermann et al., 1970), with a recent increase in the number of plasticity studies using behavioral readouts. This increase has been accompanied by more sophisticated analyses of the complex movements that are associated with learned behaviors. Recent advances in machine learning have been applied to behavioral readouts (Mathis & Mathis, 2020; Robie et al., 2017), with classification performance at human accuracy with relatively little training data. These types of approaches are now widely used and help standardize analyses of behavioral data and the changes in behavior associated with learning paradigms, which can then be linked to neuronal measurements of plasticity.

Computational Approaches

Computational approaches are used in the study of neural plasticity, both in the development of novel analyses of experimental data and in the generation of models based on existing data. First, with the increased magnitude of data that is collected in a given experiment, including combinations of behavioral, genetic, imaging, or electrophysiology readouts across numerous brain regions, advanced computational analyses are necessary to examine the interactions between these variables. Advances in machine-learning approaches have been critical in dimensionality reduction of data and identification of key features of the data (Mitchell-Heggs et al., 2023). Deep neural network analyses are now being applied to neural data and will likely play a large role in future analyses of large-scale plasticity data across multiple paradigms and brain regions (Richards et al., 2019).

Second, computational models are often used to investigate and characterize neuronal plasticity, working from existing data in the field or accompanying novel data to propose potential explanations and theoretical frameworks. Computational models have proposed theories for underlying learning rules in the brain, which can then be tested experimentally as methodologies and tools advance to allow for the appropriate experiments. Neural models of plasticity have provided insights into many areas, for example, learning rules that are implemented in cells and networks, and the importance of compensatory mechanisms in plasticity paradigms, which are difficult to eliminate in experimental preparations (Zenke et al., 2013). As novel computational approaches are developed, these models will continue to evolve to provide frameworks and theories about neuronal plasticity that both influence and are influenced by experimental results.

Omics Approaches

Omics approaches analyze genes, gene expression, and proteins (Armand et al., 2021; Hosp & Mann, 2017; Jung & Kim, 2023) in animals that have undergone plasticity induction and their control counterparts. These omics approaches can be applied in single cells, with numerous combinations of multiomics approaches, or using spatial multiomics approaches in blocks of tissue (Armand et al., 2021; Hosp & Mann, 2017; Jung & Kim, 2023). These approaches are important for understanding the changes in genes, gene expression, and protein translation in the brain. They can also be useful in finding genetically identifiable cell types that are undergoing plasticity and can therefore be targeted with methodological tools to measure changes and manipulate activity in plasticity experiments.

Combining Methods and Tools

Studying neural plasticity requires mixing these tools and methods in different combinations to best address the spatial and temporal scales of plasticity in question, as well as triangulate results across methods with different advantages and limitations. Many of the most powerful plasticity studies use a combination of behavioral and *in vivo* recordings (either electrophysiology or imaging), with manipulations of activity or measurements in genetically defined cell types, together with *in vitro* and molecular characterizations of plasticity mechanisms associated with changes in activity/behavior and modelling of outcomes to develop theories and general rules of plasticity. These combinations have allowed scientists studying plasticity to start to disentangle the many aspects of plasticity and causally test hypotheses and theories of plasticity. The further development of methodologies, tools, and analytical approaches will facilitate future experiments that deepen our understanding of neuronal plasticity and its implementation in the brain and nervous system.

Animal Models for Studying Neuronal Plasticity

A wide range of animal models have been used in the study of plasticity. Here, we outline many of the commonly used animal model systems, highlighting their advantages and challenges.

- *Aplysia* was famously used in early studies of neuronal plasticity and memory, examining the role of circuit plasticity in facilitating the gill and siphon withdrawal reflex (Kupfermann et al., 1970). These were some of the earliest experiments to combine neurophysiology to measure neuronal changes associated with plasticity, with changes in behavioral outcomes for the animal. This model continues to be used to examine aspects of compulsive behavior related to feeding and types of associative learning.

- *Drosophila* have been used for decades in biomedical research, with the benefits of a short lifespan and relative ease in manipulating gene expression—for example, using the GAL4-UAS system (Brand & Perrimon, 1993). There are a number of natural behavioral readouts in *Drosophila* (Neckameyer & Bhatt, 2016), which allows for a model where measures of gene expression can be combined with behavioral measures throughout the lifespan to gain insights into plasticity mechanisms.

- Larval zebrafish have been used in several neuronal plasticity experiments (Orger & de Polavieja, 2017) due to their transparent nature, which allows for imaging of a large number of neurons, dendrites, or synapses in a single experiment. This imaging can be combined with (1) genetic manipulations (Brand & Perrimon, 1993), both for labeling of cell types with structural or functional optical markers and for manipulating gene expression to understand its role in plasticity, and (2) natural behavior (e.g., related to prey hunting; Zhu & Goodhill, 2023), which allow for powerful measures of plasticity during development.

- Zebra finch songbirds are another commonly used model for developmental plasticity, specifically related to the acquisition of speech and early experience (Mello, 2014). They also are an excellent model for neurogenesis, as new neurons are added to the circuit throughout the lifespan of the animal. As a larger animal model, they are ideal for electrophysiology and multiphoton imaging experiments during behavior, and recent advances in the understanding of their genetics now allow for targeting genetic manipulations to specific subsets of neurons in the brain.

• Mice are often used in the study of plasticity due to the wide range of genetic tools available for the manipulation of neural circuits and labeling of specific subsets of cells in the brain, as well as the ease of measuring molecular, synaptic, cellular, and network activity using *in vivo* electrophysiology and imaging approaches (Navabpour et al., 2020). They are also well suited to *ex vivo* measurements using electrophysiology in acute slice preparations. Mouse behavioral methodologies have expanded over the past decades, and mice can be used in numerous learning paradigms to study behavioral outcomes of plasticity.

• Rats are also a commonly used animal model, but because fewer genetically modified rat lines have been developed and imaging techniques are limited in depth with the larger rat brain, rats are less frequently used than mice in some imaging experiments (Ellenbroek & Youn, 2016). Their larger brains and head size can be an advantage for chronic electrophysiology experiments, where larger electrophysiology head fixtures allow for recording from additional channels. Rats are also a commonly used model system for studying plasticity in acute slice preparations and cultured neurons, utilizing electrophysiology, uncaging, and immunohistochemistry techniques, particularly during developmental stages.

• Cats have historically been used in the study of plasticity, particularly developmental plasticity (Wiesel & Hubel, 1963). They have been used extensively in experiments utilizing electrophysiological measures of the activity of individual neurons and more recently have been used in some imaging experiments, particularly in the study of visual cortical plasticity.

• Similarly, ferrets have been used in studying visual developmental cortical plasticity (Issa et al., 1999) due to their relatively slow developmental time course. Experiments in ferrets include measures of cellular plasticity, using both electrophysiology and multiphoton imaging, but with fewer approaches for genetic manipulation.

• Finally, nonhuman primates have long been used for learning and memory tasks, as they can learn high-level tasks similar to those used in humans, with concurrent electrophysiology or imaging measurements from synapses, cells, or networks of cells. Recently, more genetic tools have been optimized in nonhuman primates, allowing for the targeting of specific cell type manipulations or testing the impact of manipulating gene expression (Feng et al., 2020).

Conclusion

This chapter highlights the key approaches for studying neuronal plasticity in a range of animal models, discussing the ways in which plasticity is typically induced—through manipulation of sensory input, learning, or manipulation of activity—and the methodologies to measure plasticity, such as imaging, *in vivo* and *in vitro* electrophysiology, behavioral readouts, computational approaches, and omics approaches. Further discussion highlights the important tools that have facilitated advances in our understanding of plasticity over the past decades, including novel ways to manipulate activity in specific cell types using optogenetic and chemogenetic tools, as well as label molecules, synapses, and cells with structural or functional fluorescent markers. Finally, the chapter highlights how these tools and methodologies can be powerfully combined to manipulate and measure plasticity and expand our understanding of the underlying mechanisms of plasticity in the brain.

REFERENCES

Alexander, G. M., Rogan, S. C., Abbas, A. I., Armbruster, B. N., Pei, Y., Allen, J. A., et al. (2009). Remote control of neuronal activity in transgenic mice expressing evolved G protein-coupled receptors. *Neuron, 63*, 27–39.

Armand, E. J., Li, J., Xie, F., Luo, C., & Mukamel, E. A. (2021). Single-cell sequencing of brain cell transcriptomes and epigenomes. *Neuron, 109*, 11–26.

Bando, Y., Grimm, C., Cornejo, V. H., & Yuste, R. (2019). Genetic voltage indicators. *BMC Biology, 17*, 71.

Barnes, S. J., & Finnerty, G. T. (2010). Sensory experience and cortical rewiring. *Neuroscientist, 16*, 186–198.

Barnes, S. J., Keller, G. B., & Keck, T. (2022). Homeostatic regulation through strengthening of neuronal network-correlated synaptic inputs. *eLife, 11*, e81958.

Barnes, S. J., Sammons, R. P., Jacobsen, R. I., Mackie, J., Keller, G. B., & Keck, T. (2015). Subnetwork-specific homeostatic plasticity in mouse visual cortex in vivo. *Neuron, 86*, 1290–1303.

Bear, M. F., & Abraham, W. C. (1996). Long-term depression in hippocampus. *Annual Review of Neuroscience, 19*, 437–462.

Bliss, T. V., & Lomo, T. (1973). Long-lasting potentiation of synaptic transmission in the dentate area of the anaesthetized rabbit following stimulation of the perforant path. *Journal of Physiology, 232*, 331–56.

Bourne, J. N., & Harris, K. M. (2012). Nanoscale analysis of structural synaptic plasticity. *Current Opinion in Neurobiology, 22*, 372–382.

Branco, T., Clark, B. A., & Häusser, M. (2010). Dendritic discrimination of temporal input sequences in cortical neurons. *Science, 329*, 1671–1675.

Brand, A. H., & Perrimon, N. (1993). Targeted gene expression as a means of altering cell fates and generating dominant phenotypes. *Development, 118*, 401–415.

Bugeon, S., Duffield, J., Dipoppa, M., Ritoux, A., Prankerd, I., Nicoloutsopoulos, D., et al. (2022). A transcriptomic axis predicts state modulation of cortical interneurons. *Nature, 607*, 330–338.

Campbell, E. J., & Marchant, N. J. (2018). The use of chemogenetics in behavioural neuroscience: Receptor variants, targeting approaches and caveats. *British Journal of Pharmacology, 175*, 994–1003.

Cisek, P., & Green, A. M. (2024). Toward a neuroscience of natural behavior. *Current Opinion in Neurobiology, 86*, 102859.

Day-Cooney, J., Dalangin, R., Zhong, H., & Mao, T. (2023). Genetically encoded fluorescent sensors for imaging neuronal dynamics in vivo. *Journal of Neurochemistry, 164*, 284–308.

Denk, W., Horstmann, H. (2004). Serial block-face scanning electron microscopy to reconstruct three-dimensional tissue nanostructure. *PLoS Biology, 2*, e329.

Ellenbroek, B., & Youn, J. (2016). Rodent models in neuroscience research: Is it a rat race? *Disease Models & Mechanisms, 9*, 1079–1087.

Emiliani, V., Entcheva, E., Hedrich, R., Hegemann, P., Konrad, K. R., Lüscher, C., et al.

(2022). Optogenetics for light control of biological systems. *Nature Reviews Methods Primer, 2*, 55.

Fabian, B., & Sachse, S. (2023). Experience-dependent plasticity in the olfactory system of *Drosophila melanogaster* and other insects. *Frontiers in Cellular Neuroscience, 17*, 1130091.

Fang, H., Bygrave, A. M., Roth, R. H., Johnson, R. C., & Huganir, R. L. (2021). An optimized CRISPR/Cas9 approach for precise genome editing in neurons. *eLife, 10*, e65202.

Feng, G., Jensen, F. E., Greely, H. T., Okano, H., Treue, S., Roberts, A. C., et al. (2020). Opportunities and limitations of genetically modified nonhuman primate models for neuroscience research. *Proceedings of the National Academy of Sciences, 117*, 24022–24031.

Fenno, L., Yizhar, O., & Deisseroth, K. (2011). The development and application of optogenetics. *Annual Review of Neuroscience, 34*, 389–412.

Gavériaux-Ruff, C., & Kieffer, B. L. (2007). Conditional gene targeting in the mouse nervous system: Insights into brain function and diseases. *Pharmacology & Therapeutics, 113*, 619–634.

Ghosh, K. K., Burns, L. D., Cocker, E. D., Nimmerjahn, A., Ziv, Y., Gamal, A. E., et al. (2011). Miniaturized integration of a fluorescence microscope. *Nature Methods, 8*, 871–878.

Grinvald, A., Lieke, E., Frostig, R. D., Gilbert, C. D., & Wiesel, T. N. (1986). Functional architecture of cortex revealed by optical imaging of intrinsic signals. *Nature, 324*, 361–364.

Grinvald, A., Omer, D. B., Sharon, D., Vanzetta, I., & Hildesheim, R. (2016). Voltage-sensitive dye imaging of neocortical activity. *Cold Spring Harbor Protocols, 2016*(1), pdb.top089367.

Hille, B. (2001). *Ion channels of excitable membranes* (3rd ed.). Sinauer.

Holtmaat, A., & Svoboda, K. (2009). Experience-dependent structural synaptic plasticity in the mammalian brain. *Nature Reviews Neuroscience, 10*, 647–658.

Hosp, F., & Mann, M. (2017). A primer on concepts and applications of proteomics in neuroscience. *Neuron, 96*, 558–571.

Hubbard, I. J., Parsons, M. W., Neilson, C., & Carey, L. M. (2009). Task-specific training: Evidence for and translation to clinical practice. *Occupational Therapy International, 16*(3–4), 175–189.

Huber, D., Gutnisky, D. A., Peron, S., O'Connor, D. H., Wiegert, J. S., Tian, L., et al. (2012). Multiple dynamic representations in the motor cortex during sensorimotor learning. *Nature, 484*, 473–478.

Issa, N. P., Trachtenberg, J. T., Chapman, B., Zahs, K. R., & Stryker, M. P. (1999). The critical period for ocular dominance plasticity in the Ferret's visual cortex. *Journal of Neuroscience, 19*, 6965–6978.

Jiang, J., Cui, H., & Rahmouni, K. (2017). Optogenetics and pharmacogenetics: Principles and applications. *American Journal of Physiology—Regulatory, Integrative and Comparative Physiology, 313*, R633–R645.

Jun, J. J., Steinmetz, N. A., Siegle, J. H., Denman, D. J., Bauza, M., Barbarits, B., et al. (2017). Fully integrated silicon probes for high-density recording of neural activity. *Nature, 551*, 232–236.

Jung, N., & Kim, T.-K. (2023). Spatial transcriptomics in neuroscience. *Experimental & Molecular Medicine, 55*, 2105–2115.

Keck, T., Keller, G. B., Jacobsen, R. I., Eysel, U. T., Bonhoeffer, T., & Hübener, M. (2013). Synaptic scaling and homeostatic plasticity in the mouse visual cortex in vivo. *Neuron, 80*, 327–334.

Keck, T., Mrsic-Flogel, T. D., Afonso, M. V., Eysel, U. T., Bonhoeffer, T., & Hübener, M. (2008). Massive restructuring of neuronal circuits during functional reorganization of adult visual cortex. *Nature Neuroscience, 11*, 1162–1167.

Kerlin, A. M., Andermann, M. L., Berezovskii, V. K., & Reid, R. C. (2010). Broadly tuned response properties of diverse inhibitory neuron subtypes in mouse visual cortex. *Neuron, 67*, 858–871.

Kim, C. K., Adhikari, A., & Deisseroth, K. (2017). Integration of optogenetics with complementary methodologies in systems neuroscience. *Nature Reviews Neuroscience, 18*, 222–235.

Kim, T. H., & Schnitzer, M. J. (2022). Fluorescence imaging of large-scale neural ensemble dynamics. *Cell, 185*, 9–41.

Kupfermann, I., Castellucci, V., Pinsker, H., & Kandel, E. (1970). Neuronal correlates of habituation and dishabituation of the gill-withdrawal reflex in Aplysia. *Science, 167*, 1743–1745.

Lee, W. C., Huang, H., Feng, G., Sanes, J. R., Brown, E. N., So, P. T., et al. (2006). Dynamic remodeling of dendritic arbors in GABAergic interneurons of adult visual cortex. *PLoS Biology, 4*, e29.

Madisen, L., Zwingman, T. A., Sunkin, S. M., Oh, S. W., Zariwala, H. A., Gu, H., et al. (2010). A robust and high-throughput Cre reporting and characterization system for the whole mouse brain. *Nature Neuroscience, 13*, 133–140.

Mathis, M. W., & Mathis, A. (2020). Deep learning tools for the measurement of animal behavior in neuroscience. *Current Opinion in Neurobiology, 60*, 1–11.

Matsuzaki, M., & Kasai, H. (2011). Two-photon uncaging microscopy. *Cold Spring Harbor Protocols, 2011*(5), pdb.prot5620.

Mello, C. V. (2014). The zebra finch, *Taeniopygia guttata*: An avian model for investigating the neurobiological basis of vocal learning. *Cold Spring Harbor Protocols, 2014*(12), 1237–1242.

Mitchell-Heggs, R., Prado, S., Gava, G. P., Go, M. A., & Schultz, S. R. (2023). Neural manifold analysis of brain circuit dynamics in health and disease. *Journal of Computational Neuroscience, 51*, 1–21.

Navabpour, S., Kwapis, J. L., & Jarome, T. J. (2020). A neuroscientist's guide to transgenic mice and other genetic tools. *Neuroscience & Biobehavioral Reviews, 108*, 732–748.

Neckameyer, W. S., & Bhatt, P. (2016). Protocols to study behavior in *Drosophila. Methods in Molecular Biology (Clifton NJ), 1478*, 303–320.

O'Keefe, J., & Recce, M. L. (1993). Phase relationship between hippocampal place units and the EEG theta rhythm. *Hippocampus, 3*, 317–330.

Orger, M. B., & de Polavieja, G. G. (2017). Zebrafish behavior: Opportunities and challenges. *Annual Review of Neuroscience, 40*, 125–147.

Reed, W. A., Yan, M. F., & Schnitzer, M. J. (2002). Gradient-index fiber-optic microprobes for minimally invasive in vivo low-coherence interferometry. *Optics Letters, 27*, 1794–1796.

Richards, B. A., Lillicrap, T. P., Beaudoin, P., Bengio, Y., Bogacz, R., Christensen, A., et al. (2019). A deep learning framework for neuroscience. *Nature Neuroscience, 22*, 1761–1770.

Robie, A. A., Seagraves, K. M., Egnor, S. E. R., & Branson, K. (2017). Machine vision methods for analyzing social interactions. *Journal of Experimental Biology, 220*, 25–34.

Rose, T., Jaepel, J., Hübener, M., & Bonhoeffer, T. (2016). Cell-specific restoration of stimulus preference after monocular deprivation in the visual cortex. *Science, 352*, 1319–1322.

Rost, B. R., Schneider-Warme, F., Schmitz, D., & Hegemann, P. (2017). Optogenetic tools for subcellular applications in neuroscience. *Neuron, 96*, 572–603.

Scott, B. B., Thiberge, S. Y., Guo, C., Tervo, D. G. R., Brody, C. D., Karpova, A. Y., et al. (2018). Imaging cortical dynamics in GCaMP transgenic rats with a head-mounted widefield macroscope. *Neuron, 100*(5), 1045–1058.e5.

Shemesh, O. A., Tanese, D., Zampini, V., Linghu, C., Piatkevich, K., Ronzitti, E., et al. (2017). Temporally precise single-cell-resolution optogenetics. *Nature Neuroscience, 20*, 1796–1806.

Simpson, J. H., & Looger, L. L. (2018). Functional imaging and optogenetics in *Drosophila. Genetics, 208*, 1291–1309.

Svoboda, K., & Yasuda, R. (2006). Principles of two-photon excitation microscopy and its applications to neuroscience. *Neuron, 50*, 823–839.

Tao, C., Zhang, G., Xiong, Y., & Zhou, Y. (2015). Functional dissection of synaptic circuits: In vivo patch-clamp recording in neuroscience. *Frontiers in Neural Circuits, 9*, 23.

Tønnesen, J., & Nägerl, U. V. (2013). Superresolution imaging for neuroscience. *Experimental Neurology, 242*, 33–40.

Trachtenberg, J. T., Chen, B. E., Knott, G. W., Feng, G., Sanes, J. R., Welker, E., et al. (2002). Long-term in vivo imaging of experience-dependent synaptic plasticity in adult cortex. *Nature, 420*, 788–94.

Turrigiano, G. G., & Nelson, S. B. (2000). Hebb and homeostasis in neuronal plasticity. *Current Opinion in Neurobiology, 10*, 358–364.

Ueda, H. R., Ertürk, A., Chung, K., Gradinaru, V., Chédotal, A., Tomancak, P., et al. (2020). Tissue clearing and its applications in neuroscience. *Nature Reviews Neuroscience, 21*, 61–79.

Wickersham, I. R., Lyon, D. C., Barnard, R. J. O., Mori, T., Finke, S., Conzelmann, K.-K., et al. (2007). Monosynaptic restriction of transsynaptic tracing from single, genetically targeted neurons. *Neuron, 53*, 639–647.

Wiesel, T. N., & Hubel, D. H. (1963). Single-cell responses in striate cortex of kittens deprived of vision in one eye. *Journal of Neurophysiology, 26*, 1003–1017.

Wilson, M. A., & McNaughton, B. L. (1993). Dynamics of the hippocampal ensemble code for space. *Science, 261*, 1055–1058.

Yang, W., & Yuste, R. (2017). In vivo imaging of neural activity. *Nature Methods, 14*, 349–359.

Zenke, F., Hennequin, G., & Gerstner, W. (2013). Synaptic plasticity in neural networks needs homeostasis with a fast rate detector. *PLoS Computational Biology, 9*, e1003330.

Zhang, S., Gumpper, R. H., Huang, X.-P., Liu, Y., Krumm, B. E., Cao, C., et al. (2022). Molecular basis for selective activation of DREADD-based chemogenetics. *Nature, 612*, 354–362.

Zhang, Y., & Looger, L. L. (2024). Fast and sensitive GCaMP calcium indicators for neuronal imaging. *Journal of Physiology, 602*, 1595–1604.

Zhang, Y., Rózsa, M., Liang, Y., Bushey, D., Wei, Z., Zheng, J., et al. (2023). Fast and sensitive GCaMP calcium indicators for imaging neural populations. *Nature, 615*, 884–891.

Zhu, S. I., & Goodhill, G. J. (2023). From perception to behavior: The neural circuits underlying prey hunting in larval zebrafish. *Frontiers in Neural Circuits, 17*, 1087993.

Zong, W., Obenhaus, H. A., Skytøen, E. R., Eneqvist, H., de Jong, N. L., Vale, R., et al. (2022). Large-scale two-photon calcium imaging in freely moving mice. *Cell, 185*, 1240–1256.e30.

Zucker, R. S., & Regehr, W. G. (2002). Short-term synaptic plasticity. *Annual Review of Physiology, 64*, 355–405.

CHAPTER 3

Methods for Studying Brain Plasticity in Humans

Christine J. Charvet

Introduction

Experience, skill learning, injury, and life-changing events cause functional, molecular, and structural reorganization of the brain, which are here defined as brain plasticity. Such experiences can induce reorganization at multiple scales, including modifications in cortical representation fields, synapse formation and elimination, change in neuron morphology, and the production of new neurons (Baroncelli et al., 2011; Burke & Barnes, 2006; Fawcett, 2009; Mora et al., 2007; Murphy et al., 2014; Ungerleider et al., 2002). It is evident that there is lifelong brain plasticity. Different forms of plasticity predominate different life stages, which impact disease risk as well as rates of aging (Kramer et al., 2004).

Several techniques are available to study brain plasticity. Some methods focus on genetic and molecular scales, whereas other methods collect information at anatomical and behavioral scales. Some of the methods used to probe brain plasticity can be studied directly in humans, whereas others are unsuitable for humans. Instead, they are suited for model systems such as mice and macaques. Neuroimaging techniques are well suited for the study of human brain plasticity because they are noninvasive. In addition, some molecular and histological techniques can be applied to the study of postmortem humans (Axer & Amunts, 2022; Bassett & Sporns, 2017; Park & Friston, 2013; Yeh et al., 2018). Human brain samples are generally limited for study. These limitations make model systems well suited for certain assays that are not tractable in humans. The necessity to rely on model systems means that there is a need to map findings from model systems to humans. This has traditionally been a complex problem because of the large gap in biology and behavior between traditional model systems (e.g., mice) and humans (Clancy et al., 2001). Translating Time is a project that finds corresponding ages across species and bridges the gap across model systems to humans.

Model systems are typically used to probe brain plasticity at the microscale and as a surrogate to understand how the human brain changes in response to environmental input. There are significant biological and behavioral differences between humans and model systems. Mice are, by far, the most studied model systems (de Sousa et al., 2023). Other model systems, which include rats, macaques, and marmosets, are used to study biological processes in health and disease states. While there has been much focus on using mice as models for human biology, different model systems may be best suited to address different kinds of questions and study different processes and disease states. The necessity to rely on model systems to learn about human brain plasticity raises several important issues and questions. Which model system is best suited to study human brain plasticity? Which model system is most suitable to study specific kinds of plasticity? What is the most appropriate age to study a given biological process in humans? The following chapter addresses these questions. I concentrate on a resource called Translating Time, which relies on the collection of time points to find corresponding ages across humans and model systems (Charvet, 2021; Clancy et al., 2001; Cottam et al., 2025). I discuss how Translating Time can be used to evaluate which model system is best suited for which process in health or disease states.

I review several types of brain plasticity that stretch across the lifespan. The Translating Time tool can inform the most appropriate age of model systems and guide the most suitable model system selection (Charvet et al., 2023; Clancy et al., 2001; Cottam et al., 2025). One important lesson from these comparative analyses is that different species evolved species-specific sensory and cognitive specializations (Hunt et al., 2006; Krubitzer et al., 1995, 1997). Accordingly, different model systems are subject to different kinds of environmental input and forms of plasticity. Therefore, integrating information across diverse model systems will be pivotal to fully understanding human brain plasticity.

Neuroplasticity Varies across the Lifespan

The environment shapes the brain and behavior across the lifespan, but the type of input an animal is ready to process varies across its lifetime. Different forms of plasticity exist throughout an animal's lifespan, and they are specific to each species. The brain is plastic before birth.

During prenatal brain development, the neural tube closes, and proliferative cells generate neurons and glial cells (Clemenson et al., 2015). The environment can target developmental processes that span these fetal stages of life. At those ages, major processes include neuron production, synapse formation, and establishing long- and short-range connections. For example, exposure to music during the prenatal period shapes the development of the auditory system and neural responses to music (Marzola et al., 2023; Partanen et al., 2013). While prenatal experiences may enrich specific developmental processes, these same developmental processes are susceptible to damage. For example, prenatal exposure to toxins (e.g., alcohol, lead) causes a lasting impact on brain function, and exposure to these toxins results in major brain damage and developmental delays that persists throughout the lifespan (Wasserman et al., 2004). Therefore, environmental exposure, whether adverse or favorable, has a lasting impact on brain structure and function and will impact subsequent plasticity in the individual's lifespan.

How the brain responds to these environmental stimuli changes with age. Shortly after birth, the external environment shapes the development of sensory and motor capacities. The brain also goes through several critical periods. At these ages, the brain expects experiences to function appropriately at subsequent ages. Some of these critical periods impact sensory systems (e.g., binocular vision), while others impact sensory–motor systems (e.g., language, socialization), though these critical periods ultimately impact behavior (Gordon & Stryker, 1996; Hunt et al., 2006; Kramer et al., 2004; Murphy et al., 2014; Walker, 1981). In species with some degree of binocular vision (e.g., cats, nonhuman primates, humans, mice), there is a critical period for binocular vision. Input from two eyes must be integrated to process visual information. Suppose that one eye is prevented from receiving sensory input through occlusion during the critical period. In that case, the visual cortex will shift to favor the representation of the uncovered eye, leading to a persistent loss of vision in the occluded eye (i.e., lazy eye). Uncovering the occluded eye during the critical period can restore function and interaction across the eyes. However, sensory stimulation of the occluded eye must occur within a critical period (i.e., time window) for restoration to occur (Gordon et al., 1996; Wang et al., 2010). Another important critical period is language in humans. If language input does not occur at around 2–13 years of age in humans, it is unlikely that the individual will ever achieve full command of language in adulthood (Walker, 1981). These examples show that neural circuits are experience-expectant. Environmental stimulation must occur within a critical period for optimal functioning of neural circuits subserving those behaviors, and many of these processes are species-specific. This is the case for language, which is often considered uniquely human. The presence of shared timelines of brain plasticity is an important attribute when selecting a model system to be used as a surrogate for human brain functioning.

Environment shapes brain structure through postnatal ages. Some classic experiments come from studying rats that were raised in different environments. These showed the importance of environment on brain structure and function. Rats (ages 22–25 days) were exposed to varying amounts of stimuli (e.g., toys) within their cage (Volkmar & Greenough, 1972). Rats in the environmentally enriched condition developed changes in neuronal morphology (e.g., increased branches per neuron) within their visual cortex compared with rats raised alone without the toys. Similar types of enrichment are thought to apply to humans, but we cannot probe human brains like we can those of rats (Sale et al., 2014). Therefore, model systems are needed to understand how environment shapes brain structure.

Several forms of neuroplasticity are observed in adults and older individuals. We know that novel experiences, physical exercise, and sleep shape brain structure and function throughout the lifespan (Davidson & McEwen, 2012; Mahncke et al.,

2006a, 2006b). For example, neurogenesis (i.e., the production of new neurons), long-term potentiation, long-term depression, and brain remapping occur during development, but the extent of plasticity is thought to diminish with aging (Marzola et al., 2023). Different model systems are well suited to study human biology. It is not always clear which model system is best suited to study human plastic changes. Another important consideration in selecting an animal model is its age. Different species mature and age at different rates, so they are subject to different forms of plasticity at different ages (Charvet et al., 2023; Clancy et al., 2001; Workman et al., 2013). Therefore, there is a need to identify the optimal model system for studying human processes. In the following section, I discuss the Translating Time resource, which finds corresponding ages across humans and a diverse model system, and how this resource can help identify the most appropriate model system to study human brain plasticity.

Translating Time

Translating Time is a resource, which relies on time points to find corresponding ages across species. The resource has grown over the past 25 years (Charvet & Finlay, 2018; Charvet et al., 2023; Clancy et al., 2001; Cottam et al., 2025; Finlay & Darlington, 1995; Workman et al., 2013). The resource is housed on a website (*www.translatingtime.org*), enabling researchers to quickly find corresponding ages across humans and model systems. Initially, the database focused on prenatal development across select species, but it has now started to stretch across the lifespan of different species (Charvet et al., 2023; Clancy et al., 2001). For some time, the website is based on a model that includes 18 species, and 271 time points (i.e., events), which extended up to approximately 2 years of age in humans and their correspondence in model systems. This resource has been helpful in finding corresponding ages across developmental ages in model systems.

The website currently includes time points collected from different kinds of data. Early in the project, the team collected time points from neurogenesis of different cell classes (e.g., cerebellar Purkinje cells, layer II–III neurons; Finlay & Darlington, 1995). Time points are also extracted from the process of synaptogenesis (e.g., peak synaptogenesis), myelination (e.g., myelination of optic nerve), and behavioral development (e.g., walking). These time points are abrupt in that there was a rapid change throughout development, but other time points span longer scales and vary gradually rather than abruptly. More recently, we extracted time points from several metrics, which include temporal variation in transcription, and brain volumetric changes (Charvet et al., 2023; Cottam et al., 2025). Integrating information from structural, transcriptional, and behavioral scales permits finding corresponding ages across the lifespan of humans and some nonhuman primate species (Charvet et al., 2023). We have been able to acquire time points from abrupt and gradual changes in time points to find corresponding ages across species (Charvet et al., 2023) and expand the range of ages with which we can find corresponding ages across species.

There are several steps needed to align ages across species. Notably, some time points are not systematically available across all species. Therefore, time points are imputed to generate an "event scale," which is an average ordering of time points across species. Time points are regressed against an event scale. We used a linear model (but other models can be used) to generate age alignments across different species and identify corresponding ages at any of the ages and across any of the species in the model (Charvet et al., 2023; Workman et al., 2013). We can use these models to identify how the pace of development and aging varies across species.

There is variation in the pace of development across species. Some species take longer to develop than others. Humans take much longer to develop than many traditional species, including mice and macaques (Charvet, 2021; Cottam et al., 2025). Early in development, humans are roughly similar to chimpanzees, but humans take slightly longer to develop than chimpanzees (Charvet, 2021). As development progresses into aging, human development and aging still proceed for relatively longer than in chimpanzees. One important difference between humans and chimpanzees is their lifespan. It is rare for chimpanzees to live past their 40s (which maps onto humans in their 50s), but many humans can live past their 80s (Charvet et al., 2023). Therefore, there is a phase of life (i.e., old age) in humans with no counterparts in chimpanzees. Whether some species live to the equivalent age of a human octogenarian is an open question. This is an important question to tackle because it informs which model system lives sufficiently long to recapitulate geriatric-related changes. Those animals would be well suited to further our understanding of human aging (de Sousa et al., 2023).

The Translating Time model has grown immensely over the past 25 years. The resource serves as a bridge across species. In the next section, I describe past work where Translating Time has been instrumental in mapping brain plasticity from model systems to humans, though the resource can be used to study many forms of plasticity.

Translating Time to Select the Most Appropriate Model System

Many processes can be mapped from model systems to humans. The Translating Time resource can translate many developmental processes in different brain regions (e.g., hippocampus, cerebellum). Not all time points are conserved across species (Clancy et al., 2001). The resource permits identifying developmental processes that occur for an unusually long or short time relative to other processes. For example, past work showed that the primate cortex neurogenesis is unusually extended compared with rodents. The extension of cortical neurogenesis accounts for the expansion of the primate cortex relative to mice and rats once variation in brain size is accounted for (Cahalane et al., 2014). These important species differences in brain structure and developmental processes mean that mice may not be the best-suited model system to study human cortical development. Other animals, such as companion animals (e.g., cats and dogs) or nonhuman primates, show relative extensions in cortical neurogenesis compared with rodents, and they may be better suited to understand cortical neurogenesis in humans (Workman et al., 2013). The identification of conserved and deviant developmental programs may identify which model system is best suited to study a particular process.

Translating Time to Map Brain Plasticity from Model System to Humans

The Translating Time resource can predict the timetable of many forms of plasticity in humans. For example, the resource can indicate the timeframe of ocular dominance development, synaptogenesis, and neurogenesis in humans and any species studied. We previously investigated the temporal pattern of hippocampal neurogenesis in humans. While there is much interest in identifying whether a supply of progenitor neurons can be recruited for repair in humans, it is unclear whether new neurons are produced in the adult human brain. There should be some decline in progenitor population with age, but many studies investigating adult neurogenesis have yielded controversial findings because there are few human samples available for study and because of the limitations of the methods available (Lee & Thuret, 2018). Gold standards for tracking progenitor cell populations are not available in humans. Moreover, human hippocampal neurogenesis is, at best, low at postnatal ages, making it challenging to study.

Age alignments from model systems can be used to test whether the temporal decline in hippocampal neurogenesis of humans follows that of model systems (Charvet & Finlay, 2018). In many studied animals, there is extensive hippocampal neurogenesis during prenatal development, which declines postnatally. Various methods can be used to study neurogenesis. Some of these methods, directly or indirectly, can be used to study neurogenesis. Notably, the gold standard methods are birthdating experiments, which involve infusing a substitute of DNA in proliferating cells and tracking them as they exit the cell cycle and migrate to their final destination in the brain. These methods are not available in humans because they are invasive. Only a restricted set of tools is available to make indirect inferences about temporal patterns of hippocampal neurogenesis in humans (Sorrells et al., 2018). This makes studying hippocampal neurogenesis a challenge in humans.

The expression of proteins is available for study in postmortem human brains. Doublecortin is expressed in neurons that have recently been "born," but doublecortin is not expressed in fully mature neurons. The expression of this protein can be used to label recently generated neurons, and quantitative analyses of the relative number of doublecortin neurons can be used to compare the amount of hippocampal neurogenesis at different ages and in different animals (Sorrells et al., 2018). However, false positives and false negatives are a normal part of studying immunohistochemistry. In mice, as in many other model systems, doublecortin is strongly expressed at prenatal ages in hippocampal granule cells, and the expression of doublecortin declines rapidly within the first postnatal months. According to our Translating Time tool, mice in their first two postnatal months (e.g., P60) equate to human teenage years, which would suggest that human hippocampal neurogenesis should decline rapidly during childhood and adolescence (Charvet & Finlay, 2018; Cottam et al., 2025). Human hippocampal neurogenesis may continue beyond adolescence, but the amount of hippocampal neurogenesis is expected to occur at relatively low levels. Examples such as these show the utility of the Translating Time resource to frame whether the temporal changes in biological processes in humans are unusual relative to those of other species.

Conclusion

Translating Time is a useful resource for mapping findings from model systems to humans. We have discussed a few examples, but there is still much work to do to bridge the gap between model systems and humans. More cross-species comparisons are needed to bridge the map findings from model systems to humans.

REFERENCES

Axer, M., & Amunts, K. (2022). Scale matters: The nested human connectome. *Science, 378*, 500–504.

Baroncelli, L., Braschi, C., Spolidoro, M., Begenisic, T., Maffei, L., & Sale, A. (2011). Brain plasticity and disease: A matter of inhibition. *Neural Plasticity, 2011*, 286073.

Bassett, D. S., & Sporns, O. (2017). Network neuroscience. *Nature Neuroscience, 20*(3), 353–364.

Burke, S. N., & Barnes, C. A. (2006). Neural plasticity in the ageing brain. *Nature Reviews Neuroscience, 7*(1), 30–40.

Cahalane, D. J., Charvet, C. J., & Finlay, B. L. (2014). Modeling local and cross-species neuron number variations in the cerebral cortex as arising from a common mechanism. *Proceedings of the National Academy of Sciences, 111*(49), 17642–17647.

Charvet, C. J. (2021). Cutting across structural and transcriptomic scales translates time across the lifespan in humans and chimpanzees. *Proceedings of the Royal Society B: Biological Sciences, 288*, 20202987.

Charvet, C. J., & Finlay, B. L. (2018). Comparing adult hippocampal neurogenesis across species: Translating time to predict the tempo in humans. *Frontiers in Neuroscience, 5*(12), 706.

Charvet, C. J., Ofori, K., Falcone, C., & Rigby Dames, B. A. (2023). Transcription, structure, and organoids translate time across the lifespan of humans and great apes. *PNAS Nexus, 2*(8), pgad230.

Cottam, N., Ofori, K., Stoll, K. T., Bryant, M., Rogge, J., Hekmatyar. K., et al. (2025). From circuits to lifespan: Translating mouse and human timelines with neuroimaging based tractography. *Journal of Neuroscience, 45*(12), e1429242025.

Clancy, B., Darlington, R. B., & Finlay, B. L. (2001). Translating developmental time across mammalian species. *Neuroscience, 105*(1), 7–17.

Clemenson, G. D., Deng, W., & Gage, F. H. (2015). Environmental enrichment and neurogenesis: From mice to humans. *Current Opinion in Behavioral Sciences, 4*, 56–62.

Davidson, R. J., & McEwen, B. (2012). Social influences on neuroplasticity: Stress and interventions to promote well-being. *Nature Neuroscience, 15*, 689–695.

de Sousa, A. A, Rigby Dames, B. A., Graff, E. C., Mohamedelhassan, R., Vassilopoulos, T., & Charvet, C. J. (2023). Going beyond established model systems of Alzheimer's disease: Companion animals provide novel insights into the neurobiology of aging. *Communications Biology, 6*(1), 655.

Fawcett, J. (2009). Molecular control of brain plasticity and repair. *Progress in Brain Research*, 175, 501–509.

Finlay, B. L., & Darlington, R. B. (1995). Linked regularities in the development and evolution of mammalian brains. *Science, 268*, 1578–1584.

Gordon, J. A., & Stryker, M. P. (1996). Experience-dependent plasticity of binocular responses in the primary visual cortex of the mouse. *Journal of Neuroscience, 16*(10), 3274–3286.

Hunt, D. L., Yamoah, E. N., & Krubitzer, L. (2006). Multisensory plasticity in congenitally deaf mice: How are cortical areas functionally specified? *Neuroscience, 139*(4), 1507–1524.

Kramer, A. F., Bherer, L., Colcombe, S. J., Dong, W., & Greenough, W. T. (2004). Environmental influences on cognitive and brain plasticity during aging. *Journals of Gerontology Series A: Biological Sciences and Medical Sciences, 59*(9), M940–957.

Krubitzer, L., Künzle, H., & Kaas, J. (1997). Organization of sensory cortex in a Madagascan insectivore, the tenrec (*Echinops telfairi*). *Journal of Comparative Neurology, 379*(3), 399–414.

Krubitzer, L., Manger, P., Pettigrew, J., & Calford, M. (1995). Organization of somatosensory cortex in monotremes: In search of the prototypical plan. *Journal of Comparative Neurology, 351*(2), 261–306.

Lee, H., & Thuret, S. (2018). Adult human hippocampal neurogenesis: Controversy and evidence. *Trends in Molecular Medicine, 24*(6), 521–522.

Mahncke, H., Bronstone, A., & Merzenich, M. M. (2006a). Brain plasticity and functional losses in the aged: Scientific bases for a novel intervention. *Progress in Brain Research, 157*, 81–109.

Mahncke, H., Connor, B., Appelman, J., Ahsanuddin, O., Hardy, J., Joyce, N., et al. (2006b). Memory enhancement in healthy older adults using a brain plasticity-based training program: A randomized, controlled study. *Proceedings of the National Academy of Sciences, 103*, 12523–12528.

Marzola, P., Melzer, T., Pavesi, E., Gil-Mohapel, J., & Brocardo, P. S. (2023). Exploring the role of neuroplasticity in development, aging, and neurodegeneration. *Brain Sciences, 13*(12), 1610.

Mora, F., Segovia, G., & del Arco, A. (2007). Aging, plasticity and environmental enrichment: Structural changes and neurotransmitter dynamics in several areas of the brain. *Brain Research Review, 55*(1),78–88.

Murphy, T., Dias, G. P., & Thuret, S. (2014). Effects of diet on brain plasticity in animal and human studies: Mind the gap. *Neural Plasticity, 2014*, 563160.

Park, H. J., & Friston, K. (2013). Structural and functional brain networks: From connections to cognition. *Science, 342*, 1238411.

Partanen, E., Kujala, T., Tervaniemi, M., & Huotilainen, M. (2013). Prenatal music exposure induces long-term neural effects. *PLOS ONE, 8*(10), e78946.

Sale, A., Berardi, N., & Maffei, L. (2014). Environment and brain plasticity: Towards an endogenous pharmacotherapy (2014). *Physiological Reviews, 94*(1), 189–234.

Sorrells, S. F., Paredes, M. F., Cebrian-Silla, A., Sandoval, K., Qi, D., & Kelley, K. W. (2018). Human hippocampal neurogenesis drops sharply in children to undetectable levels in adults. *Nature, 555*, 377–381.

Ungerleider, L. G., Doyon, J., & Karni, A. (2002). Imaging brain plasticity during motor skill learning. *Neurobiology of Learning and Memory, 78*(3), 553–564.

Volkmar, F. R., & Greenough, W. T. (1972). Rearing complexity affects branching of dendrites in the visual cortex of the rat. *Science, 176*, 1445–1447.

Walker, L. C. (1981). The ontogeny of the neural substrate for language. *Journal of Human Evolution, 10*(5), 429–441.

Wang, B. S., Sarnaik, R., & Cang, J. (2010). Critical period plasticity matches binocular orientation preference in the visual cortex. *Neuron, 65*(2), 246–256.

Wasserman, G. A., Liu, X., Parvez, F., Ahsan, H., Factor-Litvak, P., van Geen, A., et al.

(2004). Water arsenic exposure and children's intellectual function in Araihazar, Bangladesh. *Environmental Health Perspectives, 112*(13), 1329–1333.

Workman, A. D., Charvet, C. J., Clancy, B., Darlington, R. B., & Finlay, B. L. (2013). Modeling transformations of neurodevelopmental sequences across mammalian species. *Journal of Neuroscience, 33*(17), 7368–7383.

Yeh, F. C, Panesar, S., Fernandes, D., Meola, A., Yoshino, M., Fernandez-Miranda J. C., et al. (2018). Population-averaged atlas of the macroscale human structural connectome and its network topology. *NeuroImage, 178*, 57–68.

CHAPTER 4

Different Levels of Plasticity

Luca Bonfanti

Brain Plasticity: Theme and Variations

Brain plasticity is one of the most studied topics in the neurosciences (>80,000 articles in PubMed), due to its involvement in the postnatal development/refinement of neural circuits and in the perspective of brain repair. The more it is discovered on brain plasticity, the more we unravel its heterogeneity, at least on two main levels: the different forms of neural structural changes that can coexist and the evolutionary adaptation of these processes from mice to humans (Bonfanti et al., 2024; Morizet & Bally-Cuif, 2025; Paredes et al., 2016b; Figure 4.1D*). The heterogeneity of brain plasticity also extends to further levels, involving the specific features of plastic changes at the cellular level, the cell populations involved, their regional location, the interspecies differences in the animal world, and their functions. As a result, different brains can produce/use plasticity in different ways, basically as an adaptation, which makes it more difficult to study plasticity, sometimes becoming a source of confusion, especially when the research is only focused on laboratory rodents (Amrein, 2015; Barker et al., 2011; Duque et al., 2022).

In biomedical research, the perception of plasticity also depends on the technical approach used to detect it: from physiological aspects of synaptic strengthening to ultrastructural visualization of single synapses, from the study of plasticity modulation by environmental cues at the cellular and molecular level to the demonstration of wide brain areas undergoing functional changes involving millions of neurons in noninvasive neuroimaging (see Chapters 2 and 3, this volume). Despite huge advancements in each research direction, some gaps between different approaches should still be overcome to gain a full picture of brain plasticity in humans.

---

* Figure 4.1 appears on the separate color insert.

Before entering the specific types of neural plasticity, a distinction can be made between functional or structural levels of plastic changes, which can be semantically questionable since molecular changes can lead to structural modifications. Functional plasticity is associated with molecular changes that occur at the cell/synaptic level, including modification in presynaptic transmitter release, postsynaptic receptor tracking, signal transduction pathways, gene activation, and synthesis of new proteins, which ultimately can change the magnitude of synaptic transmission (Chen et al., 2018; Figure 4.1A, left). Beyond these steps, the formation/elimination of synapses can be considered a form of structural plasticity involving microscopic modifications of the cell shape at the dendritic spine level (Holtmaat & Svoboda, 2009; see Figure 4.1A, right, and below). More complex modifications can affect the whole cell structure, including changes in the entire cell morphology and maturation, cell reprogramming and transdifferentiation (Robel et al., 2011), up to the genesis of new neurons and glial elements, known as neurogenesis and gliogenesis (Bond et al., 2015; Lim & Alvarez-Buylla, 2016; Paolicelli et al., 2022; Yeung et al., 2014).

All types of plastic changes can coexist and add up to each other, exerting their effects from the molecule to the system level, thus allowing the neural circuits to adapt to environmental challenges throughout the lifetime by producing learning, memory, and reactive responses. These latter, when not counterproductive for tissue repair or regeneration (e.g., some aspects of reactive gliosis), can lead to compensatory responses to tissue damage and pathological states (cross-modal plasticity; Lee & Whitt, 2015). Finally, further levels of plasticity are the object of cutting-edge studies, encompassing metaplasticity (the modulation of the ability of neurons to express synaptic plasticity, shaping the direction, magnitude, and duration of future synaptic changes; Müller-Dahlhaus & Ziemann, 2015) and the relationship between neural plasticity, structural covariance, and functional connectivity (structural changes and temporal correlations between spatially separate brain regions occurring beyond anatomical connections; Karpati et al., 2018; Stevenson et al., 2009).

Before addressing the specific types of plasticity at the cellular level, some general considerations on the possible roles of these processes are needed.

Role(s) of Brain Plasticity: Development or Repair?

The potential for structural remodeling provided by brain plasticity (affecting either neuronal/glial morphology, the specificity of interneuronal contacts, or the number of neurons) can be useful in two main contexts: (1) the refinement of neural networks in healthy individuals based on internal and external stimuli, to adapt to physiological or environmental changes, mostly finalized to learning and to refining the neural circuits and (2) the compensation for the loss of structure/function as a consequence of lesion, injury, pathological states, and in some cases also producing cell/tissue repair. Over the years, most neurodevelopmental studies have been focused on the second point. Nevertheless, the potential for brain repair is quite reduced in mammals (Weil et al., 2008). In general, the reduction of nerve cell renewal capacity (and, consequently, neural repair/regeneration) seems to follow the increase in brain complexity/size and the increased capability to perform complex cognitive functions (Alunni & Bally-Cuif, 2016; Bonfanti, 2011; Paredes et al., 2016b). This trend is evident when comparing distant animal groups, such as nonmammalian vertebrates (e.g., fish and salamanders) and mammals (Bonfanti, 2011). The former group of animals displays multiple neurogenic sites endowed with active stem cell niches in widespread regions of the brain and spinal cord, allowing substantial neuronal renewal and regeneration throughout life (Alunni & Bally-Cuif, 2016; Ganz & Brand, 2016; Grandel et al., 2006). On the other hand, stem cell–driven neurogenesis is spatially and temporally restricted in mammals (Bond et al., 2015; Lim & Alvarez-Buylla, 2016), wherein most regenerative processes are confined to postnatal stages when plasticity and tissue permissiveness are still high (Montero & Huang, 2022).

In addition to the availability, amount, location, and properties of the stem cell pool, the potential for structural plasticity is also highly defined by the tissue environment, including extracellular matrix components, myelin-associated molecules, and the glial scars that frequently form after brain injury (Adams & Gallo, 2018; Cope & Gould, 2019). Interspecies differences concerning the glial cell types (Falcone et al., 2019), as well as the animal age (Ben Abdallah et al., 2010; Ghibaudi et al., 2023; Snyder, 2019), are also important. A large bulk of research indicates that the injured nervous tissue does not favor a strategy of regeneration, but rather one of minimizing further damage, because of unavoidable evolutionary constraints (Weil et al., 2008).

Unlike the remarkable adaptation of brain plasticity reparative potential during evolution in different animal groups, the "developmental" role of plasticity seems to be a common feature in all nervous systems (Cushman et al., 2021; Semënov, 2019). All forms of plasticity, though granting neural dynamic changes through life, are particularly intense during juvenile stages, leading to a progressive stabilization around adolescence and ultimately providing a "vision of the world" based on experience. This "developmental" role of plasticity appears to be particularly true for adult neurogenesis, which is substantially different if compared with other adult stem cell–supported processes in the body. Due to progressive stem cell depletion/quiescence, the rate of neurogenesis decreases exponentially during adult life (to a lesser extent in mice, more evidently in humans; Ben Abdallah et al., 2010; Sanai et al., 2011; Sorrells et al., 2018), never reaching a steady rate and thus in sharp contrast with blood, epidermis, and small intestine epithelia, in which a steady renewal of all cells pursues at high rates throughout the lifespan (Potten & Loeffler, 1990). In the so-called "sculpting hypothesis," it has been suggested that the contribution of juvenile neurogenesis is to allow the behavioral experience to refine neural circuit connectivity such that sensory attributes that are relevant to the individual's environment are more strongly represented (Cushman et al., 2021).

In summary, while both developmental and reparative roles can be the outcome of brain structural plasticity, the former appears to be a primary, transversal feature, while the latter, especially in mammals, might be considered as a byproduct of evolution.

Specific Types of Brain Structural Plasticity

In this section, the main types of structural changes occurring in the mammalian brain will be briefly described (summarized in Figure 4.1A–C). Since remarkable interspecies differences affecting neural plasticity have emerged from mice to humans, they will be addressed in a separate section (summarized in Figure 4.1D).

Synaptic Plasticity

Beyond the activity-dependent change in neuronal connection strength (functional synaptic plasticity; Magee & Grienberger, 2020), the neural network structure can be changed through the physical modification of contacts between neurons (formation and elimination of synapses; Holtmaat & Svoboda, 2009). In healthy individuals, these processes are thought to be ubiquitous in the nervous system (Bufill et al., 2011; DeFelipe et al., 2002; Sherwood et al., 2020) and considering that the 10^{11} neurons of the human brain are connected by 10^{15} synapses, the potential for activity-dependent changes through synaptic plasticity is huge, mainly overtaking that of other forms of plasticity. Changes at the synaptic level enable the brains to produce learned or adaptive behaviors that allow individuals to thrive in complex environments and establish memories (see Chapter 6, this volume). Adaptive behaviors linked to survival are complicated, going beyond the actions determined by sensory/motor systems and requiring the capacity to make suitable decisions in the perspective of moving appropriately within the environment (Magee & Grienberger, 2020). Various types of synaptic plasticity (e.g., Hebbian long-term potentiation, long-term depression, behavioral time scale synaptic plasticity, formation and elimination of synapses) enable neuronal populations to refine their activity across postnatal development toward a target or goal pattern that is, in the end, useful to the animal in a specific behavior (Magee & Grienberger, 2020).

In pathological conditions, the spectrum of intrinsic capacities allowing the brain to react as a highly dynamic system can also be exploited for compensatory responses, such as cross-modal synaptic plasticity and compensatory plasticity in the spared sensory cortices (see Lee & Whitt, 2015, and Chapter 8, this volume). This is the basis of rehabilitation, an approach that emphasizes the relearning of functionality lost due to the injury through reorganizing neural circuits in the intact tissue (Nudo, 2006). Finally, dysfunctional plasticity can be the basis of neuropsychiatric disorders, including depression, schizophrenia, and posttraumatic stress disorder (Appelbaum et al., 2023).

Neuroglial Plasticity

For a long time, plasticity in the nervous system has been interpreted as neuronal plasticity. It is now clear that different types of glial cells, including astrocytes, oligodendrocytes, and microglia, do contribute actively to allow/induce plastic changes, involving glial precursor cell proliferation, myelination, myelin sheath remodeling, synapse functioning, synaptic pruning, stem cell–driven neurogenesis, and modulation of cell-to-cell contacts (Figure 4.1B). Most of all, a subclass of modified radial glia cells can act as stem cells, thus granting persistent neurogenesis in young and adult individuals (Doetsch et al., 1999). Recent studies using animal models revealed that, in various experimental conditions of damage, parenchymal astrocytes of nonneurogenic regions (e.g., cerebral cortex and striatum) can dedifferentiate to a stem-like cell type, giving rise to neurons (Robel et al., 2011; Sirko et al., 2023; Zamboni et al., 2020). Although astrocytic glia reprogramming is now a well-documented process, in the absence of a well-defined physiological or reparative outcome, it is not yet clear whether this process is part of a specific reactive (neurogenic) program or simply the awakening of a vestigial (ultimately abortive) potential (Alunni & Bally-Cuif, 2016). In this context, a series of repair attempts and undue reactions directed to circumscribe damage (e.g., gliosis, partial transdifferentiation and dematuration) can lead to maladaptive plasticity (also termed destructive or dysfunctional plasticity), warning that plastic processes are not limited to "constructive" mechanisms, but also imply negative consequences in various neurological disorders (Seblani et al., 2024).

Astrocytes are also involved in other forms of plasticity. They are connected by gap junctions, forming tightly regulated networks that allow remodeling (Giaume & McCarthy, 1996) and, under physiological conditions (e.g., reproduction, sensory stimulation), can participate in the so-called tripartite synapse by maintaining the synapse homeostasis and displaying plasticity in their responsiveness to neurotransmitters (Durkee & Araque, 2019; Perea et al., 2009). In addition, astrocytes can display remarkable structural changes of the distal lamellae that ensheath neurons (Theodosis et al., 2008); this plasticity can occur in a matter of minutes, allowing them to remodel the geometry of the extracellular space and the relationships with adjacent neuronal elements, including synapses (Chung et al., 2015; De Pittà et al., 2016; Theodosis et al., 2008).

Many studies have confirmed that myelin is not immutable but changing with experience through the lifespan and adapting the function of neuronal circuits (Bonetto et al., 2021; Monje, 2018; Xin & Chan, 2020). Myelination has long been viewed as a process ending in young adults; however, most of the areas in the central nervous system exhibit partial myelination and potentially become myelinated during the lifespan, thus providing a dynamic range for activity-dependent structural plasticity (Tomassy et al., 2014). Studies in animal models strongly indicate that these processes occur through oligodendrocyte progenitor cell (OPC) division and subsequent differentiation induced by manipulation of sensory experience or neuronal activity. In turn, OPC proliferation and differentiation are promoted by the performance of behavioral tasks and can lead to myelination of specific brain areas in both gray and white matter, affecting microcircuits and long-distance connections, respectively (Bonetto et al., 2021; Monje, 2018; Xin & Chan, 2020). OPCs form the largest population of dividing cells in the postnatal and adult brain parenchyma, representing themselves as a form of structural plasticity that is maintained throughout the lifespan (Boda et al., 2015; Yeung et al., 2014). Adult oligodendrogenesis and myelin remodeling represent a mechanism by which experience may modify brain connections, having an impact on circuits and systems involved in cognition and behavior and being potentially involved in brain repair (Ronzano et al., 2020). At a different scale, region-specific changes in white matter following multiple forms of learning have been shown to occur in human imaging studies (see the section "Plasticity of Large-Scale Networks").

Finally, through different actions, including phagocytosis, surveillance, and capacity for releasing soluble factors, microglia cells contribute to key biological functions involving plasticity, including synapse remodeling (e.g., developmental pruning), neurogenesis, neuronal function, myelination, inflammation, and tissue repair (Andoh & Koyama, 2021; Paolicelli et al., 2022).

Adult Neurogenesis

The genesis of new neurons in the adult mammalian brain was first suggested in rodents and monkeys in the 1960s (Altman & Das, 1965), then fully demonstrated in birds in the 1980s (Paton & Nottebohm, 1984). It was definitively confirmed in mammals at the beginning of the 1990s by using thymidine analog injections and viral vector techniques (Lois & Alvarez-Buylla, 1994); in the subsequent years, its origin from neural stem cells was established (Doetsch et al., 1999; Gage, 2000). Since then, stem cell–driven neurogenesis has been the subject of intensive research (Aimone et al., 2014; Bond et al., 2015; Lim & Alvarez-Buylla, 2016; Kempermann, 2019; Obernier & Alvarez-Buylla, 2019), raising hopes for new therapeutic strategies for neurological disorders (Bao & Song, 2018; Martino et al., 2011). Most studies were carried out on laboratory rodents, leading to the identification and cellular/molecular characterization of two "canonical" neurogenic sites: the forebrain subventricular zone, lining the walls of the lateral ventricle (Lim & Alvarez-Buylla, 2016; Obernier & Alvarez-Buylla, 2019), and the subgranular zone, in the dentate gyrus of the hippocampus (Aimone et al., 2014; Gonçalves et al., 2016). These regions contain neural stem cells derived from radial glia and hosted in remnants of the embryonic germinal layers, or "niches" (Alvarez-Buylla et al., 2001), which produce new neuronal precursors that can differentiate into region-specific types of neurons, which can functionally integrate into the olfactory bulb and hippocampal local networks (Aimone et al., 2014; Obernier et al., 2014; Figure 4.1C, top).

A third area of genesis, localized in the wall of the third ventricle and containing a population of tanycytes acting as stem cells has been identified in the hypothalamus (Kokoeva et al., 2005; Pierce & Xu, 2010). The development of specific phenotypes involved in neuroendocrine function suggests that a fraction of newly born cells might become mature; however, at present there is no clear evidence that these neurons can integrate into the hypothalamic circuitry structurally and functionally (Yoo & Blackshaw, 2018).

Other neurogenic processes have been described outside of the two/three main niches, representing the so-called "parenchymal" or "noncanonical" neurogenesis (reviewed in Feliciano et al., 2015). Yet, some of the parenchymal neurogenic processes are species-specific (Luzzati et al., 2006; Ponti et al., 2008) or lesion-induced (Lindvall & Kokaia, 2015), in some cases passing through astrocytic glia reprogramming (see the "Neuroglial Plasticity" section). Also in these processes, it is difficult to identify the outcome of the progenitor cell division in terms of a clear structural and functional integration into the neural circuits, thus suggesting that most parenchymal neurogenesis might be "incomplete" because there is no active stem cell niche to sustain them as well as evidence for a functional outcome (Bonfanti & Peretto, 2011). As a direct consequence of the highly restricted sources of protracted neurogenesis in mammals, most of the adult brain parenchyma remains a nonrenewable tissue, with most cell divisions ascribable to OPCs.

A topic that gained a lot of interest in adult neurogenesis is its possible modulation by endogenous or environmental factors. It is well known from studies carried out in laboratory rodents that aerobic physical activity, sensory stimulation, and an enriched environment can increase the production of new neurons in canonical neurogenic niches (while a lot of stress can decrease it) by affecting stem cell division and the rate of functional integration of the new neurons (Kempermann, 2019). Nevertheless, the enriched condition is only enriched relative to standard cages housing the animals in isolation, and thus far from that of animals living experiences in the wild. Similar studies carried out on natural populations of rodents living in the wild did not find the same effect (Amrein, 2015), thus suggesting that the abovementioned modulation (rapid adaptation of hippocampal neurogenesis to experimental challenges) might be induced preferably in laboratory mice that live their life in a substantially unchanging environment. Again, adult neurogenesis can be viewed as a late developmental process aimed at sculpting the "vision of the world" based on experience during youth, leading to shaping individual patterns of brain plasticity, and, ultimately, individuality (Kempermann, 2019; Semënov, 2019). In parallel, synaptic remodeling and, to a lesser extent, dendritic branching remain likely the best candidates for experience-dependent volume changes, along with an increase in vascularization induced by physical activity (see the "Plasticity of Large-Scale Networks" section).

Arrested Maturation (Dormant Neuronal Precursors and Immature Neurons)

When studying parenchymal brain regions out of the canonical stem cell niches (e.g., in the cerebral cortex and amygdala), neuronal populations expressing the markers of immaturity typically displayed by newly born neuroblasts (e.g., the cytoskeletal protein doublecortin [DCX] or the anti-adhesive, polysialylated form of the neural cell adhesion molecule [PSA-NCAM]) can also be found. Apart from specific examples of noncanonical neurogenesis (mostly linked to single nonrodent species; see the section "Adult Neurogenesis"), these immature cell populations can occur without cell division (reviewed in Bonfanti & Seki, 2021). In layer II of the paleocortex (piriform cortex), the DCX/PSA-NCAM-immunopositive cells are prenatally generated neurons continuing to exhibit markers of immaturity through adulthood (cells in arrested maturation, or cortical "immature" neurons [cINs]; Bonfanti & Nacher, 2012; Gómez-Climent et al., 2008; König et al., 2016; La Rosa et al., 2020a; Luzzati et al., 2009; Pattaro et al., 2025; Rotheneichner et al., 2018). By using a DCX-Cre-ERT2/Flox-EGFP transgenic mouse, in which a fluorescent protein is permanently expressed in DCX-positive cells and their progeny, it has been shown that most cINs are "dormant" neuronal precursors that can awake after long periods of hibernation and mature into glutamatergic neurons, becoming ultimately integrated into the preexisting neural network until very advanced ages (Benedetti et al., 2020, 2023; Rotheneichner et al., 2018; Figure 4.1C, bottom).

Most of the cINs are small, bipolar cells frozen in a state of arrested maturation, representing a reserve of nondividing, dormant precursors, some of which can awake at different time points throughout life, continuing their differentiation by increasing their size and dendritic arborization (complex cells) until complete maturation and functional integration (Benedetti et al., 2020; Rotheneichner et al., 2018). Though fully independent from the existence of stem cells/niches, in the past, these precursors were often confused with newborn neurons (Ghibaudi & Bonfanti, 2022). Their prenatal origin has been shown by the detection of 5-bromodeoxyuridine (BrdU; visualized in the progeny after embryonic injection in the mother) in rodents (Gómez-Climent et al., 2008) and sheep (Piumatti et al., 2018). Hence, the cINs can provide a sort of "neurogenesis without division" in a brain region not endowed with canonical neurogenesis (the cerebral cortex), which is extremely important for higher cognitive functions (Bonfanti et al., 2024; La Rosa et al., 2020b).

Similar DCX-positive cells not associated with the canonical stem cell niches have been described in subcortical regions (amygdala, claustrum) and in some tracts of the white matter (reviewed in Ghibaudi & Bonfanti, 2022; Page et al., 2022). Though previously interpreted as adult neurogenesis, these cells also seem to be independent of cell division, thus opening the possibility that they are dormant precursors of prenatal origin (Ghibaudi & Bonfanti, 2022; Ghibaudi et al., 2025). At present, evidence for embryonic origin has been provided in the amygdala of mice (Alderman et al., 2023) and sheep (Piumatti et al., 2018), and further knowledge is needed concerning other animal species and the exact time window in which they are produced. These immature cells also appear predominant in large-brained species (Chareyron et al., 2021; Fudge et al., 2012; Piumatti et al., 2018; Sorrells et al., 2019; see the section "Interspecies Variation in Brain Plasticity").

Hence, besides the well-characterized stem cell-driven neurogenic processes in the adult brain, some neuronal populations appear to be in a state of arrested maturation, maintaining immature marker expression and a simple morphology for a long time. Although crucial aspects of these neurons are still unknown (e.g., their functional role and the mechanism(s) leading to blocking their maturation and waking them up later), the dormant neurons can represent a reservoir of young neuronal elements in the adult brain, contributing to increasing the heterogeneity of its plasticity and to possibly representing a brain reserve (Alderman et al., 2023; La Rosa et al., 2019, 2020b; Rotheneichner et al., 2018). Their occurrence in the neocortex of gyrencephalic species might account for the maintenance of higher thickness of the upper cortical layers (II–III) typical of these species in comparison with rodents due to the higher complexity of the neuropil, which is considered to be associated with higher computational capabilities (de Sousa et al., 2023). Conversely, reduction in cortical thickness is found in most forms of dementia due to synaptic loss and reduced plasticity (see the "Plasticity of Large-Scale Networks" section). In mammals, the populations of cells in arrested maturation coexist with adult neurogenesis, and their relative occurrence, distribution, and number can remarkably vary across different species (see the section "Interspecies Variation in Brain Plasticity").

Plasticity of Large-Scale Networks

Using connectivity and tractography analysis of magnetic resonance imaging data (MRI; e.g., structural, diffusion, and functional MRI; diffusion tensor imaging and fractional anisotropy), the plasticity of large-scale networks, including measurement of the volume and thickness of brain structures or integrity of white matter and myelination, can be studied in the living human brain (Appelbaum et al., 2023; Dayan & Cohen, 2011; Lövdén et al., 2013). In structural MRI, increases in cortical gray matter thickness in adult individuals are considered indicative of neuroplasticity after task learning. These changes, believed to be secondary to synaptogenesis and dendritic arborization (or increase in the capillary network, especially after repeated physical activity), can occur over weeks to months. By measuring fractional anisotropy (a parameter based on the diffusivity of water molecules in the brain and associated with changes in white matter), it has been observed that a wide range of skilled motor and nonmotor learning (e.g., professional vs. nonprofessional musicians, or poor readers vs. good readers) can induce structural changes in specific human white matter tracts (Lövdén et al., 2013; Sampaio-Baptista & Johansen-Berg, 2017). An interesting example is provided by recent studies revealing that experiences associated with different childhood socioeconomic status can accelerate or slow down structural brain maturation, ultimately affecting the efficiency of cortical networks in adulthood (Tooley et al., 2021).

Besides the clear advantage of allowing direct investigation of changes occurring in the brain macrostructure of living human beings, it must be said that noninvasive imaging approaches do provide a general view of what is happening to "areas" of the nervous tissue, including thousands or millions of neurons, thus revealing "where" but not "how" plasticity is supposed to occur. In the study of brain plasticity, a gap still exists between the information coming from these techniques that can be applied to humans and the cellular/molecular approaches performed in animal models to reveal the neural substrates of plastic changes (Lövdén et al., 2013; Mansvelder et al., 2019).

Interspecies Variation in Brain Plasticity

The potential of the nervous tissue to perform structural modifications is highly variable depending on the species, the type of plasticity, and the brain region because of different neuroanatomical and physiological adaptations to distinct ecological niches. Most research on brain plasticity has been conducted on laboratory rodents, revealing molecular and cellular mechanisms that can be largely shared with other species (Wong et al., 2023), while differences can emerge at a system level (La Rosa et al., 2020b; Ghibaudi et al., 2025; Pattaro et al., 2025).

Maintenance of synaptic features, including synaptic types, morphology, and density, has been found in the cortex of different mammals (DeFelipe et al., 2002; Sherwood et al., 2020). On these bases, the occurrence of synaptic plasticity is estimated to be rather homogeneous and widespread across animal species, though little is known in humans, whose neuronal circuits, with neurons and synapses not readily accessible, remain a challenge (Mansvelder et al., 2019).

On the other hand, neurogenic processes can remarkably vary. It is well known that, when comparing nonmammalian vertebrates and mammals, stem cell–driven neurogenesis is highly reduced in the latter as to its rate, anatomical extension, and reparative capacity (Bonfanti, 2011; Grandel et al., 2006; see the "Brain Plasticity: Theme and Variations" section at the beginning of this chapter).

Substantial differences have also been reported among mammals, at least on three levels: (1) Neurogenesis occurring outside the canonical neurogenic sites seems to be restricted to some species and regions (e.g., the striatum and cerebellum of rabbits; Luzzati et al., 2006; Ponti et al., 2008); (2) the absence of neurogenesis (or very low levels, considered as vestigial) has been found in other species (e.g., dolphins and bats; Amrein et al., 2007; Parolisi et al., 2017; Patzke et al., 2015); and (3) a dramatic drop in canonical neurogenesis at juvenile stages has been described in humans (Sanai et al., 2011; Seki et al., 2019; Sorrells et al., 2018).

In general, adult neurogenesis relying on stem cell niches appears to be reduced in gyrencephalic, long-living mammals with respect to laboratory rodents (Bonfanti et al., 2024; Morizet & Bally-Cuif, 2025; Simard et al., 2025); this fact has been linked to early exhaustion of stem cell niche activity, stem cell depletion/quiescence, large brain size, energy-demanding costs, and evolutionary constraints (Duque et al., 2022; Encinas et al., 2011; Paredes et al., 2016b; Parolisi et al., 2018). Conversely, immature (dormant) neurons appear to be far more abundant in large-brained, highly gyrencephalic species (La Rosa et al., 2020b; Palazzo et al., 2018), including humans (Li et al., 2023).

It has been proposed that a *tradeoff* in plasticity has occurred during evolution between different types of structural changes (specifically, different types of neurogenesis), with a prevalence of stem cell–driven adult neurogenesis in rodents and a preference for delayed maturation of nondividing immature neurons in gyrencephalic species (Bonfanti et al., 2024; Figure 4.1D). The concept of a tradeoff implies that the balance of resource allocation can shift between different options, allowing evolution to favor specific processes in certain species or brain regions, depending on the ecological pressures and functional demands they face (van Noordwijdk & Jong, 1986). The tradeoff in plasticity would meet the need for mammals endowed with largely expanded neocortices to add new functional neurons during life in a region devoid of stem cells/neurogenesis, yet of paramount importance for their survival; on the other hand, rodents (characterized by a smaller, smooth cortex) would rely mostly on olfaction and the hippocampus (and their capability to add new neurons through stem cell division) for their survival (Bonfanti et al., 2024; Morizet & Bally-Cuif, 2025).

Human Brain Structural Plasticity: Evolutionary Aspects and Existing Gaps

As described in previous sections, most of the current knowledge concerning the structural substrates of brain plasticity in mammals comes from laboratory rodents, sometimes taking for granted that they might generally represent all species, the resulting information being basically translatable to humans. The human brain is composed of structures conserved through evolution and others unique to primates. The mouse brain is 0.6 gram, with a smooth cerebral cortex, reaching adult maturation in 3 months, against the 1,300 grams, highly gyrencephalic cortex, and 20 years of growth/maturation of the human brain (Arellano et al., 2024; Smaers et al., 2019; Zilles et al., 2013). Consequently, rodent models do not always recapitulate human neurobiology or pathophysiology, and some rodent-based studies can be misleading for preclinical research translation (Bolker, 2017; Brenowitz & Zakon, 2015).

Concerning brain plasticity, despite remarkable interspecies differences having been reported (Duque et al., 2022; Ghibaudi et al., 2025; La Rosa et al., 2020b; Paredes et al., 2016b; Parolisi et al., 2018; Sanai et al., 2011), researchers working exclusively on mice and rats often make claims generalizing their conclusions to humans. It is also worth mentioning that some scientists working on nonhuman primates (e.g., common marmoset, macaque) used to generalize to "primates and humans." Nevertheless, marmosets have relatively small, lissencephalic brains (brain weight: 8.5 grams; gyrification index: 1,18), which are remarkably different from other species of anthropoid primates, such as chimpanzees, with larger and highly gyrencephalic brains (brain weight: 383 grams; gyrification index: 2,31; Zilles et al., 2013).

Different forms of plasticity do coexist in most mammalian species, including humans, but with different importance and rates following a tradeoff that benefits some types of structural changes with respect to others based on evolutionary adaptations (Bonfanti et al., 2024). Brain plasticity encompasses many distinct phenomena, some of which operate across most of the lifespan (e.g., synaptic plasticity) and others that operate exclusively in postnatal development (e.g., some protracted forms of neurogenesis in humans). To fill the gap between the huge amount of knowledge gathered on brain plasticity in laboratory rodents and its possible matching in humans, several studies carried out at the cellular and molecular level on postmortem human brain tissues have provided new, valuable information (Moreno-Jiménez et al., 2019; Nascimento et al., 2023; Paredes et al., 2016a; Sanai et al., 2011; Seki et al., 2019; Sorrells et al., 2018, 2019; Zhou et al., 2022). The emerging view is that several aspects of neuronal, synapse, myelin, and white matter maturation appear to be delayed in time in humans, thus granting the maintenance of a sort of neoteny (the delaying or slowing of some developmental aspects, with retention of juvenile traits). Neotenic features can allow the experience to refine the brain circuits during postnatal life, a period whose persistence depends on the species and the lifespan, being particularly extended in humans (Workman et al., 2013; for translating times in brain developmental schedules, see Chapter 3, this volume). Comparative studies involving widely different mammals have started to reveal that gyrencephalic, long-living species endowed with high cognitive functions tend to retain neoteny at different levels, including neuronal maturation (Ciceri et al., 2024), synapse maturation (Wang et al., 2023), and the reserve of neurons in arrested maturation of the cerebral cortex layer II (Ghibaudi et al., 2023; La Rosa et al., 2020b; Li et al., 2023; Pattaro et al., 2025), somehow recapitulated in subcortical regions (Alderman et al., 2023; Fudge et al., 2012; Ghibaudi & Bonfanti, 2022; Ghibaudi et al., 2025; Piumatti et al., 2018; Sorrells et al., 2019). As a result, the pace of human brain development is protracted compared with most other species, and this can have an impact on plasticity and learning experiences associated with childhood (Tooley et al., 2021). In addition to adult neurogenesis of the canonical neurogenic sites (mostly restricted to juvenile stages), several neurodevelopmental processes continue in the human brain after birth, when not all neurons are in their final locations and neuronal migration continues throughout human infancy, allowing changes in circuit plasticity and functionality (Nascimento et al., 2023; Paredes et al., 2016a; Sorrells, 2024).

During youth, all forms of postnatal structural plasticity contribute to the substantial growth of the brain volume, a fact that has been recently linked to a rethinking of human altriciality. Since human newborns are relatively underdeveloped at birth compared with other primates, they are considered altricial. Yet, it is suggested that such altriciality is mostly driven by postnatal changes (timing of myelination and neuroplasticity) that might have evolved as a selectively advantageous trait linked to increased behavioral complexity (Gómez-Robles et al., 2024). In other words, increased adult brain size in humans is linked to longer extension of neurodevelopment, thus confirming that "larger brains need more time to grow."

Conclusion

Overall, the heterogeneous features defining plasticity of the human brain strongly support a role in terms of refinement and sculpting of the neural circuits based on experience rather than a potential for repair. Yet, the protracted postnatal neurodevelopmental plasticity might be exploited in prevention. There is emerging evidence that an appropriate neural plasticity/refinement during youth and adulthood can have an impact on the efficiency of aging brains and on the establishment of the so-called "brain reserve" or "cognitive reserve" (defined in neurology as the discrepancy between the individual level of brain pathology and the expected cognitive performance; see Chapters 9 and 12, this volume), ultimately affecting the onset/severity of neurological diseases (Barulli & Stern, 2013; Stern, 2017). According to this view, the extended neoteny and the consequent long period of time available for completing brain maturation (establishment of the above-mentioned "vision of the world"), if appropriately exploited and if followed by an appropriate training (e.g., physical activity, enriched environment, reduced sources of stress), might have a preventive effect by helping the brain to face up degeneration and damage by using preexisting cognitive processes and by recruiting compensatory processes (Darwish et al., 2018; Erten-Lyons et al., 2009; Snowdon et al., 1996).

REFERENCES

Adams, K. L., & Gallo, V. (2018). The diversity and disparity of the glial scar. *Nature Neuroscience, 21*(1), 9–15.

Aimone, J. B., Li, Y., Lee, S. W., Clemenson, G. D., Deng, W., & Gage, F. H. (2014). Regulation and function of adult neurogenesis: From genes to cognition. *Physiological Reviews, 94*, 991–1026.

Alderman, P. J., Saxon, D., Torrijos-Saiz, L. I., Sharief, M., Page, C. E., Baroudi, J. K., et al. (2023). Delayed maturation and migration of excitatory neurons in the juvenile mouse paralaminar amygdala. *Neuron, 112*(4), 574–592.e10.

Altman, J., & Das, G. D. (1965). Autoradiographic and histological evidence of postnatal hippocampal neurogenesis in rats. *Journal of Comparative Neurology, 124*, 319–335.

Alunni, A., & Bally-Cuif, L. (2016). A comparative view of regenerative neurogenesis in vertebrates. *Development, 143*, 741–753.

Alvarez-Buylla, A., García-Verdugo, J. M., & Tramontin, A. D. (2001). A unified hypothesis on the lineage of neural stem cells. *Nature Reviews Neuroscience, 2*, 287–293.

Amrein, I. (2015). Adult hippocampal neurogenesis in natural populations of mammals. *Cold Spring Harbor Perspectives in Biology, 7*, a021295.

Amrein, I., Dechmann, D. K., Winter, Y., & Lipp, H. P. (2007). Absent or low rate of adult neurogenesis in the hippocampus of bats (Chiroptera). *PLOS ONE*, 2, e455.

Andoh, M., & Koyama, R. (2021). Microglia regulate synaptic development and plasticity. *Developmental Neurobiology, 81*, 568–590.

Appelbaum, L. G., Shenasa, M. A., Stolz, L., & Daskalakis, Z. (2023). Synaptic plasticity and mental health: Methods, challenges and opportunities. *Neuropsychopharmacology, 48*(1), 113–120.

Arellano, J. I., Duque, A., & Rakic, P. (2024). A coming-of-age story: Adult neurogenesis or adolescent neurogenesis in rodents? *Frontiers in Neuroscience, 18*, 1383728.

Bao, H., & Song, J. (2018). Treating brain disorders by targeting adult neural stem cells. *Trends in Molecular Medicine, 24*(12), 991–1006.

Barker, J. M., Boonstra, R., & Wojtowicz, J. M. (2011). From pattern to purpose: How comparative studies contribute to understanding the function of adult neurogenesis. *European Journal of Neuroscience, 34*, 963–977.

Barulli, D., & Stern, Y. (2013). Efficiency, capacity, compensation, maintenance, plasticity: Emerging concepts in cognitive reserve. *Trends in Cognitive Sciences, 17*, 502–509.

Ben Abdallah, N. M., Slomianka, L., Vyssotski, A. L., & Lipp, H. P. (2010). Early age-related changes in adult hippocampal neurogenesis in C57 mice. *Neurobiology of Aging, 31*, 151–161.

Benedetti, B., Dannehl, D., König, R., Coviello, S., Kreutzer, C., Zaunmair, P., et al. (2020). Functional integration of neuronal precursors in the adult murine piriform cortex. *Cerebral Cortex, 30*(3), 1499–1515.

Benedetti, B., Reisinger, M., Hochwartner, M., Gabriele, G., Jakubecova, D., Benedetti, A., et al. (2023). The awakening of dormant neuronal precursors in the adult and aged brain. *Aging Cell, 22*(12), e13974.

Boda, E., Di Maria, S., Rosa, P., Taylor, V., Abbracchio, M. P., & Buffo, A. (2015). Early phenotypic asymmetry of sister oligodendrocyte progenitor cells after mitosis and its modulation by aging and extrinsic factors. *Glia, 63*, 271–286.

Bolker, J. A. (2017). Animal models in translational research: Rosetta stone or stumbling block? *Bioessays, 39*, 1700089.

Bond, A. M., Ming, G., & Song, H. (2015). Adult mammalian neural stem cells and neurogenesis: Five decades later. *Cell Stem Cell, 17*, 385–395.

Bonetto, G., Belin, D., & Thóra Káradóttir, R. (2021). Myelin: A gatekeeper of activity-dependent circuit plasticity? *Science, 374*, eaba6905.

Bonfanti, L. (2011). From hydra regeneration to human brain structural plasticity: A long trip through narrowing roads. *Scientific World Journal, 11*, 1270–1299.

Bonfanti, L., La Rosa, C., Ghibaudi, M., & Sherwood, C. C. (2024). Adult neurogenesis and "immature" neurons in mammals: An evolutionary trade-off in plasticity? *Brain Structure & Function, 229*(8), 1775–1793.

Bonfanti, L., & Nacher, J. (2012). New scenarios for neuronal structural plasticity in non-neurogenic brain parenchyma: The case of cortical layer II immature neurons. *Progress in Neurobiology, 98*, 1–15.

Bonfanti, L., & Peretto, P. (2011). Adult neurogenesis in mammals: A theme with many variations. *European Journal of Neuroscience, 34*, 930–950.

Bonfanti, L., & Seki, T. (2021). The PSA-NCAM-positive "immature" neurons: An old discovery providing new vistas on brain structural plasticity. *Cells, 10*, 2542.

Brenowitz, E. A., & Zakon, H. H. (2015). Emerging from the bottleneck: Benefits of the comparative approach to modern neuroscience. *Trends in Neurosciences, 38*(5), 273–278.

Bufill, E., Agustì, J., & Blesa, R. (2011). Human neoteny revisited: The case of synaptic plasticity. *American Journal of Human Biology, 23*, 729–773.

Chareyron, L. J., Banta Lavenex, P., Amaral, D. G., & Lavenex, P. (2021). Life and death of immature neurons in the juvenile and adult primate amygdala. *International Journal of Molecular Sciences, 22*, 6691.

Chen, H., Tang, A., & Blanpied, T. A. (2018). Subsynaptic spatial organization as a regulator of synaptic strength and plasticity. *Current Opinion Neurobiology, 51*, 147–153.

Chung, W.-S., Allen, N. J., & Eroglu, C. (2015). Astrocytes control synapse formation, function, and elimination. *Cold Spring Harbor Perspectives in Biology, 7*, a020370.

Ciceri, G., Baggiolini, A., Cho, H. S., Kshirsagar, M., Benito-Kwiecinski, S., Walsh, R. M., et al. (2024). An epigenetic barrier sets the timing of human neuronal maturation. *Nature, 626*, 881–890.

Cope, E. C., & Gould, E. (2019). Adult neurogenesis, glia, and the extracellular matrix. *Cell Stem Cell, 24*(5), 690–705.

Cushman, J. D., Drew, M. R., & Krasne, F. B. (2021). The environmental sculpting hypothesis of juvenile and adult hippocampal neurogenesis. *Progress in Neurobiology, 199*, 101961.

Darwish, H., Farran, N., Assaad, S., & Chaaya, M. (2018). Cognitive reserve factors in a developing country: Education and occupational attainment lower the risk of dementia in a sample of Lebanese older adults. *Frontiers in Aging Neuroscience, 10*, 277.

Dayan, E., & Cohen, L. G. (2011). Neuroplasticity subserving motor skill learning. *Neuron, 72*(3), 443–454.

DeFelipe, J., Alonso-Nanclares, L., & Arellano, J. I. (2002). Microstructure of the neocortex: Comparative aspects. *Journal of Neurocytology, 31*, 299–316.

de Sousa, A. A., Rigby Dames, D. A., Graff, E. C., Mohamedelhassan, R., Vassilopoulos, T., & Charvet, C. J. (2023). Going beyond established model systems of Alzheimer's disease: Companion animals provide novel insights into the neurobiology of aging. *Communications Biology, 6*(1), 655.

De Pittà, M., Brunel, N., & Volterra, A. (2016). Astrocytes: Orchestrating synaptic plasticity? *Neuroscience, 323*, 43–61.

Doetsch, F., Caille, I., Lim, D. A., Garcìa-Verdugo, J. M., & Alvarez-Buylla, A. (1999). Subventricular zone astrocytes are neural stem cells in the adult mammalian brain. *Cell, 97*, 703–716.

Duque, A., Arellano, J. I., & Rakic, P. (2022). An assessment of the existence of adult neurogenesis in humans and value of its rodent models for neuropsychiatric diseases. *Molecular Psychiatry, 27*(1), 377–382.

Durkee, C. A., & Araque, A. (2019). Diversity and specificity of astrocyte–neuron communication. *Neuroscience, 396*, 73–78.

Encinas, J. M., Michurina, T. V., Peunova, N., Park, J.-H., Tordo, J., Peterson, D. A., et al. (2011). Division-coupled astrocytic differentiation and age-related depletion of neural stem cells in the adult hippocampus. *Cell Stem Cell, 8*, 566–579.

Erten-Lyons, D., Woltjer, R. L., Dodge, H., Nixon, R., Vorobik, R., Calvert, J. F., et al. (2009). Factors associated with resistance to dementia despite high Alzheimer disease pathology. *Neurology, 72*, 354–360.

Falcone, C., Wolf-Ochoa, M., Amina, S., Hong, T., Vakilzadeh, G., Hopkins, W. D., et al. (2019). Cortical interlaminar astrocytes across the therian mammal radiation. *Journal of Comparative Neurology, 527*(10), 1654–1674.

Feliciano, D. M., Bordey, A., & Bonfanti, L. (2015). Noncanonical sites of adult neurogenesis in the mammalian brain. *Cold Spring Harbor Perspectives in Biology, 7*, a018846.

Fudge, J. L., Decampo, D. M., & Becoats, K. T. (2012). Revisiting the hippocampal-amygdala pathway in primates: Association with immature-appearing neurons. *Neuroscience, 212*, 104–119.

Gage, F. H. (2000). Mammalian neural stem cells. *Science, 287*, 1433–1438.

Ganz, J., & Brand, M. (2016). Adult neurogenesis in fish. *Cold Spring Harbor Perspectives in Biology, 8*(7), a019018.

Ghibaudi, M., & Bonfanti, L. (2022). How widespread are the "young" neurons of the mammalian brain? *Frontiers in Neuroscience, 16*, 918616.

Ghibaudi, M., Marchetti, N., Vergnano, E., La Rosa, C., Benedetti, B., Couillard-Despres, S., et al. (2023). Age-related changes in layer II immature neurons of the murine piriform cortex. *Frontiers in Cellular Neuroscience, 17*, 1205173.

Ghibaudi, M., La Rosa, C., Telitsyn, N., Graïc, J.-M., Faulkes, C. G., Sherwood, C. C., et al. (2025). Multispecies characterization of immature neurons in the mammalian amygdala reveals their expansion in primates. *PLoS Biology, 23*(8), e3003322.

Giaume, C., & McCarthy, K. D. (1996). Control of gap-junctional communication in astrocytic networks. *Trends in Neurosciences, 19*(8), 319–325.

Gómez-Climent, M. A., Castillo-Gómez, E., Varea, E., Guirado, R., Blasco-Ibáñez, J. M., Crespo, C., et al. (2008). A population of prenatally generated cells in the rat paleocortex maintains an immature neuronal phenotype into adulthood. *Cerebral Cortex, 18*, 2229–2240.

Gómez-Robles, A., Nicolaou, C., Smaers, J. B., & Sherwood, C. C. (2024). The evolution of human altriciality and brain development in comparative context. *Nature, 8*(1), 133–146.

Gonçalves, J. T., Schafer, S. T., & Gage, F. H. (2016). Adult neurogenesis in the hippocampus: From stem cells to behavior. *Cell, 167*, 897–914.

Grandel, H., Kaslin, J., Ganz, J., Wenzel, I., & Brand, M. (2006). Neural stem cells and neurogenesis in the adult zebrafish brain: Origin, proliferation dynamics, migration and cell fate. *Developmental Biology, 295*, 263–277.

Holtmaat, A., & Svoboda, K. (2009). Experience-dependent structural synaptic plasticity in the mammalian brain. *Nature Reviews Neuroscience, 10*(9), 647–658.

Karpati, F. J., Giacosa, C., Foster, N. E. V., Penhune, V. B., & Hyde, K. L. (2018). Structural covariance analysis reveals differences between dancers and untrained controls. *Frontiers in Human Neuroscience, 12*, 373.

Kempermann, G. (2019). Environmental enrichment, new neurons and the neurobiology of individuality. *Nature Reviews Neuroscience, 20*(4), 235–245.

Kokoeva, M. V., Yin, H., & Flier, J. S. (2005). Neurogenesis in the hypothalamus of adult mice: Potential role in energy balance. *Science, 310*, 679–683.

König, R., Benedetti, B., Rotheneichner, P., O'Sullivan, A., Kreutzer, C., Belles, M., et al. (2016). Distribution and fate of DCX/PSA-NCAM expressing cells in the adult mammalian cortex: A local reservoir for adult cortical neuroplasticity? *Frontiers in Biology, 11*, 193–213.

La Rosa, C., Cavallo, F., Pecora, A., Chincarini, M., Ala, U., Faulkes, C. G., et al. (2020a). Phylogenetic variation in cortical layer II immature neuron reservoir of mammals. *eLife, 9*, e55456.

La Rosa, C., Ghibaudi, M., & Bonfanti, L. (2019). Newly generated and non-newly generated "immature" neurons in the mammalian brain: A possible reservoir of young cells to prevent brain ageing and disease? *Journal of Clinical Medicine, 8*, 685.

La Rosa, C., Parolisi, R., & Bonfanti, L. (2020b). Brain structural plasticity: From adult neurogenesis to immature neurons. *Frontiers in Neuroscience, 14*, 75.

Lee, H.-K., & Whitt, J. L. (2015). Cross-modal synaptic plasticity in adult primary sensory cortices. *Current Opinion in Neurobiology, 35*, 119–126.

Li, Y.-N., Hu, D.-D., Cai, X.-L., Wang, Y., Yang, C., Jiang, J., et al. (2023). Doublecortin expressing neurons in human cerebral cortex layer II and amygdala from infancy to 100-year-old. *Molecular Neurobiology, 60*(6), 3464–3485.

Lim, D. A., & Alvarez-Buylla, A. (2016). The adult ventricular-subventricular zone (V-SVZ) and olfactory bulb (OB) neurogenesis. *Cold Spring Harbor Perspectives in Biology, 8*, a018820.

Lindvall, O., & Kokaia, Z. (2015). Neurogenesis following stroke affecting the adult brain. *Cold Spring Harbor Perspectives in Biology, 7*, a019034.

Lois, C., & Alvarez-Buylla, A. (1994). Long-distance neuronal migration in the adult mammalian brain. *Science, 264*, 1145–1148.

Lövdén, M., Wenger, E., Mårtensson, J., Lindenberger, U., & Bäckman, L. (2013). Structural brain plasticity in adult learning and development. *Neuroscience & Biobehavioral Reviews, 37*(9, Pt. B), 2296–2310.

Luzzati, F., Bonfanti, L., Fasolo, A., & Peretto, P. (2009). DCX and PSA-NCAM expression identifies a population of neurons preferentially distributed in associative areas of different pallial derivatives and vertebrate species. *Cerebral Cortex, 19*, 1028–1041.

Luzzati, F., De Marchis, S., Fasolo, A., & Peretto, P. (2006). Neurogenesis in the caudate nucleus of the adult rabbit. *Journal of Neuroscience, 26*, 609–621.

Magee, J. C., & Grienberger, C. (2020). Synaptic plasticity forms and functions. *Annual Review of Neuroscience, 43*, 95–117.

Mansvelder, H. D., Matthijs, B., Verhoog, M. B., & Goriounova, N. A. (2019). Synaptic plasticity in human cortical circuits: Cellular mechanisms of learning and memory in the human brain? *Current Opinion in Neurobiology, 54*, 186–193.

Martino, G., Pluchino, S., Bonfanti, L., & Schwartz, M. (2011). Brain regeneration in physiology and pathology: The immune signature driving therapeutic plasticity of neural stem cells. *Physiological Reviews, 91*, 1281–1304.

Monje, M. (2018). Myelin plasticity and nervous system function. *Annual Review of Neuroscience, 41*, 61–76.

Montero, A. M., & Huang, A. H. (2022). The regenerative capacity of neonatal tissues. *Development, 149*, dev199819.

Moreno-Jimenéz, E. P., Flor-Garcia, M., Terreros-Roncal, J., Rabano, A., Cafini, F., Pallas-Bazarra, N., et al. (2019). Adult hippocampal neurogenesis is abundant in neurologically healthy subjects and drops sharply in patients with Alzheimer's disease. *Nature Medicine, 25*, 554–560.

Morizet, D., & Bally-Cuif, L. (2025). Reduced adult neurogenesis in humans results from a tradeoff rather than direct negative selection. *Bioessays, 47*(9), e70041.

Müller-Dahlhaus, F., & Ziemann, U. (2015). Metaplasticity in human cortex. *The Neuroscientist, 21*(2), 185–202.

Nascimento, M. A., Biagiotti, S., Herranz-Pérez, V., Santiago, S., Bueno, R., Ye, C. J., et al. (2023). Protracted neuronal recruitment in the temporal lobe of young children. *Nature, 626*, 1056–1065.

Nudo, R. J. (2006). Mechanisms for recovery of motor function following cortical damage. *Current Opinion in Neurobiology, 16*, 638–644.

Obernier, K., & Alvarez-Buylla, A. (2019). Neural stem cells: Origin, heterogeneity and regulation in the adult mammalian brain. *Development, 146*(4), 156059.

Obernier, K., Tong, C. K., & Alvarez-Buylla, A. (2014). Restricted nature of adult neural stem cells: Re-evaluation of their potential for brain repair. *Frontiers in Neuroscience, 8*, 162.

Page, C. E., Biagiotti, S. W., Alderman, P. J., & Sorrells, S. F. (2022). Immature excitatory neurons in the amygdala come of age during puberty. *Developmental Cognitive Neuroscience, 56*, 101133.

Palazzo, O., La Rosa, C., Piumatti, M., & Bonfanti, L. (2018). Do large brains of long-living mammals prefer non-newly generated, immature neurons? *Neural Regeneration Research, 13*, 633–634.

Paolicelli, R. C., Sierra, A., Stevens, B., Tremblay, M.-E., Aguzzi, A., Ajami, B., et al. (2022). Microglia states and nomenclature: A field at its crossroads. *Neuron, 110*(21), 3458–3483.

Paredes, M. F., James, D., Gil-Perotin, S., Kim, H., Cotter, J. A., Ng, C., et al. (2016a). Extensive migration of young neurons into the infant human frontal lobe. *Science, 354*, aaf7073.

Paredes, M. F., Sorrells, S. F., Garcia-Verdugo, J.-M., & Alvarez-Buylla, A. (2016b). Brain size and limits to adult neurogenesis. *Journal of Comparative Neurology, 524*, 646–664.

Parolisi, R., Cozzi, B., & Bonfanti, L. (2017). Non-neurogenic SVZ-like niche in dolphins, mammals devoid of olfaction. *Brain Structure & Function, 222*, 2625–2639.

Parolisi, R., Cozzi, B., & Bonfanti, L. (2018). Humans and dolphins: Decline and fall of adult neurogenesis. *Frontiers in Neuroscience, 12*, 497.

Paton, J. A., & Nottebohm, F. N. (1984). Neurons generated in the adult brain are recruited into functional circuits. *Science, 225*, 1046–1048.

Pattaro, A., Ghibaudi, M., Corrente, C., Telitsyn, N, Graic, J.-M., Aresu, L., et al. (2025). Phylogenetic variation of layer II cortical immature neurons in dog and horse confirms covariance with brain size and neocortical surface. *Brain Structure & Function, 230*(6), 115.

Patzke, N., Spocter, M. A., Karlsson, K. Æ., Bertelsen, M. F., Haagensen, M., Chawana, R., et al. (2015). In contrast to many other mammals, cetaceans have relatively small hippocampi that appear to lack adult neurogenesis. *Brain Structure & Function, 220*, 361–383.

Perea, G., Navarrete, M., & Araque, A. (2009). Tripartite synapses: Astrocytes process and control synaptic information. *Trends in Neurosciences, 32*(8), 421–431.

Pierce, A. A., & Xu, A. W. (2010). De novo neurogenesis in adult hypothalamus as a compensatory mechanism to regulate energy balance. *Journal of Neuroscience, 30*, 723–730.

Piumatti, M., Palazzo, O., La Rosa, C., Crociara, P., Parolisi, R., Luzzati, F., et al. (2018). Non-newly generated, "immature" neurons in the sheep brain are not restricted to cerebral cortex. *Journal of Neuroscience, 38*, 826–842.

Ponti, G., Peretto, P., & Bonfanti, L. (2008). Genesis of neuronal and glial progenitors in the cerebellar cortex of peripuberal and adult rabbits. *PLOS ONE, 3*(6), e2366.

Potten, C. S., & Loeffler, M. (1990). Stem cells: Attributes, cycles, spirals, pitfalls and uncertainties: Lessons for and from the crypt. *Development, 110*, 1001–1020.

Robel, S., Berninger, B., & Götz, M. (2011). The stem cell potential of glia: Lessons from reactive gliosis. *Nature Reviews Neuroscience, 12*(2), 88–104.

Ronzano, R., Thetiot, M., Lubetzki, C., & Desmazieres, A. (2020). Myelin plasticity and repair: Neuro-glial choir sets the tuning. *Frontiers in Cellular Neuroscience, 14*, 42.

Rotheneichner, P., Belles, M., Benedetti, B., König, R., Dannehl, D., Kreutzer, C., et al. (2018). Cellular plasticity in the adult murine piriform cortex: Continuous maturation of dormant precursors into excitatory neurons. *Cerebral Cortex, 28*, 2610–2621.

Sampaio-Baptista, C., & Johansen-Berg, H. (2017). White matter plasticity in the adult brain.. *Neuron, 96*, 1239–1251.

Sanai, N., Nguyen, T., Ihrie, R. A., Mirzadeh, Z., Tsai, H.-H., Wong, M., et al. (2011). Corridors of migrating neurons in the human brain and their decline during infancy. *Nature, 478*, 382–386.

Seblani, M., Brezun, J.-M., Féron, F., & Hoquet, T. (2024). Rethinking plasticity: Analysing the concept of "destructive plasticity" in the light of neuroscience definitions. *European Journal of Neuroscience, 60*, 4798–4812.

Seki, T. (2020). Understanding the real state of human adult hippocampal neurogenesis from studies of rodents and non-human primates. *Frontiers in Neuroscience, 14*, 839.

Seki, T., Hori, T., Miyata, H., Maehara, M., & Namba, T. (2019). Analysis of proliferating neuronal progenitors and immature neurons in the human hippocampus surgically removed from control and epileptic patients. *Scientific Reports, 9*, 18194.

Semënov, M. V. (2019). Adult hippocampal neurogenesis is a developmental process involved in cognitive development. *Frontiers in Neuroscience, 13*, 159.

Sherwood, C. C., Miller, S. B., Molly, M., Stimpson, C. D., Phillips, K. A., Jacobs, B., et al. (2020). Invariant synapse density and neuronal connectivity scaling in primate neocortical evolution. *Cerebral Cortex, 30*, 5604–5615.

Simard, S., Matosin, N., & Mechawar, N. (2025). Adult hippocampal neurogenesis in the human brain: Updates, challenges, and perspectives. *Neuroscientist, 31*(2), 141–158.

Sirko, S., Schichor, C., Della Vecchia, P., Metzger, F., Sonsalla, G., Simon, T., et al. (2023). Injury-specific factors in the cerebrospinal fluid regulate astrocyte plasticity in the human brain. *Nature Medicine, 29*, 3149–3161.

Smaers, J. B., Mongle, C. S., Safi, K., & Dechmann, D. K. N. (2019). Allometry, evolution and development of neocortex size in mammals. *Progress in Brain Research, 250*, 83–107.

Snowdon, D. A., Kemper, S. J., Mortimer, J. A., Greiner, L. H., Wekstein, D. R., & Markesbery, W. R. (1996). Linguistic ability in early life and cognitive function and Alzheimer's disease in late life: Findings from the Nun Study. *Journal of the American Medical Association, 275*, 528–532.

Snyder, J. S. (2019). Recalibrating the relevance of adult neurogenesis. *Trends in Neurosciences, 42*(3), 164–178.

Sorrells, S. F. (2024). Which neurodevelopmental processes continue in humans after birth? *Frontiers in Neuroscience, 18*, 1434508.

Sorrells, S. F., Paredes, M. F., Cebrian-Silla, A., Sandoval, K., Qi, D., Kelley, K. W., et al. (2018). Human hippocampal neurogenesis drops sharply in children to undetectable levels in adults. *Nature, 555*, 377–381.

Sorrells, S. F., Paredes, M. F., Velmeshev, D., Herranz-Pérez, V., Sandoval, K., Mayer, S., et al. (2019). Immature excitatory neurons develop during adolescence in the human amygdala. *Nature Communications, 10*(1), 2748.

Stern, Y. (2017). An approach to studying the neural correlates of reserve. *Brain Imaging Behavior, 11*, 410–416.

Stevenson, I. H., Rebesco, J. M., Hatsopoulos, N. G., Haga, Z., Miller, L. E., & Körding, K. P. (2009). Bayesian inference of functional connectivity and network structure from spikes. *IEEE Transactions on Neural Systems and Rehabilitation Engineering, 17*(3), 203–213.

Theodosis, D. T., Poulain, D. A., & Oliet, S. H. (2008). Activity-dependent structural and functional plasticity of astrocyte-neuron interactions. *Physiological Reviews, 88*(3), 983–1008.

Tomassy, G. S., Srubek Tomassy, G., Berger, D. R., Chen, H.-H., Kasthuri, N., Hayworth, K. J., et al. (2014). Distinct profiles of myelin distribution along single axons of pyramidal neurons in the neocortex. *Science, 344*, 319–324.

Tooley, U. A., Bassett, D. S., & Mackey, A. P. (2021). Environmental influences on the pace of brain development. *Nature Reviews Neuroscience, 22*(6), 372–384.

van Noordwijdk, A. J., & Jong, G. (1986). Acquisition and allocation of resources: Their influence on variation in life history tactics. *The American Naturalist, 128*, 137–142.

Wang, L., Pang, K., Zhou, L., Cebrián-Silla, A., González-Granero, S., Wang, S., et al. (2023). A cross-species proteomic map reveals neoteny of human synapse development. *Nature, 622*, 112–119.

Weil, Z. M., Norman, G. J., De Vries, A. C., & Nelson, R. J. (2008). The injured nervous system: A Darwinian perspective. *Progress in Neurobiology, 86*, 48–59.

Wong, H. H.-W., Chien Chou, C. U., Watt, A. J., & Sjöström P. J. (2023). Comparing mouse and human brains. *eLife, 12*, e90017.

Workman, A. D., Charvet, C. J., Clancy, B., Darlington, R. B., & Finlay, B. L. (2013). Modeling transformations of neurodevelopmental sequences across mammalian species. *Journal of Neuroscience, 33*, 7368–7383.

Xin, W., & Chan, J. R. (2020). Myelin plasticity: Sculpting circuits in learning and memory. *Nature Reviews Neuroscience, 21*(12), 682–694.

Yeung, M. S., Zdunek, S., Bergmann, O., Bernard, S., Salehpour, M., Alkass, K., et al. (2014). Dynamics of oligodendrocyte generation and myelination in the human brain. *Cell, 159*(4), 766–774.

Yoo, S., & Blackshaw, S. (2018). Regulation and function of neurogenesis in the adult mammalian hypothalamus. *Progress in Neurobiology, 170*, 53–66.

Zamboni, M., Llorens-Bobadilla, E., Magnusson, J. P., & Frisen, J. (2020). A widespread neurogenic potential of neocortical astrocytes is induced by injury. *Cell Stem Cell, 27*, 605–617.

Zhou, Y., Su, Y., Li, S., Kennedy, B. C., Zhang, D. Y., Bond, A. M., et al. (2022). Molecular landscapes of human hippocampal immature neurons across lifespan. *Nature, 607*, 527–533.

Zilles, K., Palomero-Gallagher, N., & Amunts, K. (2013). Development of cortical folding during evolution and ontogeny. *Trends in Neurosciences, 36*, 275–284.

CHAPTER 5

Basic Mechanisms of Plasticity in Learning and Memory

Dustin Fetterhoff, Manuela Costa, and Bryan Strange

Introduction

In our lives, certain episodes associated with intense emotions, such as a marriage proposal or surviving a car accident, have a remarkable ability to etch themselves into our memories for extended periods. Conversely, every day, mundane events tend to easily be forgotten, a vital mechanism for the proper functioning of a healthy brain (Gravitz, 2019), just as significant as the capacity to retain memories. The human brain tends to prioritize the retention of events associated with both negative and positive outcomes (Dolcos et al., 2017; Hamann, 2001; McGaugh et al., 1996; Phelps, 2004; Richardson et al., 2004; Rouhani et al., 2023; Strange & Dolan, 2006), effectively facilitating the ability to anticipate and choose appropriate responses for analogous situations in the future. Such selective memory enhancement has extensive implications across diverse domains, including eyewitness testimonies, education, social interactions, cultural preservation, decision making, and sports performance. The emotional enhancement of memory can, however, become maladaptive in the context of aversive memories. Understanding the mechanisms behind emotional memory enhancement can provide insights into psychiatric disorders such as posttraumatic stress disorder (PTSD), characterized, among other symptoms, by intrusive memories (Pitman et al., 2012) and distressing recollections of past experiences (Burback et al., 2023). This understanding is also essential for pathologies marked by anxiety or depression, which frequently manifest as a consistent negative emotional bias.

Dustin Fetterhoff and Manuela Costa share senior authorship.

This chapter first offers a historical perspective on emotional memory by revisiting important findings from rodent and human studies. This is followed by the most current evidence, including direct recordings from the human amygdala and the hippocampus. The chapter is presented while assuming that synaptic plasticity, such as long-term potentiation (LTP; Bliss & Collingridge, 1993), is the underlying neural mechanism of learning on a synaptic level via coincidence detection and occurs in both the hippocampus and amygdala (Abraham et al., 2019). Studies altering neuroplasticity with behavioral paradigms such as fear conditioning or via both optical and electrical stimulation are summarized. Lastly, novel therapeutic interventions offered by pharmacological interventions and electrical stimulation are explored to provide insights into potential future research directions and therapeutic development.

Understanding Memory and Emotion through the Study of Brain Lesions

The amygdala, a brain structure resembling an almond shape, resides in the medial temporal lobe and has been remarkably conserved throughout evolution (Janak & Tye, 2015). Presently, we understand that the amygdala is involved in a myriad of processes, encompassing emotions, social behaviors, attention, learning, and memory (Gothard, 2020; Pryluk et al., 2021). Direct lesions to the amygdala result in a range of social and nonsocial deficits, also known as Klüver–Bucy syndrome (Janku et al., 2023; Klüver & Bucy, 1937; Sander et al., 2003; Terzian & Ore, 1955). This chapter focuses on the amygdala's role in enhancing memory. With its distinctive seahorse-shaped structure, the hippocampus also resides in the medial temporal lobe, with its anterior portion adjacent to the amygdala. While it has been attributed various functions, including spatial navigation (O'Keefe & Nadel, 1978; Shapiro et al., 1997) and social processing (Wirth et al., 2021), with a proposed functional organization along its longitudinal axis (Strange et al., 2014), our primary focus here is on its pivotal role in episodic memory, and specifically for emotional events.

Patients with amygdala or hippocampus lesions have been instrumental in advancing our knowledge of the brain's memory systems and the specific roles of these brain areas, leaving an enduring impact on the fields of neuroscience and psychology. Our understanding of the amygdala's role in emotional processing was significantly enhanced through studies on patient S. M., who suffered from Urbach–Wiethe disease, resulting in near-complete bilateral amygdala lesions while sparing the hippocampus (Adolphs et al., 1994). These studies revealed that S. M. struggled to recognize fear in facial expressions but could still recognize personal identities, suggesting preserved long-term memory. When exposed to fear-inducing situations, she didn't exhibit overt fear behaviors but displayed an unusual curiosity and approached fear-provoking stimuli (Feinstein et al., 2011). This led to the conclusion that the amygdala plays a pivotal role in inducing a state of fear, and its dysfunction precludes the experience of fear itself (Bechara et al., 1995; LaBar et al., 1995).

On the other hand, patients with hippocampus lesions, exemplified by patient H. M., experience severe anterograde amnesia and graded, variable retrograde amnesia. While H. M. retained short-term and procedural memory, he couldn't create new long-term memories, shedding light on the hippocampus' role in forming new episodic memories and distinguishing between different memory systems. Notably, while selective amygdala lesions in humans leave neutral memory unaffected, hippocampus lesions impair neutral and emotional episodic memory (Cahill et al., 1995).

Amygdala–Hippocampus Interactions in Emotional Memory: Insights from Rodent Studies

Learning causes behavioral modifications by modulating synapses via neuroplasticity (Abraham et al., 2019), and evidence suggests that neuroplasticity-inducing interactions between the amygdala and hippocampus underlie emotional memory. Research in rodents has demonstrated essential interactions between the amygdala and hippocampus during emotional memory, primarily using fear-conditioning paradigms (LeDoux, 2003). Fear conditioning, a form of Pavlovian learning, involves pairing an aversive stimulus (e.g., an electric shock) with a neutral stimulus (e.g., a tone or context) to ultimately create fear responses to the originally neutral stimulus (Maren, 2003). Electrophysiological recordings have shown that amygdala neurons undergo *N*-methyl-D-aspartate (NMDA)-receptor-dependent LTP during fear conditioning (Johansen et al., 2011; Sah et al., 2008), while amygdala lesions prevented fear acquisition (Maren, 1999).

Optogenetics has opened many new possibilities to inspect causality in neuronal circuit dynamics, specifically regarding emotional valence (Nieh et al., 2013). In one study, researchers paired an auditory cue with optical stimulation of lateral amygdala neurons and found that fear responses could be triggered by the auditory cue alone (Johansen et al., 2010), which validated the idea that fear learning is guided by the activation of lateral amygdala pyramidal cells through aversive stimulus exposure.

Interestingly, it has been demonstrated that the hippocampus is only involved in contextual fear conditioning and not cued conditioning (McDonald & White, 1993; Phillips & LeDoux, 1992). Amygdala lesions disrupted fear responses to both cues and context, while hippocampus lesions affected context but not cues. This indicates that the amygdala is vital for fear responses to specific and complex stimuli, while the hippocampus is involved in fear conditioning for complex situations (McDonald & White, 1993; Phillips & LeDoux, 1992). These basic principles of organization have also been observed in human functional magnetic resonance imaging (fMRI) studies (Marschner et al., 2008).

Optogenetic studies suggest a connection between basolateral amygdala (BLA) activity and memory facilitation and advance our understanding by establishing causal relationships between neural activity, plasticity, and memory. Indeed, optogenetic manipulation of BLA neuronal activity after training was found to modulate memory consolidation (Huff et al., 2013). Stimulating BLA glutamatergic neurons using gamma-frequency light pulses (40 Hz) enhanced memory retention, but 20-Hz pulses did not. Another study showed that optogenetic stimulation of the BLA enhanced hippocampal theta-modulated gamma oscillation (Ahlgrim & Manns, 2019). This is a plausible mechanism for amygdala-mediated memory enhancement via neuroplasticity because theta-burst electrical stimulation protocols induce LTP (Larson & Munkácsy, 2015). Future studies recording from the hippocampus and amygdala simultaneously while using optogenetics to target specific subpopulations of neurons would be critical for determining circuit dynamics involved in emotional memory.

The Amygdala's Role in Shaping Emotional Memory through the Noradrenergic System

The understanding of the amygdala's role in emotional memory has been significantly advanced through extensive research, both in animals and humans. The amygdala, particularly the BLA, is recognized for its involvement in the acquisition and retention of emotional experiences as compared with neutral ones. However, the amygdala is not believed to serve as the storage site for memories but, rather, plays a significant role in shaping emotional memory processes (McGaugh, 2000, 2004, 2015; McGaugh, Cahill, & Roozendaal, 1996; McGaugh et al., 2002). James McGaugh's (2000) theory, known as the "memory modulation hypothesis," suggests that the amygdala is crucial in enhancing the consolidation of memories associated with emotionally charged experiences. Thanks to its extensive connections with brain regions responsible for memory functions, such as the hippocampus, the amygdala responds to arousing experiences. These experiences, in turn, trigger the release of norepinephrine (also known as noradrenaline) and glucocorticoid hormones to strengthen the formation of memory traces via enhanced synaptic plasticity.

Early research in animals demonstrated that electrical stimulation of the amygdala in rats could either enhance or impair aversive memory, depending on the stimulation parameters and training conditions (Gold et al., 1975). More recently, it was shown that high-frequency stimulation in the BLA induces LTP in the hippocampal dentate gyrus (Abe et al., 2003). Together, these results indicate that the amygdala can influence other brain structures, including the hippocampus, during emotional memory processing by inducing synaptic plasticity. Subsequent studies involving drug infusions into the amygdala (Ellis & Kesner, 1983; Gallagher & Kapp, 1981; Gallagher et al., 1977; Roozendaal et al., 2009) revealed that the amygdala plays a crucial role in memory consolidation. Notably, infusion of beta-adrenoceptor antagonists impaired memory retention, while concurrent infusion of norepinephrine prevented memory impairment. In parallel, studies involving systemic drug administration after training demonstrated that adrenal stress hormones, such as epinephrine and corticosterone, released during emotionally arousing training may contribute to memory consolidation. Many subsequent animal studies reported that posttraining infusions of norepinephrine or a beta-adrenoceptor agonist into the amygdala enhance memory (LaLumiere et al., 2003; Roesler et al., 2021). Human studies (Cahill et al., 1994; Strange & Dolan, 2004) have provided consistent evidence, aligning with animal research, showing that stress hormones and amygdala activation play a crucial role in emotional memory. Specifically, the essential role of beta-adrenergic receptors for human emotional enhancement of memory was demonstrated by selective blockade of this enhancement following administration of the beta-1–beta-2-adrenergic antagonist propranolol (Cahill et al., 1994). In another study, postlearning administration of yohimbine, an alpha-2-adrenergic receptor antagonist, enhanced memory recall in people with elevated postencoding norepinephrine metabolite concentrations (Southwick et al., 2002). These are two early examples of studies showcasing the crucial role of norepinephrine in long-term emotional memory processing, an area of research extended to include stress, cortisol, and other adrenergic modulators (Roozendaal et al., 2009; Schwabe et al., 2012).

Amygdala–Hippocampus Interactions in Human Emotional Memory

Not every daily experience is retained in our long-term memory, but emotional events are more likely to be remembered over time (Yonelinas & Ritchey, 2015). Increasing evidence suggests that the amygdala modulates memory consolidation and plasticity processes in the hippocampus (Roesler et al., 2021). Functional neuroimaging studies have provided evidence in humans of higher amygdala activity for emotional stimuli as compared with neutral stimuli during encoding processes (Dolcos et al., 2004; Richardson et al., 2004; Strange & Dolan, 2004). In an fMRI study by Richardson and colleagues in 2004, the extent of hippocampal pathology was found to predict memory performance for both neutral and emotional items, while amygdala pathology exclusively influenced memory performance for emotional items. Moreover, a reciprocal relationship between these two brain regions during emotional memory encoding was revealed.

In the past decade, studies utilizing direct brain recordings have provided invaluable insights into the amygdala and hippocampus' response with millisecond precision during processing emotionally charged information, such as fearful faces or aversive images. Notably, research has highlighted the dynamic interplay between these structures. Zheng and colleagues (2019), recording from drug-resistant epilepsy patients, reported amygdala and hippocampal activity while subjects viewed fearful faces and landscapes. High gamma activation for fearful faces was observed first in the amygdala and later in the hippocampus. The study also revealed enhanced low-frequency coupling between the amygdala and the hippocampus while processing fearful faces, emphasizing their connection.

In 2022, Costa and colleagues conducted a study using simultaneous amygdala and hippocampal recordings during an emotional memory task. This study demonstrated that the amygdala plays a pivotal role in coordinating hippocampal activity during aversive memory formation. Successful emotional encoding was found to depend on the amygdala's theta phase, which corresponded with the peak of hippocampal gamma activity and neuronal firing. Previous evidence suggests that hippocampal LTP can be induced by electrical stimulation delivered at the peak of a theta oscillation (Huerta & Lisman, 1995). Consistent with this, inputs arriving during distinct phases of theta oscillations may trigger varying synaptic alterations, influencing the probability of encoding those inputs into long-term memory (Hasselmo et al., 2002; Hyman et al., 2003). This notion is supported by the findings of Costa and colleagues (2022), suggesting that the specific phase of theta oscillations during which hippocampal gamma activity peaks and spikes occur determines whether aversive scenes will subsequently be remembered or forgotten. In sum, this result emphasized the amygdala's role in the temporal and phasic coordination of the hippocampus during emotional memory encoding. Single-unit activity analysis has further deepened our understanding of the amygdala and hippocampus's role in emotional and memory processes. Neurons in the amygdala encode the subjective judgment of emotions in face stimuli rather than their physical features (Wang et al., 2014). A recent study has shown a separate representation of memory and emotions at the single unit and population level within the medial temporal lobe (Fetterhoff et al., 2024).

The research findings on the oscillatory frequencies of neuronal populations associated with the processing of fearful faces and aversive memory have implications for studies involving direct electrical stimulation in humans. Inman and colleagues (2018) used brief electrical stimulation to the human amygdala, revealing the amygdala's capacity to enhance declarative memory for specific images without generating a subjective emotional response. This result shows the human amygdala has a general capacity to initiate the enhancement of specific declarative memories engaging other memory-related brain regions. A novel observation using direct recording of the amygdala and the hippocampus suggests that the direction of information flow is opposite during encoding and retrieval of aversive memory. While during encoding the amygdala influences hippocampal activity, during retrieval the hippocampus exerts unidirectional influence on the amygdala (Costa et al., 2024). This is clinically relevant given the growing interest in direct electrical neuromodulation of amygdala activity as a therapeutic route for psychiatric disease (Gill et al., 2023; Inman et al., 2018).

Similar high-frequency neuronal correlates, as compared to the above electrophysiological studies, were found in the amygdala and the hippocampus in a large cohort of participants (Qasim et al., 2023). While undergoing intracranial electroencephalographic recording, participants performed a verbal episodic memory task, with emotional parameters (valence and arousal) of words assigned post hoc using standardized ratings. In the same study, the authors also used direct electrical stimulation to the hippocampus during the encoding session and showed diminished memory for emotional words. In particular, stimulation significantly impaired the recall of both high-arousal words and negative words more than other word categories.

These studies collectively emphasize the pivotal role of the amygdala–hippocampus interaction in human emotional memory and pave the way for targeting the amygdala and hippocampus network for addressing pathologies characterized by memory dysregulation and dysfunction.

Posttraumatic Stress Disorder

Advancements in brain imaging techniques, particularly fMRI and positron emission tomography, have provided new insights into PTSD. Two decades ago, PTSD was primarily associated with hippocampal-related atrophy based on structural imaging, but more recently, the understanding has shifted toward a disorder of emotional regulation (Vermetten & Lanius, 2012). Current understanding acknowledges a range of interconnected brain regions contributing to PTSD, expanding beyond the traditional frontolimbic model that emphasized the limbic system components, such as the hippocampus, amygdala, parahippocampal gyrus, and prefrontal cortex, to include the insula and anterior cingulate cortex (Burback et al., 2023).

Key findings in PTSD include hyperactivation of the amygdala and dorsal anterior cingulate cortex, reduced activity in the ventromedial prefrontal cortex (vmPFC), and hippocampal atrophy (Kamiya & Abe, 2020). PTSD is linked to reduced hippocampal volume in addition to decreased overall brain volume (Bromis et al., 2018; Burback et al., 2023). Other notable findings in PTSD involve overactive insulae and diminished volume in the insulae, medial prefrontal cortex (mPFC), and anterior cingulate (Bromis et al., 2018), which are collectively involved in attention and emotion regulation.

Fear extinction involves learning that a previously feared stimulus is no longer associated with a negative outcome, leading to reduced fear responses. It relies on inhibitory processes and new learning that competes with the original fear memory, but this process is impaired in PTSD patients. Studies on fear conditioning and extinction using fMRI have revealed heightened activation in specific brain regions of PTSD patients relative to control participants, including the hippocampus and amygdala (Alvarez et al., 2008). A meta-analysis of human fear conditioning fMRI studies showed that PTSD patients have heightened activity in the anterior hippocampus and amygdala during both conditioning and extinction learning compared with healthy controls experimentally exposed to trauma (Suarez-Jimenez et al., 2020). During conditioning, the anterior hippocampus (extending to the amygdala) and mPFC exhibit increased activation in PTSD patients compared to controls. In contrast, during extinction learning, the anterior hippocampus-amygdala regions were more active (Suarez-Jimenez et al., 2020). During extinction recall, similar areas, along with the mPFC, are activated, whereas the thalamus shows decreased activation. This indicates that PTSD involves intensified activation in regions related to detecting threats and significance, reduced thalamic activity (a crucial hub for subcortical–cortical connections), and vmPFC dysfunction (Burback et al., 2023; Suarez-Jimenez et al., 2020). These factors are thought to contribute to a failure to inhibit conditioned fear responses and difficulty distinguishing safety from threat due to impaired contextual processing involving the vmPFC, hippocampus, and thalamus (Burback et al., 2023).

Despite these advancements, our knowledge of amygdala and hippocampal dynamics in patients with PTSD remains limited. However, a case study from 2016 by Langevin and colleagues and a recent clinical trial led by the same group (Gill et al., 2023) are beginning to explore oscillatory activity in this patient population. In the clinical trial, the researchers conducted a longitudinal study involving treatment-resistant PTSD patients. They aimed to identify electrophysiological patterns associated with emotionally distressing and clinically significant states. They achieved this by examining neural activity during three distinct scenarios: viewing negative emotional images, listening to recordings of trauma-related memories specific to each participant, and monitoring periods of symptom intensification in the patients' everyday lives. Across all three negative experiences, the researchers observed a specific increase in the amygdala theta (5–9-Hz) band. To address symptoms associated with this amplified theta power, they employed a closed-loop neuromodulation technique. This technique records brain activity and initiates stimulation when certain predefined parameters are met. They used increased low-frequency amygdala power as a trigger signal for closed-loop neuromodulation and found a significant reduction in symptoms among the two treatment-resistant PTSD patients tested. This research offers valuable insights into the potential therapeutic benefits of closed-loop neuromodulation for individuals with PTSD.

Pharmacological Modulation of Fear Extinction

One of the primary objectives of emotional memory research is to develop pharmacological compounds to reduce ingrained fear responses to specific stimuli in people suffering from psychiatric conditions. Here, we will focus on PTSD while acknowledging that the principles also extend to other conditions, such as phobias. Currently, two different selective serotonin reuptake inhibitors (SSRIs), sertraline and paroxetine, are the only pharmacological methods approved for PTSD (Alexander, 2012), but promising results with alternative compounds are discussed below.

In both rodents and humans, potential PTSD treatments are examined by their ability to enhance fear extinction or impair memory reconsolidation (Raskin & Monfils, 2023). While fear extinction is believed to depend on the inhibition of fear memory, fear reconsolidation relies on reactivating a memory into a labile state where the reconsolidation process can be disrupted, weakening the original fear memory. This presumably allows for a new memory trace to form. We briefly mention some promising pharmacological methods, but the reader can refer to Burback and colleagues (2023) for an in-depth review.

One of the early pharmacological attempts to enhance fear extinction was using D-cycloserine (DCS), an antibiotic that acts as an agonist of NMDA receptors, promoting extinction learning in animals. DCS has been found to enhance fear extinction during exposure tasks in both animals (Bouton et al., 2008; Ledgerwood et al., 2004, 2005) and humans (Norberg et al., 2008). While it was hoped that DCS, by enhancing NMDA activity, could improve the impact of psychotherapy on fear extinction and facilitate neuroplasticity for long-term therapy gains, results have been mixed (Guastella et al., 2007). Some studies have shown promising effects, but overall outcomes vary from faster symptom resolution to no impact or even detrimental effects (Burback et al., 2023).

The human endocannabinoid system contains endogenous cannabinoids, such as anandamide and 2-arachidonoylglycerol, which activate cannabinoid CB1 and CB2 receptors to modulate mood, pain perception, and memory (Wotjak, 2005). CB1 receptors are found throughout the limbic system where they play a critical role in synaptic plasticity and fear extinction (Marsicano et al., 2002; Pamplona et al., 2008), and their dysfunction is linked to PTSD (Patel et al., 2017). In one study, CB1R-deficient mice displayed impaired short-term and long-term extinction in fear-conditioning tests, while memory acquisition and consolidation were unaffected (Marsicano et al., 2002). Treating normal mice with a CB1R antagonist replicated the CB1-deficient phenotype, highlighting the role of CB1R-mediated synaptic plasticity during memory extinction (Marsicano et al., 2002). During extinction trials, endocannabinoid levels increased in the basolateral amygdala complex, causing CB1R activation and leading to long-term depression of gamma-aminobutyric acid–mediated inhibitory currents (Marsicano et al., 2002). The cannabinoid receptors are also modulated by exogenous compounds present in cannabis, such as tetrahydrocannabinol and cannabidiol (CBD). CBD represents a promising compound (Lee et al., 2017) due to its ability to enhance fear extinction in both rats (Papagianni et al., 2022) and humans (Das et al., 2013), but more research is required.

Recent Phase 2 and 3 clinical trials showing that 3,4-methylenedioxymethamphetamine (MDMA; "ecstasy")–assisted psychotherapy induced significant and persistent improvements in people with severe PTSD (Mitchell et al., 2021, 2023) have led the U.S. Food and Drug Administration to designate it as a "breakthrough therapy." Like SSRIs, MDMA increases levels of serotonin in the synapse by blocking its reuptake. However, MDMA also reverses the direction of transportation, causing additional release and increased dopamine and norepinephrine levels to a lesser extent than serotonin (Young et al., 2017). The acute neuropharmacological effects ultimately lead to elevated mood, altered perception, and increased social behavior, and could facilitate the reprocessing of traumatic memories (Mitchell et al., 2021; Vizeli et al., 2022). When administered before fear extinction, MDMA augmented acquisition and retrieval of extinction memory in mice (Young et al., 2017). These behavioral effects could be driven by MDMA's ability to alter brain connectivity (Singleton et al., 2023), enhance synaptic plasticity (Ly et al., 2018), and modify social reward learning (Nardou et al., 2019). Interestingly, both chronic and acute SSRI administration before MDMA disrupted MDMA-induced enhancement of fear extinction (Young et al., 2017), possibly due to compensatory changes in serotonergic transportation, release, and receptor availability. Since chronic SSRI treatment is currently the only approved pharmacotherapy for PTSD, and previous chronic use may reduce the effectiveness of MDMA-assisted psychotherapy (Feduccia et al., 2021), it is essential to understand how this pharmacology affects neurophysiological and cognitive properties to better predict future efficacy in each patient (Mitchell et al., 2021, 2023).

Conclusion

This chapter explores the intricate landscape of neural substrates governing emotional memory, particularly focusing on interactions between the amygdala and hippocampus, and how these may lead to changes in synaptic plasticity. Through a combination of historical retrospectives, empirical investigations spanning preclinical models to human studies, and case studies, we provide evidence for how neuronal activity between the amygdala and hippocampus shapes emotional memory. Notably, the amygdala's pivotal role in modulating memory consolidation, facilitated via intricate interactions with the noradrenergic system, underscores its significance in encoding emotionally salient experiences. Moreover, insights gleaned from clinical investigations, including those examining patients with amygdala and hippocampal lesions, illuminate the indispensable contributions of these structures in human emotional processing and memory functions. Coupled with advancements in neuroimaging methodologies and direct brain recordings, our understanding of the temporal dynamics and functional connectivity within the amygdala–hippocampal circuitry during emotional memory processing has expanded substantially.

The implications of these findings transcend fundamental neuroscience, offering promising avenues for targeted therapeutic interventions in psychiatric disorders characterized by memory dysregulation. The potential for pharmacological approaches targeting fear extinction and memory reconsolidation processes to ameliorate symptoms associated with PTSD is particularly promising. Furthermore, emerging interventions such as closed-loop neuromodulation, including electrical stimulation techniques, present intriguing prospects for augmenting traditional therapeutic modalities. The current synthesis of research underscores the pivotal role of amygdala–hippocampal interactions in emotional memory processes, laying a robust foundation for continued inquiry and translational endeavors aimed at addressing memory-related pathologies and enhancing human well-being.

Plasticity plays a fundamental role in shaping our brains throughout life, enabling us to adapt in response to experiences, learn new skills, and form memories. The studies presented in this chapter provide insights into the basic mechanisms of plasticity in learning and memory, specifically focusing on the intricate interplay between the amygdala and the hippocampus during emotional memory processing. By elucidating how the amygdala modulates the hippocampus, particularly during emotional memory encoding, we gain a deeper understanding of how emotional experiences sculpt memory processes, shedding light on how emotional experiences may trigger neuroplasticity. Notably, the amygdala–hippocampal phase code proposed by Costa and colleagues (2022) suggests that the timing of the coupling between amygdala theta oscillations and hippocampal gamma peaks and neuronal spikes may dictate the likelihood of encoding aversive events into long-term memory, putatively by optimizing the phase of the hippocampal field potential to allow long-term synaptic modification (Huerta & Lisman, 1995). Furthermore, the coordination of the amygdala theta phase with transient amygdala–hippocampal gamma coherence appears to facilitate the encoding of aversive memories. Such a mechanism potentially serves as a broader framework through which the amygdala communicates emotional content to distant brain regions, potentially modulating brain plasticity underlying various aspects of cognition.

REFERENCES

Abe, K., Niikura, Y., & Misawa, M. (2003). The induction of long-term potentiation at amygdalo-hippocampal synapses *in vivo*. *Biological and Pharmaceutical Bulletin, 26*, 1560–1562.

Abraham, W. C., Jones, O. D., & Glanzman, D. L. (2019). Is plasticity of synapses the mechanism of long-term memory storage. *NPJ Science of Learning, 4*, Article 9.

Adolphs, R., Tranel, D., Damasio, H., & Damasio, A. (1994). Impaired recognition of emotion in facial expressions following bilateral damage to the human amygdala. *Nature, 372*, 669–672.

Ahlgrim, N. S., & Manns, J. R. (2019). Optogenetic stimulation of the basolateral amygdala increased theta-modulated gamma oscillations in the hippocampus. *Frontiers in Behavioral Neuroscience, 13*, 453748.

Alexander, W. (2012). Pharmacotherapy for post-traumatic stress disorder in combat veterans:

Focus on antidepressants and atypical antipsychotic agents. *Pharmacy and Therapeutics, 37,* 32.

Alvarez, R. P., Biggs, A., Chen, G., Pine, D. S., & Grillon, C. (2008). Contextual fear conditioning in humans: Cortical-hippocampal and amygdala contributions. *Journal of Neuroscience, 28,* 6211–6219.

Bechara, A., Tranel, D., Damasio, H., Adolphs, R., Rockland, C., & Damasio, A. R. (1995). Double dissociation of conditioning and declarative knowledge relative to the amygdala and hippocampus in humans. *Science, 269,* 1115–1118.

Bliss, T. V. P., & Collingridge, G. L. (1993). A synaptic model of memory: Long-term potentiation in the hippocampus. *Nature, 361,* 31–39.

Bouton, M. E., Vurbic, D., & Woods, A. M. (2008). d-Cycloserine facilitates context-specific fear extinction learning. *Neurobiology of Learning and Memory, 90,* 504–510.

Bromis, K., Calem, M., Reinders, A. A. T. S., Williams, S. C. R., & Kempton, M. J. (2018). Meta-analysis of 89 structural MRI studies in posttraumatic stress disorder and comparison with major depressive disorder. *American Journal of Psychiatry, 175,* 989–998.

Burback, L., Brémault-Phillips, S., Nijdam, M. J., McFarlane, A., & Vermetten, E. (2023). Treatment of posttraumatic stress disorder: A state-of-the-art review. *Current Neuropharmacology, 21,* 557–635.

Cahill, L., Babinsky, R., Markowitsch, H. J., & McGaugh, J. L. (1995). The amygdala and emotional memory. *Nature, 377,* 295–296.

Cahill, L., Prins, B., Weber, M., & McGaugh, J. L. (1994). Beta-adrenergic activation and memory for emotional events. *Nature, 371,* 702–704.

Costa, M., Lozano-Soldevilla, D., Gil-Nagel, A., Toledano, R., Oehrn, C. R., Kunz, L., et al. (2022). Aversive memory formation in humans involves an amygdala–hippocampus phase code. *Nature Communications, 13,* 6403.

Costa, M., Pacheco, D., Gil-Nagel, A., Toledano, R., Imbach, L., Sarnthein, J., & Strange, B. A. (2024). Retrieval of human aversive memories involves reactivation of gamma activity patterns in the hippocampus that originate in the amygdala during encoding. *BioRxiv.*

Das, R. K., Kamboj, S. K., Ramadas, M., Yogan, K., Gupta, V., Redman, E., et al. (2013). Cannabidiol enhances consolidation of explicit fear extinction in humans. *Psychopharmacology, 226,* 781–792.

Dolcos, F., Katsumi, Y., Denkova, E., Weymar, M., & Dolcos, S. (2017). Current issues and emerging directions in the impact of emotion on memory: A review of evidence from brain imaging investigations. In T. Tsukiura, & S. Umeda (Eds.), *Memory in a social context* (pp. 57–101). Springer.

Dolcos, F., LaBar, K. S., & Cabeza, R. (2004). Interaction between the amygdala and the medial temporal lobe memory system predicts better memory for emotional events. *Neuron, 42,* 855–863.

Ellis, M. E., & Kesner, R. P. (1983). The noradrenergic system of the amygdala and aversive information processing. *Behavioral Neuroscience, 97,* 399–415.

Feduccia, A. A., Jerome, L., Mithoefer, M. C., & Holland, J. (2021). Discontinuation of medications classified as reuptake inhibitors affects treatment response of MDMA-assisted psychotherapy. *Psychopharmacology, 238,* 581–588.

Feinstein, J. S., Adolphs, R., Damasio, A., & Tranel, D. (2011). The human amygdala and the induction and experience of fear. *Current Biology, 21*(1), 34.

Fetterhoff, D., Costa, M., Hellerstedt, R., Johannessen, R., Imbach, L., Sarnthein, J., & Strange, B. A. (2024). Neuronal population representation of human emotional memory. *Cell Reports, 43*(4), 114071.

Gallagher, M., & Kapp, B. S. (1981). Effect of phentolamine administration into the amygdala complex of rats on time-dependent memory processes. *Behavioral and Neural Biology, 31*, 90–95.

Gallagher, M., Kapp, B. S., Musty, R. E., & Driscoll, P. A. (1977). Memory formation: Evidence for a specific neurochemical system in the amygdala. *Science, 198*, 423–425.

Gill, J. L., Schneiders, J. A., Stangl, M., Aghajan, Z. M., Vallejo, M., Hiller, S., et al. (2023). A pilot study of closed-loop neuromodulation for treatment-resistant post-traumatic stress disorder. *Nature Communication, 14*(1), 2997.

Gold, P. E., Hankins, L., Edwards, R. M., Chester, J., & McGaugh, J. L. (1975). Memory interference and facilitation with posttrial amygdala stimulation: Effect on memory varies with footshock level. *Brain Research, 86*, 509–513.

Gothard, K. M. (2020). Multidimensional processing in the amygdala. *Nature Reviews Neuroscience, 21*, 565–575.

Gravitz, L. (2019). The forgotten part of memory. *Nature, 571*, S12–S14.

Guastella, A. J., Lovibond, P. F., Dadds, M. R., Mitchell, P., & Richardson, R. (2007). A randomized controlled trial of the effect of d-cycloserine on extinction and fear conditioning in humans. *Behaviour Research and Therapy, 45*, 663–672.

Hamann, S. (2001). Cognitive and neural mechanisms of emotional memory. *Trends in Cognitive Sciences, 5*, 394–400.

Hasselmo, M. E., Bodelón, C., & Wyble, B. P. (2002). A proposed function for hippocampal theta rhythm: Separate phases of encoding and retrieval enhance reversal of prior learning. *Neural Computation, 14*, 793–817.

Huerta, P. T., & Lisman, J. E. (1995). Bidirectional synaptic plasticity induced by a single burst during cholinergic theta oscillation in CA1 in vitro. *Neuron, 15*, 1053–1063.

Huff, M. L., Miller, R. L., Deisseroth, K., Moorman, D. E., & LaLumiere, R. T. (2013). Posttraining optogenetic manipulations of basolateral amygdala activity modulate consolidation of inhibitory avoidance memory in rats. *Proceedings of the National Academy of Sciences, 110*, 3597–3602.

Hyman, J. M., Wyble, B. P., Goyal, V., Rossi, C. A., & Hasselmo, M. E. (2003). Stimulation in hippocampal region CA1 in behaving rats yields long-term potentiation when delivered to the peak of theta and long-term depression when delivered to the trough. *Journal of Neuroscience, 23*, 11725–11731.

Inman, C. S., Manns, J. R., Bijanki, K. R., Bass, D. I., Hamann, S., Drane, D. L., et al. (2018). Direct electrical stimulation of the amygdala enhances declarative memory in humans. *Proceedings of the National Academy of Sciences, 115*, 98–103.

Janak, P. H., & Tye, K. M. (2015). From circuits to behaviour in the amygdala. *Nature, 517*, 284–292.

Janku, C., Engel, P. V, Patel, K., & Giraldo, E. (2023). The 100 most cited Klüver–Bucy research articles: A bibliometric analysis. *Cureus, 15*(9), e45382.

Johansen, J. P., Cain, C. K., Ostroff, L. E., & Ledoux, J. E. (2011). Molecular mechanisms of fear learning and memory. *Cell, 147*, 509–524.

Johansen, J. P., Hamanaka, H., Monfils, M. H., Behnia, R., Deisseroth, K., Blair, H. T., & LeDoux, J. E. (2010). Optical activation of lateral amygdala pyramidal cells instructs associative fear learning. *Proceedings of the National Academy of Sciences, 107*, 12692–12697.

Kamiya, K., & Abe, O. (2020). Imaging of posttraumatic stress disorder. *Neuroimaging Clinics of North America, 30*, 115–123.

Klüver, H., & Bucy, P. C. (1937). "Psychic blindness" and other symptoms following bilateral temporal lobectomy in Rhesus monkeys. *American Journal of Physiology, 119*, 352–353.

LaBar, K. S., LeDoux, J. E., Spencer, D. D., & Phelps, E. A. (1995). Impaired fear conditioning following unilateral temporal lobectomy in humans. *Journal of Neuroscience, 15*, 6846–6855.

LaLumiere, R. T., Buen, T. V., & McGaugh, J. L. (2003). Post-training intra-basolateral amygdala infusions of norepinephrine enhance consolidation of memory for contextual fear conditioning. *Journal of Neuroscience, 23*, 6754–6758.

Langevin, J. P., Koek, R. J., Schwartz, H. N., Chen, J. W. Y., Sultzer, D. L., Mandelkern, M. A., et al. (2016). Deep brain stimulation of the basolateral amygdala for treatment-refractory posttraumatic stress disorder. *Biological Psychiatry, 79*, e82–e84.

Larson, J., & Munkácsy, E. (2015). Theta-burst LTP. *Brain Research, 1621*, 38.

Ledgerwood, L., Richardson, R., & Cranney, J. (2004). D-cycloserine and the facilitation of extinction of conditioned fear: Consequences for reinstatement. *Behavioral Neuroscience, 118*, 505–513.

Ledgerwood, L., Richardson, R., & Cranney, J. (2005). D-cycloserine facilitates extinction of learned fear: Effects on reacquisition and generalized extinction. *Biological Psychiatry, 57*, 841–847.

LeDoux, J. E. (2003). Emotion circuits in the brain. *Annual Review of Neuroscience, 23*, 155–184.

Lee, J. L. C., Bertoglio, L. J., Guimarães, F. S., & Stevenson, C. W. (2017). Cannabidiol regulation of emotion and emotional memory processing: Relevance for treating anxiety-related and substance abuse disorders. *British Journal of Pharmacology, 174*, 3242–3256.

Ly, C., Greb, A. C., Cameron, L. P., Wong, J. M., Barragan, E. V., Wilson, P. C., et al. (2018). Psychedelics promote structural and functional neural plasticity. *Cell Reports, 23*, 3170–3182.

Maren, S. (2003). Neurobiology of Pavlovian fear conditioning. *Annual Review of Neuroscience, 24*, 897–931.

Maren, S. (1999). Neurotoxic basolateral amygdala lesions impair learning and memory but not the performance of conditional fear in rats. *Journal of Neuroscience, 19*, 8696.

Marschner, A., Kalisch, R., Vervliet, B., Vansteenwegen, D., & Büchel, C. (2008). Dissociable roles for the hippocampus and the amygdala in human cued versus context fear conditioning. *Journal of Neuroscience, 28*, 9030–9036.

Marsicano, G., Wotjak, C. T., Azad, S. C., Bisogno, T., Rammes, G., Cascio, M. G., et al. (2002). The endogenous cannabinoid system controls extinction of aversive memories. *Nature, 418*, 530–534.

McDonald, R. J., & White, N. M. (1993). A triple dissociation of memory systems: Hippocampus, amygdala, and dorsal striatum. *Behavioral Neuroscience, 107*, 3–22.

McGaugh, J. L. (2000). Memory—a century of consolidation. *Science, 287*, 248–251.

McGaugh, J. L. (2004). The amygdala modulates the consolidation of memories of emotionally arousing experiences. *Annual Review of Neuroscience, 27*, 1–28.

McGaugh, J. L. (2015). Consolidating memories. *Annual Review of Psychology, 66*, 1–24.

McGaugh, J. L., Cahill, L., & Roozendaal, B. (1996). Involvement of the amygdala in memory storage: Interaction with other brain systems. *Proceedings of the National Academy of Sciences, 93*, 13508–13514.

McGaugh, J. L., McIntyre, C. K., & Power, A. E. (2002). Amygdala modulation of memory consolidation: Interaction with other brain systems. *Neurobiology of Learning and Memory, 78*, 539–552.

Mitchell, J. M., Bogenschutz, M., Lilienstein, A., Harrison, C., Kleiman, S., Parker-Guilbert, K., et al. (2021). MDMA-assisted therapy for severe PTSD: A randomized, double-blind, placebo-controlled phase 3 study. *Nature Medicine, 27*, 1025–1033.

Mitchell, J. M., Ot'alora G, M., van der Kolk, B., Shannon, S., Bogenschutz, M., Gelfand,

Y., et al. (2023). MDMA-assisted therapy for moderate to severe PTSD: A randomized, placebo-controlled phase 3 trial. *Nature Medicine, 29*, 2473–2480.

Nardou, R., Lewis, E. M., Rothhaas, R., Xu, R., Yang, A., Boyden, E., & Dölen, G. (2019). Oxytocin-dependent reopening of a social reward learning critical period with MDMA. *Nature, 569*, 116–120.

Nieh, E. H., Kim, S. Y., Namburi, P., & Tye, K. M. (2013). Optogenetic dissection of neural circuits underlying emotional valence and motivated behaviors. *Brain Research, 1511*, 73–92.

Norberg, M. M., Krystal, J. H., & Tolin, D. F. (2008). A meta-analysis of d-cycloserine and the facilitation of fear extinction and exposure therapy. *Biological Psychiatry, 63*, 1118–1126.

O'Keefe, J., & Nadel, L. (1978). *The hippocampus as a cognitive map.* Clarendon Press.

Pamplona, F. A., Bitencourt, R. M., & Takahashi, R. N. (2008). Short- and long-term effects of cannabinoids on the extinction of contextual fear memory in rats. *Neurobiology of Learning and Memory, 90*, 290–293.

Papagianni, E. P., Warren, W. G., Cassaday, H. J., & Stevenson, C. W. (2022). Cannabidiol prevents spontaneous fear recovery after extinction and ameliorates stress-induced extinction resistance. *International Journal of Molecular Sciences, 23*(16), 9333.

Patel, S., Hill, M. N., Cheer, J. F., Wotjak, C. T., & Holmes, A. (2017). The endocannabinoid system as a target for novel anxiolytic drugs. *Neuroscience and Biobehavioral Reviews, 76*, 56–66.

Phelps, E. A. (2004). Human emotion and memory: Interactions of the amygdala and hippocampal complex. *Current Opinion in Neurobiology, 14*, 198–202.

Phillips, R. G., & LeDoux, J. E. (1992). Differential contribution of amygdala and hippocampus to cued and contextual fear conditioning. *Behavioral Neuroscience, 106*, 274–285.

Pitman, R. K., Rasmusson, A. M., Koenen, K. C., Shin, L. M., Orr, S. P., Gilbertson, M. W., et al. (2012). Biological studies of post-traumatic stress disorder. *Nature Reviews Neuroscience, 13*(11), 769–787.

Pryluk, R., Sirigu, A., & Paz, R. (2021). Two sides of the same amygdala: From shared neural mechanisms to comorbidity of social and affective disorders. *Neuron, 109*, 3908–3911.

Qasim, S. E., Mohan, U. R., Stein, J. M., & Jacobs, J. (2023). Neuronal activity in the human amygdala and hippocampus enhances emotional memory encoding. *Nature Human Behaviour, 7*(5), 754–764.

Raskin, M., & Monfils, M.-H. (2023). Reconsolidation and fear extinction: An update. *Current Topics in Behavioral Neurosciences, 64*, 307–333.

Richardson, M. P., Strange, B. A., & Dolan, R. J. (2004). Encoding of emotional memories depends on amygdala and hippocampus and their interactions. *Nature Neuroscience, 7*, 278–285.

Roesler, R., Parent, M. B., LaLumiere, R. T., & McIntyre, C. K. (2021). Amygdala-hippocampal interactions in synaptic plasticity and memory formation. *Neurobiology of Learning and Memory, 184*, 107490.

Roozendaal, B., McEwen, B. S., & Chattarji, S. (2009). Stress, memory and the amygdala. *Nature Reviews Neuroscience, 10*(6), 423–433.

Rouhani, N., Niv, Y., Frank, M. J., & Schwabe, L. (2023). Multiple routes to enhanced memory for emotionally relevant events. *Trends in Cognitive Sciences, 27*, 867–882.

Sah, P., Westbrook, R. F., & Lüthi, A. (2008). Fear conditioning and long-term potentiation in the amygdala. *Annals of the New York Academy of Sciences, 1129*, 88–95.

Sander, D., Grafman, J., & Zalla, T. (2003). The human amygdala: An evolved system for relevance detection. *Reviews in the Neurosciences, 14*, 303–316.

Schwabe, L., Joëls, M., Roozendaal, B., Wolf, O. T., & Oitzl, M. S. (2012). Stress effects on memory: An update and integration. *Neuroscience & Biobehavioral Reviews, 36*, 1740–1749.

Shapiro, M. L., Tanila, H., & Eichenbaum, H. (1997). Cues that hippocampal place cells encode: Dynamic and hierarchical representation of local and distal stimuli. *Hippocampus, 7*, 624–642.

Singleton, S. P., Wang, J. B., Mithoefer, M., Hanlon, C., George, M. S., Mithoefer, A., et al. (2023). Altered brain activity and functional connectivity after MDMA-assisted therapy for post-traumatic stress disorder. *Frontiers in Psychiatry, 13*, 947622.

Southwick, S. M., Davis, M., Horner, B., Cahill, L., Morgan, C. A., Gold, P. E., et al. (2002). Relationship of enhanced norepinephrine activity during memory consolidation to enhanced long-term memory in humans. *American Journal of Psychiatry, 159*, 1420–1422.

Strange, B. A., & Dolan, R. J. (2004). Beta-adrenergic modulation of emotional memory-evoked human amygdala and hippocampal responses. *Proceedings of the National Academy of Sciences, 101*, 11454–11458.

Strange, B. A., & Dolan, R. J. (2006). Anterior medial temporal lobe in human cognition: Memory for fear and the unexpected. *Cognitive Neuropsychiatry, 11*, 198–218.

Strange, B. A., Witter, M. P., Lein, E. S., & Moser, E. I. (2014). Functional organization of the hippocampal longitudinal axis. *Nature Reviews Neuroscience, 15*, 655–669.

Suarez-Jimenez, B., Albajes-Eizagirre, A., Lazarov, A., Zhu, X., Harrison, B. J., Radua, J., et al. (2020). Neural signatures of conditioning, extinction learning, and extinction recall in posttraumatic stress disorder: A meta-analysis of functional magnetic resonance imaging studies. *Psychological Medicine, 50*, 1442–1451.

Terzian, H., & Ore, G. D. (1955). Syndrome of Klüver and Bucy; reproduced in man by bilateral removal of the temporal lobes. *Neurology, 5*, 373–380.

Vermetten, E., & Lanius, R. A. (2012). Biological and clinical framework for posttraumatic stress disorder. *Handbook of Clinical Neurology, 106*, 291–342.

Vizeli, P., Straumann, I., Duthaler, U., Varghese, N., Eckert, A., Paulus, M. P., et al. (2022). Effects of 3,4-methylenedioxymethamphetamine on conditioned fear extinction and retention in a crossover study in healthy subjects. *Frontiers in Pharmacology, 13*, 906639.

Wang, S., Tudusciuc, O., Mamelak, A. N., Ross, I. B., Adolphs, R., & Rutishauser, U. (2014). Neurons in the human amygdala selective for perceived emotion. *Proceedings of the National Academy of Sciences, 111*(30), E3110–E3119.

Wirth, S., Soumier, A., Eliava, M., Derdikman, D., Wagner, S., Grinevich, V., & Sirigu, A. (2021). Territorial blueprint in the hippocampal system. *Trends in Cognitive Sciences, 25*, 831–842.

Wotjak, C. (2005). Role of endogenous cannabinoids in cognition and emotionality. *Mini Reviews in Medicinal Chemistry, 5*, 659–670.

Yonelinas, A. P., & Ritchey, M. (2015). The slow forgetting of emotional episodic memories: An emotional binding account. *Trends in Cognitive Sciences, 19*, 259–267.

Young, M. B., Norrholm, S. D., Khoury, L. M., Jovanovic, T., Rauch, S. A. M., Reiff, C. M., et al. (2017). Inhibition of serotonin transporters disrupts the enhancement of fear memory extinction by 3,4-methylenedioxymethamphetamine (MDMA). *Psychopharmacology, 234*, 2883–2895.

Zheng, J., Stevenson, R. F., Mander, B. A., Mnatsakanyan, L., Hsu, F. P. K., Vadera, S., et al. (2019). Multiplexing of theta and alpha rhythms in the amygdala-hippocampal circuit supports pattern separation of emotional information. *Neuron, 102*(4), 887–898.e5.

CHAPTER 6

Development and Plasticity of the Human Visual System

Maxime Bleau and Maurice Ptito

Introduction

The visual system is one of the most extensively studied sensory systems. As the main sensory channel for humans to acquire information about objects, space, and other individuals, it plays a crucial role in almost all aspects of human development. Indeed, visual functions develop rapidly in infancy and underpin the development of gross and fine motor skills, help refine and calibrate other senses (Bremner et al., 2012), and contribute to developing higher-order knowledge and skills necessary to navigate both the environment (Ekstrom, 2015) and social interactions (Klauke et al., 2023). Most of all, the visual system shows a particular ability to adapt to its sensory environment. As a result, the visual system has become a flagship model from the early beginnings of neuroscience to study and understand the brain and its plasticity.

This chapter covers the development and plasticity of the visual system. Notably, we describe the early postnatal period, a period of high neural plasticity when the brain circuits are malleable. During this time, the visual system has well-defined critical periods, or windows of time, when the brain is particularly susceptible to visual input, and visual experience can significantly shape the structure and function of the visual cortex and other associated areas. This makes the visual system an exemplary model for studying how sensory loss and other environmental factors influence neural development. Finally, we illustrate how the brain adapts to sensory loss, such as congenital blindness, by repurposing visual areas to process information from other senses, a phenomenon known as cross-modal plasticity.

The Developing Visual System

Maturation of Visual Structures

The development of visual abilities is closely linked to the anatomical and physiological maturation of all structures composing the visual system. More precisely, over the first few months of life, the rapid improvements in depth perception, motion detection, and facial recognition recorded in infants are linked to retinal maturation and the refinement of the visual pathways.

The Retina

The retina, the photoreceptive layer in the eye, is not fully developed at birth (Marcos et al., 2021; Van Cruchten et al., 2017). It undergoes significant maturation during the first few years of life. In early postnatal development, rods are better developed than cones, but as cones mature at 3 months of age, infants gain the ability to discriminate colors. Over time, the photoreceptor layer becomes more specialized (Hendrickson et al., 2012). Particularly at the fovea, the area responsible for high visual acuity, cone density also increases as they become shorter and their inner segments become thinner (Van Cruchten et al., 2017). Cones, however, do not reach their adult size until after 45 months of life (Hendrickson & Yuodelis, 1984; see Figure 6.1*). Myelination of the optic nerve, from which visual information exits the eye, begins in the seventh month of gestation, and its thickness continues to increase for 6–8 years after birth (Graw, 2010; Van Cruchten et al., 2017).

The Lateral Geniculate Nucleus and Visual Pathways

The lateral geniculate nucleus (LGN), the central thalamic retino-recipient structure, also undergoes significant development during the first months of life, as its connections to the visual cortex, although present, are still immature at birth. In the first few months after birth, the LGN undergoes substantial synaptogenesis and refinement, as projections from each eye are initially diffuse and overlapping (Stacy & Van Hooser, 2022). These connections become more precise and segregated into eye-specific layers through activity-dependent plasticity. Myelination of the optic radiations, which connect the LGN to the visual cortex, also progresses rapidly in the first few months of life (Dubois et al., 2014). This process enhances the speed and efficiency of the transmission of visual signals.

The Visual Cortex

The development of the visual cortex is an ongoing, almost lifelong process that is at its most rapid state in infancy and continues gradually into adulthood. Indeed, the primary visual cortex (V1) undergoes significant changes during early childhood as synaptic connections mature and functional circuits are established. The maturation

* All figures appear on the separate color insert.

TABLE 6.1. Postnatal Maturation of the Visual Cortex

Period	Aspects of maturation
Infancy (0–2 years)	Rapid growth and initial formation of synaptic connections. Binocular vision is crucial during this period for normal development.
Early childhood (2–5 years)	Continued growth and refinement of synaptic connections. Visual acuity and contrast sensitivity begin to improve.
Late childhood (5–12 years)	Maturation of visual circuits and further improvement in visual functions. This stage generally completes the basic functions of early sensory areas of the cortex.
Adolescence (12–19 years)	Prolonged development with significant synaptic density and myelination changes. Visual acuity and contrast sensitivity continue to mature.
Adulthood (19–55 years)	Stabilization of visual functions, with ongoing plasticity allowing for adaptation to new visual experiences.

of human V1 covers a large period from infancy to adulthood and involves mostly the structural remodeling of synaptic connectivity (Siu & Murphy, 2018; see Table 6.1).

The maturation of visual functions is also linked to changes in the expression of glutamatergic and GABA-ergic (i.e., gamma-aminobutyric acid) mechanisms during the first 6 years of postnatal development (Desgent & Ptito, 2012; Murphy et al., 2005). These changes affect spatial and temporal integration in visual cortical neurons and contribute to the prolonged critical period in human visual development. The balance between excitatory and inhibitory plasticity mechanisms, including *N*-methyl-D-aspartate receptor activation and GABA-mediated inhibition, plays a crucial role in shaping neural circuitry during this critical period (Murphy et al., 2005).

Development of Visual Abilities

Newborns have limited visual acuity due to immature retinal structures and underdeveloped visual circuits. Visual gratings acuity tests (Teller, 1997) have shown that infants have no more than 20/600 vision. This acuity and contrast sensitivity (the ability to register light and dark variations) are sufficient for visual interactions with the parents, typically happening at distances shorter than one meter (Atkinson & Braddick, 2020). Indeed, it is primarily known that infants can fixate and follow high-contrast targets and respond to face-like stimuli (Simion et al., 2011) and familiar faces like their mother's (Bushneil et al., 1989). However, the maturation of the visual cortex is required to process and make sense of more complex stimuli (Danka Mohammed & Khalil, 2020; Espinosa & Stryker, 2012; Siu & Murphy, 2018). Specific V1 functions develop postnatally between 1 and 6 months and sequentially from orientation selectivity in the first weeks of life to directional motion processing at 6–10 weeks and binocular interactions at 2.5–5 months (Atkinson & Braddick, 2020). As a result, visual acuity and contrast sensitivity continue to develop very rapidly in the first 6 months of life (Atkinson, 2002), then more slowly with aging, reaching 20/200 at 1 year (Teller, 1997), then developing toward adult values by around 3–4 years (Atkinson & Braddick, 2020). Other aspects, including contrast sensitivity, continue to develop into adolescence (Leat et al., 2009; see Figure 6.2).

Critical Periods

The gross anatomical development of the visual system and the initial establishment of the functional architecture of V1 (e.g., excitatory-inhibitory transmission, orientation selectivity, ocular dominance, and the fundamental structure of receptive fields) are controlled mainly by genetically determined molecular programs (Espinosa & Stryker, 2012; Siu & Murphy, 2018). However, a vast body of research in mammals (Balmer & Pallas, 2015; Espinosa & Stryker, 2012), and even in preterm infants (Jandó et al., 2012), has shown that the refinement and maturation of these neuronal properties occur later after birth and require visual experience. Indeed, visual development in early postnatal life is characterized by periods of a high degree of neural plasticity where the brain circuits are particularly malleable and highly sensitive to environmental stimuli, thus shaping the structure and function of the visual cortex and other associated areas. This includes the refinement of synaptic connections, as the matching of presynaptic neurons to their postsynaptic targets depends on spontaneous and sensory-driven neural activity (Goodman & Shatz, 1993; Katz & Shatz, 1996). These periods of plasticity are crucial in the proper development of visual abilities and have been rightfully named “critical periods” (Spolidoro et al., 2009). An abnormal visual experience during these periods can significantly alter the development of the visual system and lead to permanent visual deficits (Lewis & Maurer, 2005). These critical periods occur at different rates for different aspects of visual function (Lewis & Maurer, 2005), influencing the consequences of visual deprivation and the effectiveness of treatments depending on the time of deprivation (reviewed in Leat et al., 2009).

The Impact of Visual Deprivation

Vision is so important to humans that, at maturity, between 27 and 35% of the brain is involved in either visual processing or its integration with other sensory modalities. As a result, there is no doubt that early visual deprivation, if not addressed promptly, can lead to permanent deficits and significant structural and functional reorganization in different cortical and subcortical networks. Therefore, visual deprivation has been vastly used to understand the development and plasticity of the visual system. Various methods for inducing visual deprivation have been used, like dark rearing, enucleation, and eyelid suturing. Dark rearing is the process of raising an animal in complete darkness from birth, while enucleation is the complete removal of the eyeballs and eye suture, the reversible stitching of the eyelids (reviewed in Kupers & Ptito, 2014).

In one of the most impactful works in the field of visual neuroscience, Wiesel and Hubel (1963a, 1963b, 1965) used monocular deprivation in kittens to study the changes in visual responses in V1. They were the first to show the presence of critical periods for ocular dominance as visual deprivation in adult cats did not cause the same dramatic changes in V1 compared with kittens being monocularly deprived between the 4th and 8th weeks of life (Hubel & Wiesel, 1970; Wiesel & Hubel, 1963b). Furthermore, they showed that alterations of ocular dominance result from competition between inputs from the two eyes and happen in V1 but not in earlier structures of the visual pathway like the LGN (Wiesel & Hubel, 1963a, 1963b). They also used a model of divergent strabismus, keeping both eyes from working together, and found that it eliminated binocular responses in V1 neurons (Hubel & Wiesel, 1965), thus providing evidence that would shape the basis of models of development (Stent, 1973) explaining the loss of stereoscopic vision in amblyopia (see Figure 6.3).

Congenital Blindness in Humans: A Model for Cross-Modal Plasticity

Early and permanent visual deprivation has massive effects on the visual system, triggering a cascade of plastic changes across the whole brain due to the complete loss of natural inputs and overreliance on other sensory channels during critical periods of development.

Like visual deprivation in animals, congenital blindness in humans (described as a loss of vision since birth) has provided a robust model for the study of critical developmental periods, sensory integration, and compensatory plasticity (e.g., how the brain changes both at the anatomical and functional levels). The advent of neuroimaging techniques has provided means to study anatomical changes in the human blind brain, such as gray and white matter volumes, cortical thickness, white matter integrity, and metabolic activity (Paré et al., 2023) in various brain regions, leading to brain reorganization. This reorganization has also been correlated with behavior using brain activation techniques such as functional magnetic resonance imaging (fMRI) and magnetoencephalography (MEG), which allowed researchers to understand how brain regions typically devoted to vision are repurposed for other sensory modalities. These anatomical and physiological changes lead to the development of compensatory abilities and even the enhancement of other sensory and cognitive abilities. This collective work demonstrating the human brain's remarkable ability to adapt to sensory deprivation will be the focus of the remaining sections.

Anatomical Changes

Early blindness leads to substantial volumetric reductions in gray and white matter throughout the visual system, but mainly along the visual pathway from the retina to V1. This includes significant reductions in the optic nerve, optic chiasma, optic tract, LGN, optic radiations, and striate and extra-striate areas of the visual cortex (Aguirre et al., 2016; Cecchetti et al., 2016; reviewed in Kupers & Ptito, 2014; Ptito et al., 2021c). Despite these reductions, the overall structure of the visual cortex is preserved but is often found to be significantly thicker compared with normally sighted individuals (Bridge et al., 2009; Voss & Zatorre, 2012). This change in cortical thickness has been attributed to the reduction of synaptic pruning. This process eliminates aberrant synaptic connections and occurs in normal development (reviewed in Anurova et al., 2015; Kupers & Ptito, 2014). In support of this hypothesis, some studies found a significant correlation between this increase in cortical thickness and the onset of blindness (Voss & Zatorre, 2012). Atrophic changes were also reported in the ventral visual stream, connecting the occipital cortex with the anterior temporal lobe, and in the inferior frontal–occipital fasciculus, connecting the occipital cortex with the prefrontal cortex. In contrast, the dorsal stream was largely preserved (Reislev et al., 2016).

As for the rest of the brain, our group recently conducted a meta-analysis (Paré et al., 2023) to investigate morphometric changes within and beyond the visual cortex. Volume reductions in white and gray matter are consistently reported across studies. More recently, increased cortical thickness was also observed outside V1 in younger blind children. However, cortical thickness tends to normalize with age, suggesting a slight delay in the refinement of synaptic connections throughout the brain (Hasson et al., 2016; Inuggi et al., 2020). Other significant atrophies were also found in the splenium of the corpus callosum (Cavaliere et al., 2020; Ptito et al., 2008b; Tomaiuolo et al., 2014), while an enlargement was identified in the anterior commissure (Cavaliere et al., 2020; see Figure 6.4).

Cross-Modal Plasticity in the Visual Cortex

Due to the lack of visual input during the critical periods of development, early onset blindness significantly alters the functional architecture of the brain, mainly all parts of the visual system, but also other nondeprived areas (Huber et al., 2019). Particularly, the alteration of the formation and refinement of neural circuits usually involved in processing visual information leads to a massive reorganization of the functions and connectivity of the visual cortex (Ptito et al., 2021a). As a result, this sensory-deprived cortex in blind animals and humans is invaded by inputs from other sensory channels through plastic modifications of subcortical and cortical connections (Desgent & Ptito, 2012; reviewed in Kupers & Ptito, 2014). While these anatomical modifications were primarily described in animals (see Kupers & Ptito, 2014), they were also reported in blind humans using event-related electroencephalographic (EEG) recordings (Uhl et al., 1991) and positron emission tomography (PET) imaging (Ptito et al., 2005; Sadato et al., 1996, 1998). Today, it is widely accepted that this repurposing of the visual cortex is due to the replacement of visual information by other sensory information to perform daily tasks (i.e., Braille reading and echolocation), a process called *sensory substitution*. This overreliance on other sensory modalities allows the brain to make use of the cortical areas that would otherwise be unused, like the visual cortex.

Indeed, the vast literature on brain imaging, including EEG, PET, and fMRI studies (Kupers & Ptito, 2014; Zhang et al., 2019), has provided evidence that this cross-modal plasticity in the occipital cortex of congenitally blind subjects is in fact training-induced (Ptito et al., 2005; Sadato et al., 1996), can appear from a young age (Bedny et al., 2015), and is involved in a variety of nonvisual tasks (Kupers &

Ptito, 2014; Nau et al., 2015). These tests include sound localization (Collignon et al., 2011), auditory and tactile motion perception (Dormal et al., 2016; Matteau et al., 2010; Ptito et al., 2009), echolocation (Thaler et al., 2011), Braille reading (Büchel et al., 1998), shape perception (Arno et al., 2001), and even verb generation (Amedi et al., 2004; Ofan & Zohary, 2007). Furthermore, area hMT+ (an area linked to visual motion processing) is also consistently found to be activated in tactile and auditory motion discrimination tasks (Jiang et al., 2014; Matteau et al., 2010; Ptito et al., 2009). Consistent with these findings, transcranial magnetic stimulation (TMS) of area hMT+ led to decreased performance and increased reaction times in tactile motion discrimination (Kupers et al., 2009). Other studies using TMS have shown that stimulating the occipital cortex leads to Braille reading errors and distortions in tactile perception (i.e., missing or phantom dots) in blind, but not sighted, individuals (Cohen et al., 1997). TMS of area V1 also induces tactile sensations in the fingers of Braille readers (Ptito et al., 2008a) and on the tongue of those who were trained with a tongue display unit (TDU) translating visual information into tactile sensations (Kupers et al., 2006; see Figure 6.5). These sensations varied in intensity and topography depending on the locus of stimulation of the occipital cortex (Kupers et al., 2006; Ptito et al., 2008a), suggesting the apparition of a new somatotopy for the fingers and the tongue in the visual cortex.

Beyond the visual cortex, the visual streams have also been shown to be recruited by the same nonvisual information. For example, tactile motion activates area hMT+ in the dorsal visual stream (Bedny et al., 2010; Matteau et al., 2010; Ptito et al., 2009), whereas the ventral stream is recruited by shape information, particularly in inferior temporal (LOtv) and fusiform gyri (Ptito et al., 2012), reading in the visual word form area (Kim et al., 2017), and face expression in the medial temporal gyrus (Kitada et al., 2013). These findings provide a strong indication that both the dorsal and ventral visual streams are preserved in blind individuals (Arbel-Yaffe & Amedi, 2016; Collignon et al., 2007; Pietrini et al., 2009; Striem-Amit & Amedi, 2014) anatomically and functionally (Kupers & Ptito, 2014; Reislev et al., 2016).

Overall, this repurposing of visual areas, combined with the recruitment of the different visual pathways and multisensory areas, makes it easier for blind individuals to learn the use of multiple sensory substitution methods (Kupers & Ptito, 2014; Ptito et al., 2005), and even significantly improve their performance after limited training (Sampaio et al., 2001). These plasticity mechanisms also highlight the brain's capacity to recruit task-specific areas, regardless of the used sensory channels (Chebat et al., 2018b). This lends support to the model of a *metamodal* brain that suggests that visual areas, despite being recruited by other modalities, perform the same perceptual functions (Proulx et al., 2014). Recently, a new model of a pluripotent brain in infancy could explain how the visual cortex is repurposed for higher cognitive demands (Saccone et al., 2024). Indeed, both models are supported by several studies showing that many visual areas in the blind brain receive multisensory information (Palejwala et al., 2021). The recruitment of the visual cortical areas by other sensory modalities is probably due to either the reinforcement of preexisting corticocortical connections or the formation of new thalamocortical connections (Kupers & Ptito, 2014).

The cortico-cortical hypothesis refers to changes in the connectivity in the cerebral cortex of blind individuals, either by the formation of new pathways or by the strengthening, or "unmasking," of preexisting connections (Ptito et al., 2005). Consistent with this hypothesis, direct connections between the primary visual and other sensory cortices have been found in cats, nonhuman primates, and other mammals (reviewed in Kupers & Ptito, 2014). These preexisting connections are strengthened following enucleation close to birth (Laramée et al., 2011). In humans, fMRI studies have also found increased functional connectivity, or correlated activity, between visual areas and other sensory cortices in the blind performing various tasks (Kupers et al., 2006; Leo et al., 2012; Ptito et al., 2005).

The thalamocortical hypothesis refers to a rerouting of nonvisual input to the thalamic sensory nuclei. This new thalamocortical pathway would likely be mediated through ectopic connections between the LGN and other sensory nuclei of the thalamus (ventral posterolateral nucleus [VPL] for touch and medial geniculate nucleus for audition), allowing the nonvisual afference to be funneled to V1 through the optic radiations. This theory is based mainly on anatomical evidence from animal studies. Aberrant connections have been found between the LGN and other sensory nuclei in anophthalmic mouse strain, ZRDCT-An (Kaiserman-Abramof et al., 1980), or with the auditory inferior colliculus in the case of the blind mole rat (Doron & Wollberg, 1994), both leading to auditory responses in area V1 (Bronchti et al., 2002; Chabot et al., 2007). Furthermore, direct connections between visual cortical area 17 and the somatosensory nucleus of the thalamus were found in the enucleated opossum (Karlen et al., 2006). Finally, recent studies from our laboratory reported evidence of such a pathway in humans (Müller et al., 2019). Using MEG, we have investigated, in early blind individuals, the time course of the tactile responses in V1 and found that a first response peak occurred as early as 35-ms poststimulus, a latency that would match a fast monosynaptic pathway between the thalamus and the visual cortex (Müller et al., 2019), through a new ectopic connection between the VPL and LGN (see Figure 6.6).

Behavioral Modifications in Early Blindness

There is a large body of scientific evidence on the abilities of blind people and how blindness can enhance other sensory modalities and cognitive functions (Kupers & Ptito, 2014; Ptito et al., 2021b). These findings highlight the brain's adaptability when relying on and compensating with other senses to perform daily tasks, such as reading and navigation. Indeed, studies have consistently shown that early blind individuals have improved tactile abilities, including tactile letter recognition (Craig, 1988) and tactile acuity (Legge et al., 2008), particularly in the finger dominant for Braille reading (Goldreich & Kanics, 2003). In addition, blind individuals showed no age-related decline in their tactile acuity compared with sighted individuals, who demonstrated a decline of approximately 1% per year (Goldreich & Kanics, 2003). Furthermore, tactile acuity was not correlated to blindness onset (Goldreich & Kanics, 2003), nor Braille reading speed, amount of Braille reading, or the age at which Braille was learned (Legge et al., 2008). Therefore, it was believed that improved tactile acuity could be either induced by blindness itself or caused by extensive experience with their sense of touch.

Wong, Gnanakumaran, and Goldreich (2011) tested this idea by comparing the improvement in tactile acuity at the fingers and at the lips, an untrained part of the body. Their results showed enhanced performance from the fingers but not from the lips. They also confirmed that blind individuals performed better with the dominant reading finger than with the other fingers, and even that performance with this specific finger correlated with the amount of Braille reading. These results suggest that a more substantial reliance on the sense of touch causes higher tactile acuity in blind individuals. Along the same line, the superior tactile acuity of blind individuals was also shown to decrease, even disappear, when their sighted counterparts received additional training (Grant et al., 2000; Heller, 1989). This finding suggests that cross-modal plasticity underlying tactile superiority is experience-dependent and can occur very rapidly following training (Merabet et al., 2008).

Performance improvements in blind individuals have also been reported for audition, particularly in auditory tasks involving musical abilities, locating sounds, and tracking moving objects in space (Arnaud et al., 2018; Röder et al., 1999). However, early-onset visual deprivation does not lead to superior performance in all auditory tasks. For example, blindness has been shown to result in better speech and tone discrimination (Niemeyer & Starlinger, 1981), better absolute pitch perception for those with extensive musical training (Hamilton et al., 2004), better pitch discrimination (Gougoux et al., 2004; Wan et al., 2010), and pitch-timbre categorization, but not better pitch working memory (Wan et al., 2010). Other studies demonstrated that blind people could better localize sounds (Lessard et al., 1998; Röder et al., 1999) and use echolocation (Thaler & Goodale, 2016). Early blindness has also been associated with improved cognitive abilities (Bavelier & Neville, 2002; Kupers & Ptito, 2014), such as verbal working memory (Amedi et al., 2003) and attention (Liotti et al., 1998). This enhancement extends to both semantic and episodic memory (Tomasello et al., 2024).

As vision plays a crucial role in the calibration of other senses (Bremner et al., 2012) and in the development of other cognitive processes, such as spatial awareness (Acredolo, 1990), early-onset blindness can also lead to functional deficits. Indeed, blind infants often show significant delays in the development of gross and fine motor skills, and deficits in sound localization, distance estimation, and spatial cognition (Cappagli et al., 2017; Rieser et al., 1980; Zwiers et al., 2001). More importantly, vision is the main sense used by humans to navigate, orient themselves in their environment, maintain balance, avoid obstacles, and take shortcuts (Gandemer et al., 2017; Maheu et al., 2017). Vision mainly enables the individual to simultaneously detect numerous landmarks (Cattaneo & Vecchi, 2008) and keep track of their location in space during locomotion. This ability allows humans and other animals to build cognitive maps, or mental representations of space, that are allocentric (e.g., independent from one's location and viewpoint; Ekstrom, 2015; Epstein et al., 2017). To date, spatial navigation and orientation remain critical challenges faced by early blind humans, as they often show significant deficits in spatial orientation and allocentric coding (Espinosa & Ochaíta, 1998; Espinosa et al., 1998; Giudice, 2018; Ungar et al., 1994). Indeed, their ability to acquire spatial information is limited to what they can touch and hear and, therefore, is more limited to their proximal space (Long & Giudice, 2010). As a result, cognitive mapping is serialized and, therefore, more cognitively demanding and time-consuming (Bleau et al., 2023; Giudice, 2018; Schinazi et al., 2016). Consequently, many blind individuals will limit themselves to familiar areas and routes, and will rely on egocentric strategies (i.e., route following) against allocentric ones (e.g., cognitive-map-based navigation) that enable more improvisation and shortcuts (Iachini et al., 2014; Pasqualotto et al., 2013). Furthermore, blind individuals are more prone to errors when using allocentric strategies (Bigelow, 1996; Coluccia et al., 2009; Iachini et al., 2014; Noordzij et al., 2006; Pasqualotto et al., 2013; Rieser et al., 1980, 1986), errors attributed to distortions in their mental representations of space (Golledge et al., 2000).

In the brain, spatial navigation has been primarily associated with the hippocampus, particularly its posterior part, as its volume correlates with navigational skills (Maguire et al., 2000; Woollett & Maguire, 2011). Only a handful of studies investigated the possible alterations in this part of the brain and have either found a significant volume reduction in its posterior part (Chebat et al., 2007) or an increase in its anterior part (Fortin et al., 2008). These changes in volume correlated with behavioral performances in spatial navigation tasks (Chebat et al., 2007; Fortin et al., 2008). Future research on navigation and spatial awareness in congenitally blind individuals will need to focus on how these abilities and underlying brain networks (such as the parahippocampus, retrosplenial complex, lateral occipital cortex, and other areas in the parietal and frontal cortices) develop and can adapt to support better navigation skills, even without visual experience (Bleau et al., 2022; Sigismondi et al., 2024). Additionally, advancements in virtual environments and virtual reality hold significant potential for enhancing spatial understanding, as they can simulate complex environments and offer more opportunities to explore and practice navigation in safe and controlled spaces (Afonso-Jaco & Katz, 2022; Bleau et al., 2022; Merabet et al., 2012; Thevin et al., 2020).

Sensory Substitution Devices as Aids for the Blind

As navigation challenges negatively affect the quality of life of many blind individuals, a panoply of new technologies and assistive tools has been manufactured throughout the last century to support navigation and orientation (reviewed in Ptito et al., 2021b). More recently, sensory substitution devices (SSDs) have become very popular since it is generally accepted that senses can be switched (audition for vision or touch for vision), and by doing so, they recruit the visual cortex and associative areas (Kupers & Ptito, 2014). Early blind subjects trained in various "visual" tasks using the tactile modality with the TDU (Bach-y-Rita & Kercel, 2003) can perceive and discriminate orientation stimuli (Ptito et al., 2005), motion (Matteau et al., 2010), and shapes (Ptito et al., 2012). The same results were reported with the auditory modality using the vOICe system (Arbel et al., 2022; Striem-Amit et al., 2011). In addition, these devices can be used to locate objects in space and successfully navigate through obstacles and mazes (Bleau et al., 2021; Chebat et al., 2011, 2015, 2020b; Paré et al., 2021; Ptito et al., 2021b).

Importantly, neuroimaging studies using SSDs have been crucial in confirming cross-modal plasticity (i.e., the recruitment of the visual cortex by nonvisual stimuli; Amedi et al., 2002; Chebat et al., 2018a; Nau et al., 2015; Ptito et al., 2005; Striem-Amit & Amedi, 2014). Moreover, this cross-modal plasticity is training-dependent and can occur very rapidly in blind individuals (Kupers & Ptito, 2014; Nau et al.,

2015). This was also true when early blind individuals were performing navigation tasks in which they recruited the dorsal visual stream and parts of the navigation network (Aggius-Vella et al., 2023; Chebat et al., 2020a; Kupers et al., 2010; Maidenbaum et al., 2018). Assistive technologies such as SSDs still remain largely preferred and more successful than retinal and cortical implants (reviewed in Ptito et al., 2021a).

Conclusion

The visual system is highly sensitive to the loss of visual input in the first years of life. Congenital blindness in humans, therefore, leads to significant anatomical alterations of the visual system and deficits, or delays, in different cognitive functions. However, the visual cortex remains functional and recruited by other senses to perform many tasks. Sensory substitution and cross-modal plasticity are hence crucial in helping the blind "see." The future generation of SSDs should consider exposing blind individuals at an early age to foster cross-modal plastic processes and, hence, the development of cognitive processes such as spatial awareness and cognitive mapping.

REFERENCES

Acredolo, L. (1990). Behavioral approaches to spatial orientation in infancy. *Annals of the New York Academy of Sciences, 608*, 596–612.

Afonso-Jaco, A., & Katz, B. F. (2022). Spatial knowledge via auditory information for blind individuals spatial cognition studies and the use of audio, VR. *Sensors, 22*(13), 4794.

Aggius-Vella, E., Chebat, D.-R., Maidenbaum, S., & Amedi, A. (2023). Activation of human visual area v6 during egocentric navigation with and without visual experience. *Current Biology, 33*(7), 1211–1219.e1215.

Aguirre, G. K., Datta, R., Benson, N. C., Prasad, S., Jacobson, S. G., Cideciyan, A. V., et al. (2016). Patterns of individual variation in visual pathway structure and function in the sighted and blind. *PLOS ONE, 11*(11), e0164677.

Amedi, A., Floel, A., Knecht, S., Zohary, E., & Cohen, L. G. (2004). Transcranial magnetic stimulation of the occipital pole interferes with verbal processing in blind subjects. *Nature Neuroscience*, 7(11), 1266–1270.

Amedi, A., Jacobson, G., Hendler, T., Malach, R., & Zohary, E. (2002). Convergence of visual and tactile shape processing in the human lateral occipital complex. *Cerebral Cortex, 12*(11), 1202–1212.

Amedi, A., Raz, N., Pianka, P., Malach, R., & Zohary, E. (2003). Early "visual" cortex activation correlates with superior verbal memory performance in the blind. *Nature Neuroscience, 6*(7), 758–766.

Anurova, I., Renier, L. A., De Volder, A. G., Carlson, S., & Rauschecker, J. P. (2015). Relationship between cortical thickness and functional activation in the early blind. *Cerebral Cortex, 25*(8), 2035–2048.

Arbel, R., Heimler, B., & Amedi, A. (2022). Congenitally blind adults can learn to identify face-shapes via auditory sensory substitution and successfully generalize some of the learned features. *Scientific Reports, 12*(1), 4330.

Arbel-Yaffe, R., & Amedi, A. (2016). Auditory face identification activates selective areas within the ventral visual stream in congenitally blind. *Journal of Vision, 16*(12), 1229–1229.

Arnaud, L., Gracco, V., & Ménard, L. (2018). Enhanced perception of pitch changes in speech and music in early blind adults. *Neuropsychologia, 117*, 261–270.

Arno, P., De Volder, A. G., Vanlierde, A., Wanet-Defalque, M.-C., Streel, E., Robert, A., et al. (2001). Occipital activation by pattern recognition in the early blind using auditory substitution for vision. *NeuroImage, 13*(4), 632–645.

Atkinson, J. (2002). Newborn vision. In J. Atkinson (Ed.), *The developing visual brain* (pp. 43–57). Oxford University Press.

Atkinson, J., & Braddick, O. (2020). Visual development. In A. Gallagher, C. Bulteau, D. Cohen, & J. L. Michaud (Eds.), *Handbook of clinical neurology* (pp. 121–142). Elsevier.

Bach-y-Rita, P., & Kercel, S. W. (2003). Sensory substitution and the human–machine interface. *Trends in Cognitive Sciences, 7*(12), 541–546.

Balmer, T. S., & Pallas, S. L. (2015). Refinement but not maintenance of visual receptive fields is independent of visual experience. *Cerebral Cortex, 25*(4), 904–917.

Bavelier, D., & Neville, H. J. (2002). Cross-modal plasticity: Where and how *Nature Reviews Neuroscience, 3*(6), 443–452.

Bedny, M., Konkle, T., Pelphrey, K., Saxe, R., & Pascual-Leone, A. (2010). Sensitive period for a multimodal response in human visual motion area mt/mst. *Current Biology, 20*(21), 1900–1906.

Bedny, M., Richardson, H., & Saxe, R. (2015). "Visual" cortex responds to spoken language in blind children. *Journal of Neuroscience, 35*(33), 11674–11681.

Bigelow, A. E. (1996). Blind and sighted children's spatial knowledge of their home environments. *International Journal of Behavioral Development, 19*(4), 797–816.

Bleau, M., Pare, S., Chebat, D. R., Kupers, R., Nemargut, J. P., & Ptito, M. (2022). Neural substrates of spatial processing and navigation in blindness: An activation likelihood estimation meta-analysis. *Frontiers in Neuroscience, 16*, 1010354.

Bleau, M., Pare, S., Djerourou, I., Chebat, D. R., Kupers, R., & Ptito, M. (2021). Blindness and the reliability of downwards sensors to avoid obstacles: A study with the eyecane. *Sensors (Basel), 21*(8).

Bleau, M., van Acker, C., Martiniello, N., Nemargut, J. P., & Ptito, M. (2023). Cognitive map formation in the blind is enhanced by three-dimensional tactile information. *Scientific Reports, 13*(1), 9736.

Bremner, A. J., Lewkowicz, D. J., & Spence, C. (2012). *Multisensory development.* Oxford University Press.

Bridge, H., Cowey, A., Ragge, N., & Watkins, K. (2009). Imaging studies in congenital anophthalmia reveal preservation of brain architecture in "visual" cortex. *Brain, 132*(12), 3467–3480.

Bronchti, G., Heil, P., Sadka, R., Hess, A., Scheich, H., & Wollberg, Z. (2002). Auditory activation of "visual" cortical areas in the blind mole rat (spalax ehrenbergi). *European Journal of Neuroscience, 16*(2), 311–329.

Büchel, C., Price, C., Frackowiak, R. S., & Friston, K. (1998). Different activation patterns in the visual cortex of late and congenitally blind subjects. *Brain, 121*(3), 409–419.

Bushneil, I. W. R., Sai, F., & Mullin, J. T. (1989). Neonatal recognition of the mother's face. *British Journal of Developmental Psychology, 7*(1), 3–15.

Cappagli, G., Cocchi, E., & Gori, M. (2017). Auditory and proprioceptive spatial impairments in blind children and adults. *Developmental Science, 20*(3).

Cattaneo, Z., & Vecchi, T. (2008). Supramodality effects in visual and haptic spatial processes. *Journal of Experimental Psychology: Learning, Memory, and Cognition, 34*(3), 631.

Cavaliere, C., Aiello, M., Soddu, A., Laureys, S., Reislev, N. L., Ptito, M., et al. (2020). Organization of the commissural fiber system in congenital and late-onset blindness. *NeuroImage: Clinical, 25*, 102133.

Cecchetti, L., Ricciardi, E., Handjaras, G., Kupers, R., Ptito, M., & Pietrini, P. (2016). Congenital blindness affects diencephalic but not mesencephalic structures in the human brain. *Brain Structure and Function, 221*(3), 1465–1480.

Chabot, N., Robert, S., Tremblay, R., Miceli, D., Boire, D., & Bronchti, G. (2007). Audition differently activates the visual system in neonatally enucleated mice compared with anophthalmic mutants. *European Journal of Neuroscience, 26*(8), 2334–2348.

Chebat, D.-R., Chen, J. K., Schneider, F., Ptito, A., Kupers, R., & Ptito, M. (2007). Alterations in right posterior hippocampus in early blind individuals. *Neuroreport, 18*(4), 329–333.

Chebat, D.-R., Harrar, V., Kupers, R., Maidenbaum, S., Amedi, A., & Ptito, M. (2018a). Sensory substitution and the neural correlates of navigation in blindness. In E. Pissaloux & R. Velazquez (Eds.), *Mobility of visually impaired people: Fundamentals and ICT assistive technologies* (pp. 167–200). Springer International.

Chebat, D.-R., Heimler, B., Hofsetter, S., & Amedi, A. (2018b). The implications of brain plasticity and task selectivity for visual rehabilitation of blind and visually impaired individuals. In C. Habas (Ed.), *The neuroimaging of brain diseases: Structural and functional advances* (pp. 295–321). Springer International.

Chebat, D.-R., Maidenbaum, S., & Amedi, A. (2015). Navigation using sensory substitution in real and virtual mazes. *PLOS ONE, 10*(6).

Chebat, D.-R., Schneider, F. C., Kupers, R., & Ptito, M. (2011). Navigation with a sensory substitution device in congenitally blind individuals. *Neuroreport, 22*(7), 342–347.

Chebat, D.-R., Schneider, F. C., & Ptito, M. (2020a). Neural networks mediating perceptual learning in congenital blindness. *Scientific Reports, 10*(1), 495.

Chebat, D.-R., Schneider, F. C., & Ptito, M. (2020b). Spatial competence and brain plasticity in congenital blindness via sensory substitution devices. *Frontiers in Neuroscience, 14*, 815.

Cohen, L. G., Celnik, P., Pascual-Leone, A., Corwell, B., Faiz, L., Dambrosia, J., et al. (1997). Functional relevance of cross-modal plasticity in blind humans. *Nature, 389*, 180–183.

Collignon, O., Lassonde, M., Lepore, F., Bastien, D., & Veraart, C. (2007). Functional cerebral reorganization for auditory spatial processing and auditory substitution of vision in early blind subjects. *Cerebral Cortex, 17*(2), 457–465.

Collignon, O., Vandewalle, G., Voss, P., Albouy, G., Charbonneau, G., Lassonde, M., et al. (2011). Functional specialization for auditory-spatial processing in the occipital cortex of congenitally blind humans. *Proceedings of the National Academy of Sciences, 108*(11), 4435–4440.

Coluccia, E., Mammarella, I. C., & Cornoldi, C. (2009). Centred egocentric, decentred egocentric, and allocentric spatial representations in the peripersonal space of congenital total blindness. *Perception, 38*(5), 679–693.

Craig, J. C. (1988). The role of experience in tactual pattern perception: A preliminary report. *International Journal of Rehabilitation Research, 11*(2), 167–171.

Danka Mohammed, C. P., & Khalil, R. (2020). Postnatal development of visual cortical function in the mammalian brain. *Frontiers in Systems Neuroscience, 14*, 29.

Desgent, S., & Ptito, M. (2012). Cortical GABAergic interneurons in cross-modal plasticity following early blindness. *Neural Plasticity, 2012*(1), 590725.

Dormal, G., Rezk, M., Yakobov, E., Lepore, F., & Collignon, O. (2016). Auditory motion in the sighted and blind: Early visual deprivation triggers a large-scale imbalance between auditory and "visual" brain regions. *NeuroImage, 134*, 630–644.

Doron, N., & Wollberg, Z. (1994). Cross-modal neuroplasticity in the blind mole rat Spalax ehrenbergi: A WGA-HRP tracing study. *Neuroreport, 5*(18), 2697–2702.

Dubois, J., Dehaene-Lambertz, G., Kulikova, S., Poupon, C., Hüppi, P. S., & Hertz-Pannier, L. (2014). The early development of brain white matter: A review of imaging studies in fetuses, newborns and infants. *Neuroscience, 276*, 48–71.

Ekstrom, A. D. (2015). Why vision is important to how we navigate. *Hippocampus, 25*(6), 731–735.

Epstein, R. A., Patai, E. Z., Julian, J. B., & Spiers, H. J. (2017). The cognitive map in humans: Spatial navigation and beyond. *Nature Neuroscience, 20*(11), 1504–1513.

Espinosa, J. S., & Stryker, M. P. (2012). Development and plasticity of the primary visual cortex. *Neuron, 75*(2), 230–249.

Espinosa, M. A., & Ochaíta, E. (1998). Using tactile maps to improve the practical spatial knowledge of adults who are blind. *Journal of Visual Impairment & Blindness, 92*(5), 338–345.

Espinosa, M. A., Ungar, S., Ochaíta, E., Blades, M., & Spencer, C. (1998). Comparing methods for introducing blind and visually impaired people to unfamiliar urban environments. *Journal of Environmental Psychology, 18*(3), 277–287.

Fortin, M., Voss, P., Lord, C., Lassonde, M., Pruessner, J., Saint-Amour, D., et al. (2008). Wayfinding in the blind: Larger hippocampal volume and supranormal spatial navigation. *Brain, 131*(Pt. 11), 2995–3005.

Gandemer, L., Parseihian, G., Kronland-Martinet, R., & Bourdin, C. (2017). Spatial cues provided by sound improve postural stabilization: Evidence of a spatial auditory map? *Frontiers in Neuroscience, 11*, 357.

Giudice, N. A. (2018). Navigating without vision: Principles of blind spatial cognition. In D. R. Montello (Ed.), *Handbook of behavioral and cognitive geography* (pp. 260–288). Edward Elgar.

Goldreich, D., & Kanics, I. M. (2003). Tactile acuity is enhanced in blindness. *Journal of Neuroscience, 23*(8), 3439–3445.

Golledge, R. G., Jacobson, R. D., Kitchin, R., & Blades, M. (2000). Cognitive maps, spatial abilities, and human wayfinding. *Geographical Review of Japan, Series B, 73*(2), 93–104.

Goodman, C. S., & Shatz, C. J. (1993). Developmental mechanisms that generate precise patterns of neuronal connectivity. *Cell, 72*, 77–98.

Gougoux, F., Lepore, F., Lassonde, M., Voss, P., Zatorre, R. J., & Belin, P. (2004). Neuropsychology: Pitch discrimination in the early blind. *Nature, 430*, 309.

Grant, A. C., Thiagarajah, M. C., & Sathian, K. (2000). Tactile perception in blind Braille readers: A psychophysical study of acuity and hyperacuity using gratings and dot patterns. *Perception & Psychophysics, 62*(2), 301–312.

Graw, J. (2010). Eye development. In P. Koopman (Ed.), *Current topics in developmental biology* (pp. 343–386). Academic Press.

Gregory-Evans, C. Y., & Gregory-Evans, K. (2011). Foveal hypoplasia: The case for arrested development. *Expert Review of Ophthalmology, 6*(5), 565–574.

Hamilton, R. H., Pascual-Leone, A., & Schlaug, G. (2004). Absolute pitch in blind musicians. *Neuroreport, 15*(5).

Hasson, U., Andric, M., Atilgan, H., & Collignon, O. (2016). Congenital blindness is associated with large-scale reorganization of anatomical networks. *NeuroImage, 128*, 362–372.

Heller, M. A. (1989). Picture and pattern perception in the sighted and the blind: The advantage of the late blind. *Perception, 18*(3), 379–389.

Hendrickson, A., Possin, D., Vajzovic, L., & Toth, C. A. (2012). Histologic development of the human fovea from midgestation to maturity. *American Journal of Ophthalmology, 154*(5), 767–778.e762.

Hendrickson, A. E., & Yuodelis, C. (1984). The morphological development of the human fovea. *Ophthalmology, 91*(6), 603–612.

Hubel, D. H., & Wiesel, T. N. (1965). Binocular interaction in striate cortex of kittens reared with artificial squint. *Journal of Neurophysiology, 28*(6), 1041–1059.

Hubel, D. H., & Wiesel, T. N. (1970). The period of susceptibility to the physiological effects of unilateral eye closure in kittens. *Journal of Physiology, 206*(2), 419–436.

Huber, E., Chang, K., Alvarez, I., Hundle, A., Bridge, H., & Fine, I. (2019). Early blindness shapes cortical representations of auditory frequency within auditory cortex. *Journal of Neuroscience, 39*(26), 5143–5152.

Iachini, T., Ruggiero, G., & Ruotolo, F. (2014). Does blindness affect egocentric and allocentric frames of reference in small and large scale spaces? *Behavioural Brain Research, 273*, 73–81.

Inuggi, A., Pichiecchio, A., Ciacchini, B., Signorini, S., Morelli, F., & Gori, M. (2020). Multisystemic increment of cortical thickness in congenital blind children. *Cerebral Cortex Communications, 1*(1), tgaa071.

Jandó, G., Mikó-Baráth, E., Markó, K., Hollódy, K., Török, B., & Kovacs, I. (2012). Early-onset binocularity in preterm infants reveals experience-dependent visual development in humans. *Proceedings of the National Academy of Sciences, 109*(27), 11049–11052.

Jiang, F., Stecker, G. C., & Fine, I. (2014). Auditory motion processing after early blindness. *Journal of Vision, 14*(13), 4.

Kaiserman-Abramof, I. R., Graybiel, A. M., & Nauta, W. J. H. (1980). The thalamic projection to cortical area 17 in a congenitally anophthalmic mouse strain. *Neuroscience, 5*(1), 41–52.

Karlen, S. J., Kahn, D. M., & Krubitzer, L. (2006). Early blindness results in abnormal corticocortical and thalamocortical connections. *Neuroscience, 142*(3), 843–858.

Katz, L. C., & Shatz, C. J. (1996). Synaptic activity and the construction of cortical circuits. *Science, 274*, 1133–1138.

Kim, J. S., Kanjlia, S., Merabet, L. B., & Bedny, M. (2017). Development of the visual word form area requires visual experience: Evidence from blind Braille readers. *Journal of Neuroscience, 37*(47), 11495.

Kitada, R., Okamoto, Y., Sasaki, A. T., Kochiyama, T., Miyahara, M., Lederman, S. J., et al. (2013). Early visual experience and the recognition of basic facial expressions: Involvement of the middle temporal and inferior frontal gyri during haptic identification by the early blind. *Frontiers in Human Neuroscience, 7*, 7.

Klauke, S., Sondocie, C., & Fine, I. (2023). The impact of low vision on social function: The potential importance of lost visual social cues. *Journal of Optometry, 16*(1), 3–11.

Kupers, R., Baeck, A., Matteau, I., Melillo, M., Madsen, K., Nielsen, J. B., et al. (2009). rTMS of area MT impairs motion discrimination performance in a tactile vision sensory substitution task in blind but not in seeing subjects. *NeuroImage, 47*, S107.

Kupers, R., Chebat, D. R., Madsen, K. H., Paulson, O. B., & Ptito, M. (2010). Neural correlates of virtual route recognition in congenital blindness. *Proceedings of the National Academy of Sciences, 107*(28), 12716–12721.

Kupers, R., Fumal, A., De Noordhout, A. M., Gjedde, A., Schoenen, J., & Ptito, M. (2006). Transcranial magnetic stimulation of the visual cortex induces somatotopically organized qualia in blind subjects. *Proceedings of the National Academy of Sciences, 103*(35), 13256–13260.

Kupers, R., & Ptito, M. (2014). Compensatory plasticity and cross-modal reorganization following early visual deprivation. *Neuroscience & Biobehavioral Revews, 41*, 36–52.

Laramée, M. E., Kurotani, T., Rockland, K. S., Bronchti, G., & Boire, D. (2011). Indirect pathway between the primary auditory and visual cortices through layer V pyramidal neurons in V2L in mouse and the effects of bilateral enucleation. *European Journal of Neuroscience, 34*(1), 65–78.

Leat, S. J., Yadav, N. K., & Irving, E. L. (2009). Development of visual acuity and contrast sensitivity in children. *Journal of Optometry, 2*(1), 19–26.

Legge, G. E., Madison, C., Vaughn, B. N., Cheong, A. M. Y., & Miller, J. C. (2008). Retention of high tactile acuity throughout the life span in blindness. *Perception & Psychophysics, 70*(8), 1471–1488.

Leo, A., Bernardi, G., Handjaras, G., Bonino, D., Ricciardi, E., & Pietrini, P. (2012). Increased bold variability in the parietal cortex and enhanced parieto-occipital connectivity during tactile perception in congenitally blind individuals. *Neural Plasticity, 2012*(1), 720278.

Lessard, N., Paré, M., Lepore, F., & Lassonde, M. (1998). Early-blind human subjects localize sound sources better than sighted subjects. *Nature, 395*, 278–280.

Lewis, T. L., & Maurer, D. (2005). Multiple sensitive periods in human visual development: Evidence from visually deprived children. *Developmental Psychobiology, 46*(3), 163–183.

Liotti, M., Ryder, K., & Woldorff, M. G. (1998). Auditory attention in the congenitally blind: Where, when and what gets reorganized? *Neuroreport, 9*(6).

Long, R. G., & Giudice, N. A. (2010). Establishing and maintaining orientation for mobility. In W. R. Wiener, R. L. Welsh, & B. B. Blasch (Eds.), *Foundations of orientation and mobility* (pp. 45–62). American Foundation for the Blind.

Maguire, E. A., Gadian, D. G., Johnsrude, I. S., Good, C. D., Ashburner, J., Frackowiak, R. S. J., et al. (2000). Navigation-related structural change in the hippocampi of taxi drivers. *Proceedings of the National Academy of Sciences, 97*(8), 4398–4403.

Maheu, M., Sharp, A., Landry, S. P., & Champoux, F. (2017). Sensory reweighting after loss of auditory cues in healthy adults. *Gait & Posture, 53*, 151–154.

Maidenbaum, S., Chebat, D.-R., & Amedi, A. (2018). Human navigation without and with vision—the role of visual experience and visual regions. *bioRxiv*, 480558.

Marcos, L. F., Wilson, S. L., & Roach, P. (2021). Tissue engineering of the retina: From organoids to microfluidic chips. *Journal of Tissue Engineering, 12*, 20417314211059876.

Matteau, I., Kupers, R., Ricciardi, E., Pietrini, P., & Ptito, M. (2010). Beyond visual, aural and haptic movement perception: hMT+ is activated by electrotactile motion stimulation of the tongue in sighted and in congenitally blind individuals. *Brain Research Bulletin, 82*(5–6), 264–270.

Merabet, L. B., Connors, E. C., Halko, M. A., & Sanchez, J. (2012). Teaching the blind to find their way by playing video games. *PLOS ONE, 7*(9).

Merabet, L. B., Hamilton, R., Schlaug, G., Swisher, J. D., Kiriakopoulos, E. T., Pitskel, N. B., et al. (2008). Rapid and reversible recruitment of early visual cortex for touch. *PLOS ONE, 3*(8), e3046.

Müller, F., Niso, G., Samiee, S., Ptito, M., Baillet, S., & Kupers, R. (2019). A thalamocortical pathway for fast rerouting of tactile information to occipital cortex in congenital blindness. *Nature Communications, 10*(1), 5154.

Murphy, K. M., Beston, B. R., Boley, P. M., & Jones, D. G. (2005). Development of human visual cortex: A balance between excitatory and inhibitory plasticity mechanisms. *Developmental Psychobiology, 46*(3), 209–221.

Nau, A. C., Murphy, M. C., & Chan, K. C. (2015). Use of sensory substitution devices as a model system for investigating cross-modal neuroplasticity in humans. *Neural Regeneration Research, 10*(11).

Niemeyer, W., & Starlinger, I. (1981). Do the blind hear better? Investigations on auditory processing in congenital or early acquired blindness II. Central functions. *Audiology, 20*(6), 510–515.

Noordzij, M. L., Zuidhoek, S., & Postma, A. (2006). The influence of visual experience on the ability to form spatial mental models based on route and survey descriptions. *Cognition, 100*(2), 321–342.

Ofan, R. H., & Zohary, E. (2007). Visual cortex activation in bilingual blind individuals during use of native and second language. *Cerebral Cortex, 17*(6), 1249–1259.

Palejwala, A. H., Dadario, N. B., Young, I. M., O'Connor, K., Briggs, R. G., Conner, A. K., et al. (2021). Anatomy and white matter connections of the lingual gyrus and cuneus. *World Neurosurgery, 151*, e426–e437.

Paré, S., Bleau, M., Djerourou, I., Malotaux, V., Kupers, R., & Ptito, M. (2021). Spatial navigation with horizontally spatialized sounds in early and late blind individuals. *PLOS ONE, 16*(2), e0247448.

Paré, S., Bleau, M., Dricot, L., Ptito, M., & Kupers, R. (2023). Brain structural changes in blindness: A systematic review and an anatomical likelihood estimation (ale) meta-analysis. *Neuroscience & Biobehavioral Reviews, 150*, 105165.

Pasqualotto, A., Spiller, M. J., Jansari, A. S., & Proulx, M. J. (2013). Visual experience facilitates allocentric spatial representation. *Behavioural Brain Research, 236*(1), 175–179.

Pietrini, P., Ptito, M., & Kupers, R. (2009). Blindness and consciousness: New light from the dark. In S. Laureys, O. Gosseries, & G. Tononi (Eds.), *The neurology of conciousness* (2nd ed., pp. 393–406). Academic Press.

Proulx, M. J., Brown, D. J., Pasqualotto, A., & Meijer, P. (2014). Multisensory perceptual learning and sensory substitution. *Neuroscience & Biobehavioral Reviews, 41*, 16–25.

Ptito, M., Bleau, M., & Bouskila, J. (2021a). The retina: A window into the brain. *Cells, 10*(12).

Ptito, M., Bleau, M., Djerourou, I., Paré, S., Schneider, F. C., & Chebat, D. R. (2021b). Brain-machine interfaces to assist the blind. *Frontiers in Human Neuroscience, 15*, 638887.

Ptito, M., Fumal, A., de Noordhout, A. M., Schoenen, J., Gjedde, A., & Kupers, R. (2008a). TMS of the occipital cortex induces tactile sensations in the fingers of blind Braille readers. *Experimental Brain Research, 184*(2), 193–200.

Ptito, M., Matteau, I., Gjedde, A., & Kupers, R. (2009). Recruitment of the middle temporal area by tactile motion in congenital blindness. *Neuroreport, 20*(6), 543–547.

Ptito, M., Matteau, I., Zhi Wang, A., Paulson, O. B., Siebner, H. R., & Kupers, R. (2012). Crossmodal recruitment of the ventral visual stream in congenital blindness. *Neural Plasticity, 2012*.

Ptito, M., Moesgaard, S. M., Gjedde, A., & Kupers, R. (2005). Cross-modal plasticity revealed by electrotactile stimulation of the tongue in the congenitally blind. *Brain, 128*(3), 606–614.

Ptito, M., Paré, S., Dricot, L., Cavaliere, C., Tomaiuolo, F., & Kupers, R. (2021c). A quantitative analysis of the retinofugal projections in congenital and late-onset blindness. *NeuroImage: Clinical, 32*, 102809.

Ptito, M., Schneider, F. C. G., Paulson, O. B., & Kupers, R. (2008b). Alterations of the visual pathways in congenital blindness. *Experimental Brain Research, 187*(1), 41–49.

Reislev, N. L., Kupers, R., Siebner, H. R., Ptito, M., & Dyrby, T. B. (2016). Blindness alters the microstructure of the ventral but not the dorsal visual stream. *Brain Structure and Function, 221*(6), 2891–2903.

Rieser, J. J., Guth, D. A., & Hill, E. W. (1986). Sensitivity to perspective structure while walking without vision. *Perception, 15*(2), 173–188.

Rieser, J. J., Lockman, J. J., & Pick, H. L. (1980). The role of visual experience in knowledge of spatial layout. *Perception & Psychophysics, 28*(3), 185–190.

Röder, B., Teder-Sälejärvi, W., Sterr, A., Rösler, F., Hillyard, S. A., & Neville, H. J. (1999). Improved auditory spatial tuning in blind humans. *Nature, 400*, 162–166.

Saccone, E. J., Tian, M., & Bedny, M. (2024). Developing cortex is functionally pluripotent: Evidence from blindness. *Developmental Cognitive Neuroscience, 66*, 101360.

Sadato, N., Pascual-Leone, A., Grafman, J., Deiber, M.-P., Ibanez, V., & Hallett, M. (1998). Neural networks for Braille reading by the blind. *Brain, 121*(7), 1213–1229.

Sadato, N., Pascual-Leone, A., Grafman, J., Ibañez, V., Deiber, M.-P., Dold, G., et al. (1996). Activation of the primary visual cortex by Braille reading in blind subjects. *Nature, 380*, 526–528.

Sampaio, E., Maris, S., & Bach-y-Rita, P. (2001). Brain plasticity: 'Visual' acuity of blind persons via the tongue. *Brain Research, 908*(2), 204–207.

Schinazi, V. R., Thrash, T., & Chebat, D. R. (2016). Spatial navigation by congenitally blind individuals. *Cognitive Science, 7*(1), 37–58.

Sigismondi, F., Xu, Y., Silvestri, M., & Bottini, R. (2024). Altered grid-like coding in early blind people. *Nature Communications, 15*(1), 3476.

Simion, F., Di Giorgio, E., Leo, I., & Bardi, L. (2011). The processing of social stimuli in early infancy: From faces to biological motion perception. In O. Braddick, J. Atkinson, & G. M. Innocenti (Eds.), *Progress in brain research* (pp. 173–193). Elsevier.

Siu, C. R., & Murphy, K. M. (2018). The development of human visual cortex and clinical implications. *Eye and Brain, 10*, 25–36.

Spolidoro, M., Sale, A., Berardi, N., & Maffei, L. (2009). Plasticity in the adult brain: Lessons from the visual system. *Experimental Brain Research, 192*(3), 335–341.

Stacy, A. K., & Van Hooser, S. D. (2022). Development of functional properties in the early visual system: New appreciations of the roles of lateral geniculate nucleus. In S. L. Andersen (Ed.), *Sensitive periods of brain development and preventive interventions* (pp. 3–35). Springer International.

Stent, G. S. (1973). A physiological mechanism for Hebb's postulate of learning. *Proceedings of the National Academy of Sciences, 70*(4), 997–1001.

Striem-Amit, E., & Amedi, A. (2014). Visual cortex extrastriate body-selective area activation in congenitally blind people "seeing" by using sounds. *Current Biology, 24*(6), 687–692.

Striem-Amit, E., Dakwar, O., Hertz, U., Meijer, P., Stern, W., Pascual-Leone, A., et al. (2011). The neural network of sensory-substitution object shape recognition. *Functional Neurology, Rehabilitation and Ergonomics, 1*(2), 271–278.

Teller, D. Y. (1997). First glances: The vision of infants. The friedenwald lecture. *Investigative Ophthalmology & Visual Science, 38*(11), 2183–2203.

Thaler, L., Arnott, S. R., & Goodale, M. A. (2011). Neural correlates of natural human echolocation in early and late blind echolocation experts. *PLOS ONE, 6*(5), e20162.

Thaler, L., & Goodale, M. A. (2016). Echolocation in humans: An overview. *Wiley interdisciplinary reviews. Cognitive Science, 7*(6), 382–393.

Thevin, L., Briant, C., & Brock, A. M. (2020). X-road: Virtual reality glasses for orientation and mobility training of people with visual impairments. *ACM Transactions on Accessible Computing, 13*(2), 1–47.

Tomaiuolo, F., Campana, S., Collins, D. L., Fonov, V. S., Ricciardi, E., Sartori, G., et al. (2014). Morphometric changes of the corpus callosum in congenital blindness. *PLOS ONE, 9*(9), e107871.

Tomasello, R., Carriere, M., & Pulvermüller, F. (2024). The impact of early and late blindness on language and verbal working memory: A brain-constrained neural model. *Neuropsychologia, 196*, 108816.

Uhl, F., Franzen, P., Lindinger, G., Lang, W., & Deecke, L. (1991). On the functionality of the visually deprived occipital cortex in early blind persons. *Neuroscience Letters, 124*(2), 256–259.

Ungar, S., Blades, M., Spencer, C., & Morsley, K. (1994). Can visually impaired children use tactile maps to estimate directions? *Journal of Visual Impairment & Blindness, 88*(3), 221–233.

Van Cruchten, S., Vrolyk, V., Perron Lepage, M.-F., Baudon, M., Voute, H., Schoofs, S., et al. (2017). Pre- and postnatal development of the eye: A species comparison. *Birth Defects Research, 109*(19), 1540–1567.

Voss, P., & Zatorre, R. J. (2012). Occipital cortical thickness predicts performance on pitch and musical tasks in blind individuals. *Cerebral Cortex, 22*(11), 2455–2465.

Wan, C. Y., Wood, A. G., Reutens, D. C., & Wilson, S. J. (2010). Early but not late-blindness leads to enhanced auditory perception. *Neuropsychologia, 48*(1), 344–348.

Wiesel, T. N., & Hubel, D. H. (1963a). Effects of visual deprivation on morphology and physiology of cells in the cat's lateral geniculate body. *Journal of Neurophysiology, 26*(6), 978–993.

Wiesel, T. N., & Hubel, D. H. (1963b). Single-cell responses in striate cortex of kittens deprived of vision in one eye. *Journal of Neurophysiology, 26*(6), 1003–1017.

Wiesel, T. N., & Hubel, D. H. (1965). Comparison of the effects of unilateral and bilateral eye closure on cortical unit responses in kittens. *Journal of Neurophysiology, 28*(6), 1029–1040.

Wong, M., Gnanakumaran, V., & Goldreich, D. (2011). Tactile spatial acuity enhancement in blindness: Evidence for experience-dependent mechanisms. *Journal of Neuroscience, 31*(19), 7028–7037.

Woollett, K., & Maguire, E. A. (2011). Acquiring "the knowledge" of london's layout drives structural brain changes. *Current Biology, 21*(24), 2109–2114.

Zhang, C., Lee, T. M. C., Fu, Y., Ren, C., Chan, C. C. H., & Tao, Q. (2019). Properties of cross-modal occipital responses in early blindness: An ALE meta-analysis. *NeuroImage: Clinical, 24*, 102041.

Zwiers, M. P., Van Opstal, A. J., & Cruysberg, J. R. (2001). A spatial hearing deficit in early-blind humans. *Jornal of Neuroscience, 21*(9), RC142.

CHAPTER 7

Adaptive Plasticity

Davide Bottari and Elena Nava

Introduction

Traditionally, vision has been considered the preferred modality for investigating the effects of sensory experience on neural representations, especially in early developmental stages (Hubel & Wiesel, 1970; for reviews, see Levelt & Hubener, 2012; Morishita & Hensch, 2008). However, in recent decades, research on human auditory and somatosensory systems has revealed fundamental knowledge about plastic adaptive mechanisms. Studies that have systematically distorted the acoustic environment of developing animals (Dahmen & King, 2007; Persic et al., 2020) and research in newborns have contributed to the notion that early sound exposure is crucial for the emergence of functional representations in the auditory cortex. Furthermore, the success of cochlear implants has provided a causal model for understanding the impact of a period of auditory deprivation in life (Pavani & Bottari, 2022). Moreover, some of the most definitive effects of perceptual learning on neuronal response properties have been observed in the auditory cortex by training procedures (Polley et al., 2006) and cortical reorganization after selective damage to the cochlea demonstrated plasticity throughout life. Similarly, the investigation of the somatosensory system has spurred research revealing the high plasticity of the primary somatosensory cortex (S1; Feldman & Brecht, 2005) in cases of extensive use and response to peripheral injuries, such as amputation (Weiss et al., 2000). The intersection of the study of plasticity in case of limb absence or amputation, brain functional development, and phantom pain has provided fundamental findings concerning sensory representations and their experience of dependence (Schone et al., 2022).

This chapter aims to briefly summarize the past, present, and future of adaptive plasticity in the auditory and somatosensory cortices.

Plasticity of the Auditory Cortex

Early-Experience-Dependent Plasticity of the Auditory Cortex

Sensory systems comprise functionally specialized maps in which close neurons represent similar aspects in sensory feature space. As processing progresses through the hierarchy, these maps tend to shift from precise, point-to-point representations of receptor activity toward computations optimized for task-solving rather than detailed stimulus representation (Schreiner et al., 2007). Following the organization of the organ of Corti in the cochlea, cochleotopic or tonotopic maps are organized neuronal response preferences to sound frequencies across the cortical space. This is typically observed in all mammals' primary auditory cortex (A1). The organization of the tonotopic maps is genetically preset and initially formed with a coarse scaffolding during prenatal development. This organization is refined through activity-dependent mechanisms: first, with spontaneous neural activity and, after hearing begins, through sound-evoked activity. Thus, early life profoundly affects map organization in adults through experience-dependent plasticity mechanisms, which allow individuals to adapt to diverse environments that cannot be fully anticipated by their genetic predispositions (Rauschecker, 1999). Orthogonally organized to tonotopic representations, periodotopic gradients have been measured, representing the temporal characteristics of sounds (Brewer & Barton 2016).

The plasticity of the tonotopic map in A1 is currently the primary model for investigating the critical periods (CPs) in the auditory system, brief postnatal periods of heightened nervous system adaptability (Hensch, 2004; Wiesel & Hubel, 1965). During these periods, tonotopic maps are formed for frequency tuning, and auditory experiences strongly shape their organization (Keuroghlian & Knudsen, 2007; Sanes & Woolley, 2011). For instance, rat pups exposed only to pulsed single-tone stimuli develop an overrepresentation of that specific sound frequency and a reduced representation of the other frequencies (Zhang et al., 2001). In rats, this remarkable plasticity is limited to a short CP lasting 3 days (Barkat et al., 2011; de Villers-Sidani et al., 2007). Crucially, the timing of CPs in the auditory cortex is flexible, and the quality of sensory input is crucial for CP dynamics, to an extent that noisy environments with unstructured sounds and sensory deprivation delay the closure of CPs (Bose et al., 2010; Bureš et al., 2018; Cai et al., 2010; Chang & Merzenich, 2003). Moreover, CP changes are specific to the types of sounds to which animals are exposed; for example, rearing rats in an environment with a particular band of noise delays the CP closure only in A1 noise-exposed regions, keeping them in an immature state without affecting other A1 regions (de Villers-Sidani et al., 2008).

In humans, environmental sounds such as vocalizations elicit neural responses and discrimination abilities well before birth, suggesting a robust biological predisposition. However, a newborn's brain is profoundly shaped by sound exposure. Infants born prematurely (before 32 weeks of gestation) and exposed to maternal sounds during the first months of life exhibit significantly larger auditory cortices compared with infants exposed to standard hospital noise in the same period, providing evidence that the auditory cortex is highly responsive to very early auditory experiences (Webb et al., 2015). Moreover, it has recently been found that newborns' electrophysiological activity shows increased temporal correlations only with the language heard prenatally, indicating early emergence of brain specialization for the native language (Mariani et al., 2023).

Research has revealed that the timing of these sensitive periods, at least to some extent, depends on the processing hierarchy so that sensitive periods for basic auditory functions end earlier than those for more complex ones (Sanes & Woolley, 2011). For example, frequency resolution (detecting a tone among other tones) reaches adult performance by about 6 months of age, coinciding with the completion of cochlear development (Schneider et al., 1990; Spetner & Olsho, 1990). In contrast, frequency discrimination (the ability to differentiate two sequential tones) has a protracted development that ends around age 10 (Maxon & Hochberg, 1982; Moore et al., 2011).

In sum, the interaction between genetic predisposition, comprising prenatal scaffolding and orchestrated periods of enhanced experience-dependent plasticity depending on the processing hierarchy, and the environment's statistics characterize the early functional organization of the auditory cortex.

Cochlear Implants

A cochlear implant (CI) is a prosthetic device that converts sounds into electrical impulses delivered directly to the auditory nerve via electrodes implanted in the cochlea, bypassing damaged hair cells. This process approximates natural hearing; however, unlike normal hearing, which relies on thousands of inner hair cells, CIs employ up to 22 electrodes, providing limited sound resolution. Despite this limitation, CIs are successful neural prostheses and the preferred treatment for sensorineural deafness in children and adults. Numerous studies have shown that CIs enable users to understand speech without visual cues and some music perception and improve spatial hearing, especially with bilateral implants (Fallon et al., 2009; Nava et al., 2009; Pavani & Bottari, 2022; Wilson & Dorman, 2008).

Cochlear implantation in animal models has provided important information concerning the adaptive plasticity of the auditory cortex, particularly because animal models allow the inducing of deafness and the restoration of auditory input through a cochlear implant at any desired moment. Similarly to the case of noise rearing, intracortical recordings from deafened animals have revealed that, without early auditory input, the auditory cortex remains in an immature state, further strengthening the role of experience for cortical refinement (Kral et al., 2019). Due to the high degree of experience-dependent plasticity in early development, different outcomes are determined when the period of deprivation occurs. For instance, inhibitory synaptic properties, essential for stimulus processing (Isaacson & Scanziani, 2011; Takesian et al., 2018), can be permanently impaired by early hearing loss, and hearing restoration does not fully recover typical activity, indicating a critical period for this functional development. In contrast, adult hearing loss does not exhibit the same adverse effects.

A basic form of tonotopy was observed at both cortical and subcortical levels in cats with no prior auditory experience tested immediately after cochlear implantation (Hartmann et al., 1997; Kral et al., 2001, 2002; Raggio & Schreiner, 1999; Shepherd et al., 1997; Tillein et al., 2010). This observation indicated that the auditory cortex could form a proto-organization to represent sound frequencies, even in the absence of sensory input. Importantly, when implantation occurred precociously (at 8 weeks of age) and was followed by prolonged stimulation (up to 7 months), the tonotopic organization of the A1 in cats became much more refined (e.g., Fallon et al., 2009, 2014). As these studies suggest, the onset of the auditory deprivation period, the timing of cochlear implantation, and the duration of auditory experience are crucial for the effectiveness of cochlear implants on auditory cortex functionality and adaptation.

Longitudinal studies on large groups of early deaf children have shown significant alterations in auditory evoked responses (measured with the electroencephalogram) after cochlear implantation (Sharma et al., 2002, 2005, 2007). These studies highlighted the critical role of age at implantation, supporting the presence of a sensitive period for optimal auditory cortex responsiveness to sound, consistent with animal model findings. Sharma and colleagues (2002) found that children implanted early (before 3.5 years) showed auditory response latencies within the typical range, whereas those implanted later did not (Sharma et al., 2007).

Adult Perceptual Learning

Recanzone and colleagues (1992) first demonstrated changes in A1 by training monkeys in a frequency discrimination task. As the monkeys' performance improved, neurophysiological recordings showed a significant enlargement of the A1 containing neurons tuned to the frequencies used during training. This expansion specifically occurred in the cortical region representing the trained frequencies. The A1 integrates both bottom-up sensory inputs and top-down influences (Kral et al., 2019). Thus, researchers have investigated whether plasticity in the auditory cortex is driven by sensory input statistics and task-related top-down influences. For instance, adult rats were trained to focus on either frequency or intensity changes within the same set of sounds. Those trained to focus on frequency showed expanded sound frequency representations, while those focusing on intensity had larger changes in sound intensity maps. The degree of map plasticity correlated with perceptual learning suggests that top-down inputs can selectively modify specific auditory features without affecting others in interaction with bottom-up inputs and reinforcement signals (Polley et al., 2006). Furthermore, animal studies have shown that sensory representations in A1 are bidirectionally changed as a function of the behavioral relevance of sensory stimuli. Daily passive exposure to sounds causes a persistent decrease in how A1 neurons encode them due to an increase in inhibition. Conversely, tasks behaviorally guided by the same sounds determine excitatory responses to the same habituated cells to intensify, while responses of inhibition-related neurons are reduced.

Studies on human auditory perceptual learning have explored various stimulus attributes such as frequency, level, duration, and interaural disparities. The characteristics of perceptual learning, such as its time course and learning curve shape, differ depending on the specific attribute studied (Wright & Zhang, 2009). Research has shown that perceptual learning across different tasks correlates with changes in auditory cortical activity. Studies using functional magnetic resonance imaging (fMRI) showed that hemodynamic responses in the auditory cortex decrease following training and suggest a plastic reorganization of cortical representation for the trained frequencies (Jäncke et al., 2001). Similar studies employing musical training revealed reduced modulation of auditory cortex activity by pitch intervals, suggesting more efficient encoding in pitch-sensitive regions, requiring less metabolic consumption after training (Zatorre et al., 2012).

An alternative example of adult plasticity is represented by tinnitus, a phantom auditory sensation frequently associated with hearing loss, often due to noise exposure or aging. Studies in humans have shown that tinnitus pitch and quality are related to the noise exposure frequency spectrum. While in the case of perceptual learning neural representations change in response to training, in the case of tinnitus, damage to the periphery of the auditory system would lead to phantom auditory perception. The first represents a form of adaptive plasticity, as it enhances the representation of behaviorally significant information. Conversely, plasticity associated with tinnitus is typically considered maladaptive and its origin linked to homeostatic plasticity mechanisms aiming to preserve the activity of the neural circuits (e.g., Turrigiano, 2011). In case of noise-related damage, the maladaptive plasticity arises as a consequence of increased spontaneous firing rates in neurons sensitive to frequencies close to the noise exposure spectrum (Heffner & Heffner, 2012; Loeb & Smith, 1967). Studies in the animal model have shown that tinnitus is strongly linked to altered neuronal activity in the cochlear nucleus and extends up to the auditory cortex (Kaltenbach & McCaslin, 1996). Interestingly, a hypothesis exists that the tinnitus might also be due to a multisensory alteration (Wu et al., 2016). The loss of auditory inputs from the cochlea (e.g., due to damage) would disrupt the balance between auditory and somatosensory activities in the cochlear nucleus, causing hyperactivity in the circuits (Shore et al., 2016). This might explain why many tinnitus sufferers can change the loudness and pitch of their tinnitus perception by moving their face and neck. This condition, known as somatosensory or somatic tinnitus, affects up to two-thirds of people with tinnitus.

Recently, novel frontiers for the study of auditory cortex plasticity have emerged. Computational methods in auditory neuroscience enable the mathematical formalization of auditory processing. Rooted in information theory (Barlow, 1961), these approaches propose that the brain perceives sensory input based on a set of measurements, or auditory statistics. Any signal containing values that match these measurements will be perceived identically by the brain. McDermott and Simoncelli (2011) extracted auditory statistics from natural sounds using a biologically plausible model and synthesized artificial sounds that adhered to these statistical characteristics (see Kell & McDermott, 2019, for more recent versions). By applying these synthesis techniques, it is now possible to create stimuli with desired statistical properties and specifically test the degree of adaptability of different auditory computations with unprecedented control (see Berto et al., 2021).

Plasticity of the Somatosensory Cortex

Somatosensory maps in S1 are highly plastic and can adapt to different contexts, such as in response to peripheral lesions (e.g., amputation) or overuse, as studies in professional musicians (Schlaug, 2015) or Braille readers have shown (Hamilton & Pascual-Leone, 1998).

Animal studies were the first to provide insight into such plasticity, showing that the cutting of a peripheral nerve or the amputation of a digit promotes the reorganization of S1; that is, the cortical representation of the denervated or removed part gets "invaded" by the representation of adjacent parts (Kaas, 1991; Merzenich et al., 1983). For example, if digit 3 of the hand gets amputated, its cortical area will be taken over by digits 2 and 4 (Merzenich et al., 1984). Interestingly, the expansion of receptive fields of neurons in area 3b (which corresponds to S1 in monkeys) occurs immediately; in animals, it was found that following digit amputation, the receptive fields on the amputated digit had new receptive fields extending from the wound to the adjacent digits (Calford & Tweedale, 1991). The rapidity of such plastic changes has been observed in human reports, too: Following amputation of the middle and ring fingers, the neural representation of the amputated fingers gets invaded by the neighboring cell assemblies of the index and little finger of the same hand within 10 days from amputation (Weiss et al., 2000).

Extensive use of body parts leads to similar plastic changes observed following amputation; for example, heightened stimulation of digits will result in enlarged representations of those digits in S1 (Jenkins et al., 1990; Recanzone et al., 1992). The most dramatic changes occurring in S1 have been observed following the complete amputation of a body part, leading to the question of whether brain remapping can be so strong, to an extent that the boundaries between distinct body parts can reorganize. For example, following lesions of the dorsal columns of the spinal cord, face inputs expand into the deafferented hand representation in area 3b of S1 of the monkey brain, shifting the representational boundaries up to 14 mm (Jain et al., 2008; Tandon et al., 2009).

Changes in Phantom Sensations and Pain across Development

Amputated individuals represent a unique window to understand the plasticity of the somatosensory cortex and its relationship to experience and sensations. A wealth of research has been dedicated to investigating the maladaptive plastic changes that occur in association with phantom limb pain. Indeed, two sensory experiences accompany most amputees: the feeling of the presence of the amputated limb (phantom sensation) and/or the pain felt in the amputated limb. These two experiences do not necessarily go hand in hand and dissociate as a function of age of amputation and experience with a missing limb.

First, it is important to define the difference between phantom sensation and phantom pain. The first is reported by the amputees as feeling the continued presence of the amputated limb, sometimes accompanied by tingling, itching, and/or numbness (Diers et al., 2022; Kooijman et al., 2000). The sensation of the phantom limb is so strong in some amputees that they report being able to move it voluntarily (Shukla et al., 1982). More recently, a transcranial magnetic stimulation (TMS) study corroborated this report: Three traumatic above-elbow amputees received TMS pulses over their hand area of the motor cortex, which elicited sensations of movement of the phantom hand.

Phantom limb pain, on the contrary, is typically described as feeling like burning, aching, cramping, and stabbing, and is usually intermittent and lasting from seconds to hours, but sometimes also permanently (Ehde et al., 2000). Contrary to phantom sensations, phantom pain occurs in 80% of adult surgical amputees but is almost absent in congenital amputees. A recent study presented data from several phantom phenomena, such as congenital amputees and individuals who underwent amputation before age 6, with or without phantom pain. Phantom limb pain was highest and more frequent in 5- and 6-year-old children but lower in comparison with other studies in which adult pain was assessed (Diers et al., 2022; Ephraim et al., 2005). Interestingly, pain was absent in congenital amputees. The fact that phantom sensations and phantom pain vary as a function of age (i.e., when the amputation took place during development) has potentially important implications for the understanding of the concept of adaptive plasticity.

The first focus should be placed on phantom sensations, especially highlighting that such sensations exist even in individuals who were born without a limb. The person with an aplastic limb reporting phantom sensations has been taken as an example to suggest that neural representations of the body are hardwired, genetically encoded, and thus not very malleable throughout experience (Brugger et al., 2000; Gallagher et al., 1998). This appears in contrast with the idea of "adaptation," as one would expect that the brain, throughout sensory experience (i.e., seeing and touching one's own body), provides the feedback necessary for the brain and body to adjust to the changes and thus eliminate the phantom sensations within the first months or years of life. However, there are other explanations for why the brain maintains such sensations. The first alternative explanation suggests that the phantom sensations may arise from the mirror image of the healthy contralateral limb. This view is supported by the observation that some amputees report movements and touch performed in both the missing limb and the healthy limb (Melzack et al., 1997; Ramachandran & Hirstein, 1998). It has also been suggested that the neural representation of the two limbs may be connected cross-cortically, thus supporting such intermanual referral.

The second alternative refers to a more general type of mirroring, namely seeing other bodies (Brugger et al., 2000). This view supports the role of vision in promoting mirroring mechanisms and the mirror neuron system, by which action preparation and observation are subserved by a specialized neural network (Bonini et al., 2022). Indeed, even in the absence of the physical body part executing an action, seeing others moving their limbs could activate the missing limb representation and give rise to phantom sensations.

Finally, a third alternative explanation frames all phantom sensations (i.e., not only phantom limb sensations, but also auditory and visual phantoms) within a Bayesian frame of reference. According to this view, the brain follows Bayesian rules; that is, the brain makes constant predictions that are updated by experience to reduce uncertainty (De Ridder et al., 2014). In this sense, sensory processing can be seen as having evolved to optimize predictions. Indeed, the Bayesian brain tests its beliefs against sensory experiences, and feedback is used to update the beliefs. If one sense is missing or a body part is amputated, the brain will have a limited (or distorted) amount of information to make sense of the world; this, in turn, will increase the uncertainty in the environment. To decrease uncertainty, the brain will try to obtain the missing information by increasing the salience of such (missing) information. The mechanisms for this can correspond to an increase in cortical excitability, widening of receptive fields, axonal rewiring, or hippocampal memory, which will, on a sensation level, correspond to the perception of the phantom limb. Thus, according to this view, the phantom limb represents a filling mechanism of the brain to reduce uncertainty, a maladaptive compensatory consequence to minimize the salience (Mohan & Vanneste, 2017).

Phantom Limb Pain: Stability versus Plasticity in the Somatosensory Cortex

As evidenced before, phantom sensations and phantom pain are different consequences of the deafferentation of a body part, and the presence of one or both strongly depends on when, during development, the deafferentation takes place. Several times, the question has been debated whether such plastic changes are also associated with sensations and pain.

There are several theories for the development of phantom limb pain, but two major views have dominated the past years. On the one hand, there is the so-called *maladaptive plasticity model* (Flor et al., 2006; Nava & Röder, 2011), which postulates that representations of body parts adjacent to the deafferented limb's representation take over the deprived cortex, leading to the reported pain. This view is supported by evidence documenting a relationship between cortical reorganization and phantom pain intensity, as reported by the amputees. For example, a series of studies reported that stimulation of the mouth in upper-extremity amputees triggered activity in the deafferented hand area in S1. Furthermore, the larger the shift, the higher the intensity of the pain reported by the patients (Flor et al., 1995). Such findings have also been shown in the deprived motor cortex (e.g., Karl et al., 2001; Raffin et al., 2016).

The main idea of the maladaptive plasticity model is that pain arises as a perceptual consequence of cortical reorganization following amputation, mainly due to a "shrinking" of the cortically represented amputated body part. According to this model, the pain results from a mismatch between the input that the nondeprived territories receive and that the adjacent deprived body area erroneously responds to. In other words, if a hand gets amputated, the cortical representation of the hand shrinks and gets invaded by the lip area. Every time the lips move or touch an object, since its cortical representation has expanded into the hand area, the latter will receive input, too, leading to a mismatch between body part representations, and in turn, to the perception of pain arising from the phantom hand.

The fact that the brain translates the input to the missing limb as pain is not so obvious. The maladaptive plasticity model has integrated the cortical reorganization view with the idea of the memory of pain experienced before amputation. Indeed, it has been reported that the pain in the phantom body part mimics the pain experienced before the amputation (Katz & Melzack, 1990; Nikolajsen et al., 1997) and that the intensity of the pain before the amputation predicts the onset of phantom limb pain (Flor, 2002). Thus, it could be that the pain experienced before the amputation "primes" the pain following amputation, thus targeting the pain before amputation could represent a way to decrease the likelihood of developing phantom limb pain following amputation.

It should also be noted that the memory of pain theory appears in line with evidence that individuals born with congenital limb abnormalities do not develop pain. Indeed, in their case, the absence of a limb was not a consequence of painful and traumatic injury, thus no painful memory was associated to the limb loss.

The main clinical implication for the maladaptive plasticity model is that, if there is a causal relationship between cortical reorganization and pain, reestablishing the missing body part representation should remove the pain. However, numerous studies have attempted to do so (for an example using the mirror box therapy, see Finn et al., 2017; Murray et al., 2006) but have obtained contrasting results (Herrador Colmenero et al., 2018), with some being extremely cautious in recommending such therapies to alleviate the pain (Barbin et al., 2016) and others presenting promising evidence that reversal of cortical reorganization correlates with a reduction in phantom pain (for a review, see Moseley & Flor, 2012).

Makin and colleagues (2013) put forward a different model for phantom limb pain in a series of works (see also Kikkert et al., 2018; Makin, 2021) in which, contrary to the maladaptive plasticity model, the authors proposed that it is the absence of reorganization of the missing limb representation that triggers the pain. In the first of their studies (Makin et al., 2013), unilateral upper-limb amputees, as well as individuals with congenital upper-limb deficiency, were instructed to move both their missing and intact hands during fMRI scanning. There was significant activation in S1 contralateral to the phantom hand in almost all amputees when they moved their missing limb. This was comparable to the activity found in controls, thus revealing a preserved representation of the missing limb.

Furthermore, no shift of lip representation in the former hand area, as well as no correlation between activation of lip movements and phantom pain intensity, was found, thus challenging the maladaptive plasticity view. Importantly, activation during phantom movements correlated with ratings of pain intensity, which is in exact contrast with what was proposed by the maladaptive plasticity model. That is, it is the persistence of the hand representation that correlates with the reported pain, and the authors proposed that the pain works as a direct experience that helps maintain the representation.

While these two views appear contradictory, it should be noted that other mechanisms can account for the cortical changes observed in the maladaptive plasticity theory, which can be a consequence of use-dependent plasticity. Indeed, compensatory behaviors, such as daily usage of intact body parts, can trigger the remapping of S1. For example, it has been observed that individuals with hand loss typically learn to (over)use the intact arm, lips, and feet (Hahamy et al., 2015, 2017). Thus, it is this daily compensatory usage of intact body parts that shapes the remapping observed in S1, leading to the expansion of, for example, arm and lips representation into the deprived hand representation.

Conclusion

In sum, the interaction between genetic predispositions, comprising prenatal scaffolding and orchestrated periods of enhanced plasticity that depend on the processing hierarchy and the environment's statistics, and therefore their absence, strongly characterizes the functional organization of both the auditory and somatosensory cortex. In Figure 7.1,* we summarize the principal mechanisms underlying adaptive plasticity and suggest that the study of models of sensory alteration, deprivation, restoration, and training represent unique opportunities to causally link atypical development and the degree of experience-dependent adaptations.

REFERENCES

Barbin, J., Seetha, V., Casillas, J. M., Paysant, J., & Perennou, D. (2016). The effects of mirror therapy on pain and motor control of phantom limb in amputees: A systematic review. *Annals of Physical and Rehabilitation Medicine, 59*, 270–275.

Barkat, T. R., Polley, D. B., & Hensch, T. K. (2011). A critical period for auditory thalamocortical connectivity. *Nature Neuroscience, 14*, 1189–1194.

Barlow, H. B. (1961). Possible principles underlying the transformation of sensory messages. *Sensory Communication, 1*(1), 217–233.

Berto, M., Ricciardi, E., Pietrini, P., & Bottari, D. (2021). Interactions between auditory statistics processing and visual experience emerge only in late development. *Iscience, 24*(11).

Bonini, L., Rotunno, C., Arcuri, E., & Gallese, V. (2022). Mirror neurons 30 years later: Implications and applications. *Trends in Cognitive Sciences, 26*(9), 767–781.

Bose, M., Muñoz-llancao, P., Roychowdhury, S., Nichols, J. A., Jakkamsetti, V., Porter, B., et al. (2010). Effect of the environment on the dendritic morphology of the rat auditory cortex. *Synapse, 64*, 97–110.

Brewer, A. A., & Barton, B. (2016). Maps of the auditory cortex. *Annual Review of Neuroscience, 39*, 385–407.

Brugger, P., Kollias, S. S., Müri, R. M., Crelier, G., Hepp-Reymond, M. C., & Regard, M. (2000). Beyond re-membering: Phantom sensations of congenitally absent limbs. *Proceedings of the National Academy of Sciences, 97*, 6167–6172.

Bureš, Z., Pysanenko, K., Lindovský, J., & Syka, J. (2018). Acoustical enrichment during early development improves response reliability in the adult auditory cortex of the rat. *Neural Plasticity, 2018*, 5903720.

Cai, R., Zhou, X., Guo, F., Xu, J., Zhang, J., & Sun, X. (2010). Maintenance of enriched environment-induced changes of auditory spatial sensitivity and expression of GABAA, NMDA, and AMPA receptor subunits in rat auditory cortex. *Neurobiology of Learning and Memory, 94*, 452–460.

Calford, M. B., & Tweedale, R. (1991). Immediate expansion of receptive fields of neurons in area 3b of macaque monkeys after digit denervation. *Somatosensory & Motor Research, 8*, 249–260.

Chang, E. F., & Merzenich, M. M. (2003). Environmental noise retards auditory cortical development. *Science, 300*, 498–502.

Dahmen, J. C., & King, A. J. (2007). Learning to hear: Plasticity of auditory cortical processing. *Current Opinion in Neurobiology, 17*, 456–464.

De Ridder, D., Vanneste, S., & Freeman, W. (2014). The Bayesian brain: Phantom percepts resolve sensory uncertainty. *Neuroscience & Biobehavioral Reviews, 44*, 4–15.

de Villers-Sidani, E., Chang, E. F., Bao, S., & Merzenich, M. M. (2007). Critical period window for spectral tuning defined in the primary auditory cortex (A1) in the rat. *Journal of Neuroscience, 27*(1), 180–189.

*Figure 7.1 appears on the separate color insert.

de Villers-Sidani, E., Simpson, K. L., Lu, Y. F., Lin, R. C., & Merzenich, M. M. (2008). Manipulating critical period closure across different sectors of the primary auditory cortex. *Nature Neuroscience, 11, 957–965.*

Diers, M., Krumm, B., Fuchs, X., Bekrater-Bodmann, R., Milde, C., Trojan, J., et al. (2022). The prevalence and characteristics of phantom limb pain and non-painful phantom phenomena in a nationwide survey of 3,374 unilateral limb amputees. *Journal of Pain, 23,* 411–423.

Ehde, D. M., Czerniecki, J. M., Smith, D. G., Campbell, K. M., Edwards, W. T., Jensen, M. P., & Robinson, L. R. (2000). Chronic phantom sensations, phantom pain, residual limb pain, and other regional pain after lower limb amputation. *Archives of Physical Medicine and Rehabilitation, 81,* 1039–1044.

Ephraim, P. L., Wegener, S. T., MacKenzie, E. J., Dillingham, T. R., & Pezzin, L. E. (2005). Phantom pain, residual limb pain, and back pain in amputees: Results of a national survey. *Archives of Physical Medicine and Rehabilitation, 86,* 1910–1919.

Fallon, J. B., Irvine, D. R., & Shepherd, R. K. (2009). Cochlear implant use following neonatal deafness influences the cochleotopic organization of the primary auditory cortex in cats. *Journal of Computational Neurology, 512,* 101–114.

Fallon, J. B., Shepherd, R. K., & Irvine, D. R. (2014). Effects of chronic cochlear electrical stimulation after an extended period of profound deafness on primary auditory cortex organization in cats. *European Journal of Neuroscience, 39,* 811–820.

Feldman, D. E., & Brecht, M. (2005). Map plasticity in somatosensory cortex. *Science, 310,* 810–815.

Finn, S. B., Perry, B. N., Clasing, J. E., Walters, L. S., Jarzombek, S. L., Curran, S., et al. (2017). A randomized, controlled trial of mirror therapy for upper extremity phantom limb pain in male amputees. *Frontiers in Neurology, 8,* 267.

Flor, H. (2002). Phantom-limb pain: Characteristics, causes, and treatment. *Lancet Neurology, 1,* 182–189.

Flor, H., Elbert, T., Knecht, S., Wienbruch, C., Pantev, C., Birbaumers, N., et al. (1995). Phantom-limb pain as a perceptual correlate of cortical reorganization following arm amputation. *Nature, 375,* 482–484.

Flor, H., Nikolajsen, L., & Staehelin Jensen, T. (2006). Phantom limb pain: A case of maladaptive CNS plasticity? *Nature Reviews Neuroscience,* 7, 873–881.

Gallagher, S., Butterworth, G. E., Lew, A., & Cole, J. (1998). Hand–mouth coordination, congenital absence of limb, and evidence for innate body schemas. *Brain and Cognition, 38,* 53–65.

Hahamy, A., MacDonald, S. N., van den Heiligenberg, F., Kieliba, P., Emir, U., Malach, R., et al. (2017). Representation of multiple body parts in the missing-hand territory of congenital one-handers. *Current Biology, 27,* 1350–1355.

Hahamy, A., Sotiropoulos, S. N., Henderson Slater, D., Malach, R., Johansen-Berg, H., & Makin, T. R. (2015). Normalisation of brain connectivity through compensatory behaviour, despite congenital hand absence. *Elife, 4,* e04605.

Hamilton, R. H., & Pascual-Leone, A. (1998). Cortical plasticity associated with Braille learning. *Trends in Cognitive Sciences, 2*(5), 168–174.

Hartmann, R., Shepherd, R. K., Heid, S., & Klinke, R. (1997). Response of the primary auditory cortex to electrical stimulation of the auditory nerve in the congenitally deaf white cat. *Hearing Research, 112,* 115–133.

Heffner, H. E., & Heffner, R. S. (2012). Behavioral tests for tinnitus in animals. In J. J. Eggermont, F.-G. Zeng, A. N. Popper, & R. R. Fay (Eds.), *Tinnitus* (pp. 21–58). Springer.

Hensch, T. K. (2004). Critical period regulation. *Annual Review of Neuroscience, 27*(1), 549–579.

Herrador Colmenero, L., Perez Marmol, J. M., Martí-García, C., Querol Zaldivar, L. Á., Tapia Haro, R. M., Castro Sánchez, A. M., & Aguilar-Ferrándiz, M. E. (2018). Effectiveness of mirror therapy, motor imagery, and virtual feedback on phantom limb pain following amputation: A systematic review. *Prosthetics and Orthotics International, 42*, 288–298.

Hubel, D. H., & Wiesel, T. N. (1970). The period of susceptibility to the physiological effects of unilateral eye closure in kittens. *Journal of Physiology, 206*, 419–436.

Isaacson, J. S., & Scanziani, M. (2011). How inhibition shapes cortical activity. *Neuron, 72*, 231–243.

Jain, N., Qi, H. X., Collins, C. E., & Kaas, J. H. (2008). Large-scale reorganization in the somatosensory cortex and thalamus after sensory loss in macaque monkeys. *Journal of Neuroscience, 28*, 11042–11060.

Jäncke, L., Gaab, N., Wüstenberg, T., Scheich, H., & Heinze, H. J. (2001). Short-term functional plasticity in the human auditory cortex: An fMRI study. *Cognitive Brain Research, 12*(3), 479–485.

Jenkins, W. M., Merzenich, M. M., Ochs, M. T., Allard, T., & Guic-Robles, E. (1990). Functional reorganization of primary somatosensory cortex in adult owl monkeys after behaviorally controlled tactile stimulation. *Journal of Neurophysiology, 63*, 82–104.

Kaas, J. H. (1991). Plasticity of sensory and motor maps in adult animals. *Annual Review of Neuroscience, 14*, 137–67.

Kaltenbach, J. A., & McCaslin, D. L. (1996). Increases in spontaneous activity in the dorsal cochlear nucleus following exposure to high intensity sound: A possible neural correlate of tinnitus. *Auditory Neuroscience, 3*, 57.

Karl, A., Birbaumer, N., Lutzenberger, W., Cohen, L. G., & Flor, H. (2001). Reorganization of motor and somatosensory cortex in upper extremity amputees with phantom limb pain. *Journal of Neuroscience, 21*, 3609–3618.

Katz, J., & Melzack, R. (1990). Pain "memories" in phantom limbs: Review and clinical observations. *Pain, 43*, 319–336.

Kell, A. J., & McDermott, J. H. (2019). Invariance to background noise as a signature of non-primary auditory cortex. *Nature Communications, 10*, 3958.

Keuroghlian, A. S., & Knudsen, E. I. (2007). Adaptive auditory plasticity in developing and adult animals. *Progress in Neurobiology, 82*, 109–121.

Kikkert, S., Johansen-Berg, H., Tracey, I., & Makin, T. R. (2018). Reaffirming the link between chronic phantom limb pain and maintained missing hand representation. *Cortex, 106*, 174–184.

Kooijman, C. M., Dijkstra, P. U., Geertzen, J. H., Elzinga, A., & Van der Schans, C. P. (2000). Phantom pain and phantom sensations in upper limb amputees: An epidemiological study. *Pain, 87*, 33–41.

Kral, A., Dorman, M. F., & Wilson, B. S. (2019). Neuronal development of hearing and language: Cochlear implants and critical periods. *Annual Review of Neuroscience, 42*, 47–65.

Kral, A., Hartmann, R., Tillein, J., Heid, S., & Klinke, R. (2001). Delayed maturation and sensitive periods in the auditory cortex. *Audiology & Neurotology, 6*, 346–362.

Kral, A., Hartmann, R., Tillein, J., Heid, S., & Klinke, R. (2002). Hearing after congenital deafness: Central auditory plasticity and sensory deprivation. *Cerebral Cortex, 12*, 797–807.

Levelt, C. N., & Hübener, M., 2012. Critical-period plasticity in the visual cortex. *Annual Review of Neuroscience, 35*, 309–330.

Loeb, M., & Smith, R. P. (1967). Relation of induced tinnitus to physical characteristics of the inducing stimuli. *Journal of the Acoustical Society of America, 42*, 453–455.

Makin, T. R. (2021). Phantom limb pain: Thinking outside the (mirror) box. *Brain, 144*, 1929–1932.

Makin, T. R., Scholz, J., Filippini, N., Henderson Slater, D., Tracey, I., & Johansen-Berg, H. (2013). Phantom pain is associated with preserved structure and function in the former hand area. *Nature Communications, 4*, 1570.

Mariani, B., Nicoletti, G., Barzon, G., Ortiz Barajas, M. C., Shukla, M., Guevara, R., et al. (2023). Prenatal experience with language shapes the brain. *Science Advances, 9*, eadj3524.

Maxon, A. B., & Hochberg, I. (1982). Development of psychoacoustic behavior: Sensitivity and discrimination. *Ear and Hearing, 3*, 301–308.

McDermott, J. H., & Simoncelli, E. P. (2011). Sound texture perception via statistics of the auditory periphery: Evidence from sound synthesis. *Neuron, 71*(5), 926–940.

Melzack, R., Israel, R., Lacroix, R., & Schultz, G. (1997). Phantom limbs in people with congenital limb deficiency or amputation in early childhood. *Brain: A Journal of Neurology, 120*, 1603–1620.

Merzenich, M. M., Kaas, J. H., Wall, J., Nelson, R. J., Sur, M., & Felleman, D. (1983). Topographic reorganization of somatosensory cortical areas 3b and 1 in adult monkeys following restricted deafferentation. *Neuroscience*, 8, 33–56.

Merzenich, M. M., Nelson, R. J., Stryker, M. P., Cynader, M. S., Schoppmann, A., & Zook, J. M. (1984). Somatosensory cortical map changes following digit amputation in adult monkeys. *Journal of Comparative Neurology, 224*, 591–605.

Mohan, A., & Vanneste, S. (2017). Adaptive and maladaptive neural compensatory consequences of sensory deprivation—From a phantom percept perspective. *Progress in Neurobiology, 153*, 1–17.

Moore, D. R., Cowan, J. A., Riley, A., Edmondson-Jones, A. M., & Ferguson, M. A. (2011). Development of auditory processing in 6- to 11-yr-old children. *Ear and Hearing, 32*, 269–285.

Morishita, H., & Hensch, T. K. (2008). Critical period revisited: Impact on vision. *Current Opinion in Neurobiology, 18*, 101–107.

Moseley, G. L., & Flor, H. (2012). Targeting cortical representations in the treatment of chronic pain: A review. *Neurorehabilitation and Neural Repair, 26*, 646–652.

Murray, C. D., Patchick, E., Pettifer, S., Howard, T., Caillette, F., Kulkarni, J., & Bamford, C. (2006). Investigating the efficacy of a virtual mirror box in treating phantom limb pain in a sample of chronic sufferers. *International Journal on Disability and Human Development, 5*, 227–234.

Nava, E., & Röder, B. (2011). Adaptation and maladaptation: Insights from brain plasticity. *Progress in Brain Research, 191*, 177–194.

Nava, E., Bottari, D., Portioli, G., Bonfioli, F., Beltrame, M. A., Formigoni, P., & Pavani, F. (2009). Hearing again with two ears: Recovery of spatial hearing after bilateral cochlear implantation. *Neuropsychologia, 47*, 928–932.

Nikolajsen, L., Ilkjaer, S., Kroner, K., Christensen, J. H., & Jensen, T. S. (1997). The influence of preamputation pain on postamputation stump and phantom pain. *Pain, 72*, 393–405.

Pavani, F., & Bottari, D. (2022). Neuroplasticity following cochlear implants. In G. Miceli, P. Bartolomeo, & V. Navarro (Eds.), *Handbook of clinical neurology: Vol. 187. The temporal lobe* (pp. 89–108). Elsevier.

Persic, D., Thomas, M. E., Pelekanos, V., Ryugo, D. K., Takesian, A. E., Krumbholz, K., & Pyott, S. J. (2020). Regulation of auditory plasticity during critical periods and following hearing loss. *Hearing Research, 397*, 107976.

Polley, D. B., Steinberg, E. E., & Merzenich, M. M. (2006). Perceptual learning directs auditory cortical map reorganization through top-down influences. *Journal of Neuroscience, 26*, 4970–4982.

Raffin, E., Richard, N., Giraux, P., & Reilly, K. T. (2016). Primary motor cortex changes after amputation correlate with phantom limb pain and the ability to move the phantom limb. *NeuroImage, 130*, 134–144.

Raggio, M. W., & Schreiner, C. E. (1999). Neuronal responses in cat primary auditory cortex to electrical cochlear stimulation. III. Activation patterns in short-and long-term deafness. *Journal of Neurophysiology, 82*, 3506–3526.

Ramachandran, V. S., & Hirstein, W. (1998). The perception of phantom limbs. The DO Hebb lecture. *Brain, 121*, 1603–1630.

Rauschecker, J. P. (1999). Auditory cortical plasticity: a comparison with other sensory systems. *Trends in Neurosciences, 22*, 74–80.

Recanzone, G. H., Jenkins, W. M., Hradek, G. T., & Merzenich, M. M. (1992). Progressive improvement in discriminative abilities in adult owl monkeys performing a tactile frequency discrimination task. *Journal of Neurophysiology, 67*, 1015–1030.

Sanes, D. H., & Woolley, S. M. (2011). A behavioral framework to guide research on central auditory development and plasticity. *Neuron, 72*, 912–929.

Schlaug, G. (2015). Musicians and music making as a model for the study of brain plasticity. *Progress in Brain Research, 217*, 37–55.

Schneider, B. A., Morrongiello, B. A., & Trehub, S. E. (1990). Size of critical band in infants, children, and adults. *Journal of Experimental Psychology: Human Perception and Performance, 16*, 642–652.

Schone, H. R., Baker, C. I., Katz, J., Nikolajsen, L., Limakatso, K., Flor, H., & Makin, T. R. (2022). Making sense of phantom limb pain. *Journal of Neurology, Neurosurgery & Psychiatry, 93*, 833–843.

Schreiner, C. E., & Winer, J. A. (2007). Auditory cortex mapmaking: Principles, projections, and plasticity. *Neuron, 56*, 356–365.

Sharma, A., Dorman, M. F., & Kral, A. (2005). The influence of a sensitive period on central auditory development in children with unilateral and bilateral cochlear implants. *Hearing Research, 203*, 134–143.

Sharma, A., Dorman, M. F., & Spahr, A. J. (2002). A sensitive period for the development of the central auditory system in children with cochlear implants: Implications for age of implantation. *Ear & Hearing, 23*, 532–539.

Sharma, A., Gilley, P. M., Dorman, M. F., & Baldwin, R. (2007). Deprivation induced cortical reorganization in children with cochlear implants. *International Journal of Audiology, 46*, 494–499.

Shepherd, R. K., Hartmann, R., Heid, S., Hardie, N., & Klinke, R. (1997). The central auditory system and auditory deprivation: Experience with cochlear implants in the congenitally deaf. *Acta Otolaryngology, 117*, 28–33.

Shore, S. E., Roberts, L. E., & Langguth, B. (2016). Maladaptive plasticity in tinnitus—triggers, mechanisms and treatment. *Nature Reviews Neurology, 12*, 150–160.

Shukla, G. D., Sahu, S. C., Tripathi, R. P., & Gupta, D. K. (1982). Phantom limb: A phenomenological study. *British Journal of Psychiatry, 141*, 54–58.

Spetner, N. B., & Olsho, L. W. (1990). Auditory frequency resolution in human infancy. *Child Development, 61*, 632–652.

Takesian, A. E., Bogart, L. J., Lichtman, J. W., & Hensch, T. K. (2018). Inhibitory circuit gating of auditory critical-period plasticity. *Nature Neuroscience, 21*, 218–227.

Tandon, S., Kambi, N., Lazar, L., Mohammed, H., & Jain, N. (2009). Large-scale expansion of the face representation in somatosensory areas of the lateral sulcus after spinal cord injuries in monkeys. *Journal of Neuroscience, 29*, 12009–12019.

Tillein, J., Hubka, P., Syed, E., Hartmann, R., Engel, A. K., & Kral, A. (2010). Cortical representation of interaural time difference in congenital deafness. *Cerebral Cortex, 20*, 492–506.

Turrigiano, G. (2012). Homeostatic synaptic plasticity: Local and global mechanisms for stabilizing neuronal function. *Cold Spring Harbor Perspectives in Biology, 4*(1), a005736.

Webb, A. R., Heller, H. T., Benson, C. B., & Lahav, A. (2015). Mother's voice and heartbeat sounds elicit auditory plasticity in the human brain before full gestation. *Proceedings of the National Academy of Sciences, 112*(10), 3152–3157.

Weiss, T., Miltner, W. H., Huonker, R., Friedel, R., Schmidt, I., & Taub, E. (2000). Rapid functional plasticity of the somatosensory cortex after finger amputation. *Experimental Brain Research, 134*, 199–203.

Wiesel, T. N., & Hubel, D. H. (1965). Comparison of the effects of unilateral and bilateral eye closure on cortical unit responses in kittens. *Journal of Neurophysiology, 28*(6), 1029–1040.

Wilson, B. S., & Dorman, M. F. (2008). Cochlear implants: A remarkable past and a brilliant future. *Hearing Research, 242*, 3–21.

Wright, B. A., & Zhang, Y. (2009). A review of the generalization of auditory learning. *Philosophical Transactions of the Royal Society B: Biological Sciences, 364*, 301–311.

Wu, C., Stefanescu, R. A., Martel, D. T., & Shore, S. E. (2016). Tinnitus: Maladaptive auditory–somatosensory plasticity. *Hearing Research, 334*, 20–29.

Zatorre, R. J., Delhommeau, K., & Zarate, J. M. (2012). Modulation of auditory cortex response to pitch variation following training with microtonal melodies. *Frontiers in Psychology, 3*, 544.

Zhang, L. I., Bao, S., & Merzenich, M. M. (2001). Persistent and specific influences of early acoustic environments on primary auditory cortex. *Nature Neuroscience, 4*, 1123–1130.

CHAPTER 8

Cortical Reorganization after Brain Damage

Valentina Azzollini and Leonardo G. Cohen

Introduction

The human brain experiences reorganizational changes throughout the lifespan (Dayan & Cohen, 2011; Quentin et al., 2019) in response to environmental challenges and learning new skills (Dayan & Cohen, 2011; Nielsen & Cohen, 2008), as well as following brain lesions (Kleim & Jones, 2008). Here, we define *plasticity* operationally as reorganizational changes in brain function or structure that occur in association with or in response to lesions, development, or environmental stimuli. In this way, plasticity could be causally related to behavior (adaptive plasticity; Amedi et al., 2007, 2004; Cohen et al., 1997; Duymuş et al., 2024) or simply be a consequence or epiphenomenon of such behavior. In other circumstances, plastic changes could be maladaptive and result in undesirable behavioral consequences (i.e., phantom limb pain; Flor, 2008; Flor et al., 2006; Ramachandran & Altschuler, 2009). While plasticity occurs at all levels of the central nervous system (CNS), here we will focus on plasticity in brain function (Hummel & Cohen, 2005). Modern interest in plasticity and cortical organization started with seminal studies by Kaas and Merzenich reporting changes in the boundary of sensory and motor representational maps in the motor and somatosensory cortices following deafferentation and amputations (Buonomano & Merzenich, 1998; Kaas, 2000; Merzenich et al., 1996; Merzenich & Jenkins, 1993).

These plastic changes develop over different time windows, within seconds and minutes during deafferentation (Werhahn, Mortensen, Kaelin-Lang, et al., 2002; Werhahn, Mortensen, Van Boven, et al., 2002) or at a slower pace during maturation and learning (Cheung et al., 2020; Penhune et al., 2005; Staudt et al., 2004; Tomblin et al., 2007). Plastic changes in cortical organization are age-dependent, more profound in young individuals, and of lesser magnitude in older subjects (Vargha-Khadem et al., 2003).

The neural mechanisms underlying these various forms of plasticity include the unmasking of previously existent connections (Hebscher et al., 2019) and the development of new synaptic contacts (Chen et al., 2002) due to sprouting. Developing insight into the mechanisms of plastic changes in cortical organization, and their causal contribution to the behavior, is crucial to designing rational, mechanistically driven strategies to promote beneficial plastic processes or downregulate maladaptive ones (Ward & Cohen, 2004).

This chapter aims to provide an overview of cortical reorganization reported after brain damage. In addition, it presents evidence supporting plasticity in situations where brain damage has occurred. Recovery of brain activity after the insult is also discussed.

Brain Damage

Brain damage encompasses a spectrum of injuries and pathologies that can profoundly impact the structure and function of the CNS. These range from acute events like stroke and traumatic brain injury to chronic conditions such as those developing in the course of neurodegenerative diseases. The consequences of brain damage vary widely, affecting individuals across the lifespan.

Stroke

Stroke, a leading cause of long-term disability, often results in localized damage to brain tissue due to ischemia (interruption of blood flow) or hemorrhage. The infarct area undergoes acute changes, triggering a cascade of molecular and cellular responses (Zhao et al., 2022). Initially, the surrounding tissue may experience hypoperfusion, metabolic stress, and inflammation, leading to secondary neuronal injury and synaptic dysfunction. Additionally, distant regions interconnected with the impaired one can experience reorganizational changes. Thus, local cell death results in cell dysfunction in surrounding connected areas (Dalise et al., 2014). Multiple reports over time have described cortical reorganization characterized by changes in synaptic connections, dendritic morphology, and neural activity patterns, both locally and in distant regions of the brain (Joy & Carmichael, 2021; Ward & Carmichael, 2020). For example, following a local brain lesion, adjacent cortical areas may expand their motor or sensory representation to include the body part previously represented by the lesioned one (Nudo, 2003; Nudo et al., 1996). Following a cortical or subcortical lesion, it is possible that alternate neural pathways unmask latent connections, contributing to functional recovery and rehabilitation of the lost or perturbed behavior.

Traumatic Brain Injury

Traumatic brain injury (TBI) encompasses a range of injuries resulting from falls, collisions, or blasts that disrupt normal brain function. The pathophysiology of TBI involves primary injury, caused by the initial mechanical trauma, and secondary injury, characterized by biochemical and cellular cascades leading to neuroinflammation, oxidative stress, and excitotoxicity (Bass et al., 2012; McAllister et al., 2006). Like in stroke, neuroplasticity mechanisms, including axonal sprouting, dendritic remodeling, and synaptogenesis, operate in the context of TBI (Fesharaki-Zadeh & Datta, 2024; VanItallie, 2019). Cortical reorganization is often influenced by the severity and location of the injury, with more significant disruptions leading to more extensive reorganization.

Neurodegenerative Disease

Neurodegenerative diseases, such as Alzheimer's disease (Bhembre et al., 2023), Parkinson's disease (Chu, 2020; Udupa et al., 2022), and amyotrophic lateral sclerosis (Gulino, 2023; Penndorf et al., 2018), involve progressive degeneration of neurons and brain structures over time. These conditions are characterized by the accumulation of misfolded proteins, oxidative stress, and neuroinflammation, leading to widespread neuronal dysfunction and death (Ransohoff, 2016; Soto & Estrada, 2008). Despite the chronic and progressive nature of neurodegenerative diseases, evidence suggests that neuroplasticity mechanisms persist throughout the course of the disease (Bhembre et al., 2023; Chu, 2020; Gulino, 2023). Cortical reorganization in neurodegenerative diseases may involve compensatory recruitment of intact brain regions and the adoption of alternative neural pathways to preserve cognitive reserve and delay functional decline. However, the capacity for plasticity may eventually become overwhelmed as the disease progresses, highlighting the importance of early intervention strategies to promote adaptive changes and preserve brain function (Simons et al., 2023).

In summary, brain damage poses significant challenges to the brain's structural and functional integrity. Evidence suggests that, in this context, the brain retains adaptive capabilities, possibly influencing recovery, compensation, and rehabilitation.

Mechanisms of Cortical Reorganization and Plasticity

The initial response of the brain to damage, its adaptation, and subsequent functional recovery are facilitated by a complex interplay of mechanisms at the cellular, synaptic, and network levels. As pointed out above, it is important to note that the occurring changes can be adaptive (leading to the restoration of a function), maladaptive (worsening the performance) or simply epiphenomenal (Dalise et al., 2014). These qualitatively different kinds of plasticity may be driven by similar neurobiological processes happening at different times and dimensional scales. Based on this idea, it is possible to define a time course for the occurring changes (acute, subacute, chronic) and a magnitude scale (macro-, meso-, micro-, and nanoscale; see Figure 8.1*).

In the acute phase following injury, there is an initial decrease in activity in the penumbra that can be reestablished after reperfusion. In the perilesional cortex, immediately following the acute event, the balance between inhibitory gamma-aminobutyric acid (GABA-ergic) and excitatory glutamatergic signaling moves

*Figure 8.1 appears on the separate color insert.

toward a state of relative inhibition (Bönstrup et al., 2019). Recovery from this state develops at the mesoscale (edema resolution), microscale (reactivation of surviving neurons, invasion of glial cell and neuroblasts), and nanoscale (inflammation resolution, secretion of growth factor) levels (Dalise et al., 2014). These processes could theoretically contribute to strengthening of functional connections relevant to the compensation of lost functions (Bestmann et al., 2010; Hammerbeck et al., 2017; Stefanou et al., 2018).

Areas anatomically distant from the lesioned one can undergo profound modifications, a phenomenon referred to as diaschisis. Diaschisis refers to the functional depression or inhibition of brain areas remote from the site of primary damage. Diaschisis engages aberrant neurotransmission, tissue hypometabolism, and neurovascular uncoupling (Carrera & Tononi, 2014). The modification of synaptic connections and reversal of diaschisis leads to a dynamic reconfiguration of neural networks and functional connectivity patterns that may potentially influence functional recovery (Dalise et al., 2014).

Imbalances in interhemispheric inhibition have been reported in the chronic stage following stroke (Duque et al., 2007; Murase et al., 2004; Xu et al., 2019). Healthy individuals exhibit a delicate balance of excitatory and inhibitory interactions between the two cerebral hemispheres thought to influence motor control, cognition, and information processing. Following unilateral damage, such as a stroke affecting the motor cortex, there is evidence of anomalous interhemispheric inhibition from the uninjured to the lesioned hemisphere when patients attempt to move the paretic hand (Duque et al., 2005). Interhemispheric inhibition from the unaffected to the affected hemisphere abnormally persists when the subject attempts to contract the paretic limb and could potentially interfere with the initiation of movement (Di Pino et al., 2014). Different interventional approaches have been proposed based on this model (Floel & Cohen, 2006). Strategies aimed at modulating interhemispheric inhibition, or increasing the excitability of specific regions, such as noninvasive brain stimulation (NIBS), have emerged as potential therapeutic interventions to rebalance hemispheric activity and promote functional recovery (Di Pino et al., 2014; Hummel & Cohen, 2005; Quentin et al., 2019). Overall, the magnitude of functional recovery induced by these approaches has been limited, and advances in these areas very slow, leading to the proposal that this form of cortical reorganization may not contribute to recovery at all (Makin & Krakauer, 2023). Despite this, several studies have shown that the increased activation of the unaffected hemisphere, such as of other ipsilesional cortical areas like the premotor cortex and the supplementary motor area, could be adaptive to functional recovery (Di Pino et al., 2014).

At the cellular level, reorganization engages the formation, modification, and elimination of synaptic connections. Initial inhibitory states that follow a brain lesion relate to a diminished reuptake of the inhibitory neurotransmitter GABA by reactive astrocytes (Gleichman & Carmichael, 2014) and a decreased number of *N*-methyl-D-aspartate receptors, an adapting response to the increased level of glutamate, potentially toxic for neuronal cells (Dalise et al., 2014).

Different molecules guide the development of plastic mechanisms after brain damage. It has been shown that basic fibroblast growth factor may attenuate thalamic degeneration following cortical infarction and enhance neuronal sprouting

(Kawamata et al., 1997; Yamada et al., 1991). Nerve growth factor has been reported to reduce dendritic atrophy in the remaining pyramidal neurons of rats (Kolb et al., 1997). Brain-derived neurotrophic factor (BDNF) may promote neuronal proliferation, survival, and differentiation, but it also affects angiogenesis in the brain (Dalise et al., 2014). It has been proposed that functional recovery after a brain lesion could rely on strengthening residual sparse and weak pathways in the cortex, brainstem, and spinal cord, or the communication between them.

Techniques Available to Evaluate and Modulate Cortical Reorganization in Humans

Neuroimaging techniques offer valuable insights into the structural and functional changes in the brain following damage, revealing widespread changes in brain activation patterns during simple movements of the affected hand after a stroke (Ball et al., 2023; Dimyan & Cohen, 2011; Tavazzi et al., 2021). Functional magnetic resonance imaging, and positron emission tomography provide spatially resolved maps of brain activity during various tasks or while at rest.

Diffusion tensor imaging (DTI) allows for the visualization and quantification of white matter tracts, providing information about the integrity and connectivity of neural pathways (Jang, 2010, 2011). The integrity of the corticospinal tract, measured by DTI, is strongly associated with functional recovery after stroke (Buch et al., 2016). It has been proposed that changes in fractional anisotropy (reflecting white matter fiber density, axonal diameter, and myelination) relate to axonal sprouting and reorganization in response to training (Quentin et al., 2019).

Magnetoencephalography (MEG) and electroencephalography (EEG) have provided essential insights into highly resolved (second by second) temporal features of functional reorganization, particularly neural oscillatory activity (Tedesco Triccas et al., 2019). MEG and EEG studies have documented anomalous neural synchronization, signal amplitude, and brain oscillatory phase coherence in both affected and unaffected brain regions after brain lesions. Measurements like lateralization of activation patterns in motor cortical regions, interhemispheric connectivity, and the strength of the beta oscillatory activity rebound predict the degree of motor recovery (Bönstrup et al., 2019).

Recent studies have shown that low-frequency oscillations (LFOs) in the motor cortex are disrupted in stroke patients (Bönstrup et al., 2019). LFOs are brief periods of delta- and lower theta-like band activity in the motor cortical areas that occur before and around movement onset. They may contribute to set a preparatory state for the execution of movement, including direction, velocity, and 3D trajectory. The acutely diminished level of LFOs is proportional to the motor deficits after stroke. With time after stroke, LFO anomalies correct. Bönstrup and colleagues (2019) recognize LFOs as a potential target for interventional therapy with neurostimulation.

Transcranial magnetic stimulation (TMS) is a noninvasive brain stimulation technique that uses magnetic fields to induce electrical currents in targeted areas of the brain (Hallett & Cohen, 1989). TMS has provided further evidence of cortical reorganization by directly modulating neural activity in specific brain regions. By applying TMS pulses over the motor cortex, researchers can assess cortical excitability, and cortical representational maps, and investigate the functional connectivity of neural networks. TMS studies have shown alterations in cortical excitability and motor-evoked potentials in individuals with stroke (Liew et al., 2014), TBI (Villamar et al., 2012), or neurodegenerative diseases (Moisello et al., 2015), reflecting changes in functional cortical organization.

Factors Influencing Cortical Reorganization

Cortical reorganization is influenced by different factors, including the size and location of the brain lesion, genetics (e.g., polymorphisms of apolipoprotein E, BDNF, and catechol-O-methyltransferase), age, race, gender, and comorbidities, as well as the timing and density of rehabilitation. The time course of cortical reorganization varies depending on factors such as the type of injury and individual characteristics (Quandt & Hummel, 2014; Wessel et al., 2021). While functional reorganization may occur rapidly in response to acute insults, others may unfold over weeks, months, or even years. Understanding the temporal dynamics of reorganization is essential for tailoring rehabilitation interventions. Postinfarct plasticity is at its highest in the first few months after a stroke, a critical period during which function is recovered faster, beginning to plateau 6 months after the stroke (Bach-y-Rita & Balliet, 1987; Duncan & Sue Min Lai, 1997). From pharmacological treatment to rehabilitation, early initiation of intervention can be more effective in improving disability. The fibrinolytic treatment with recombinant tissue plasminogen activator in ischemic stroke breaks down blood clots but could also increase BDNF levels in the site of the lesion (Chaves et al., 2000; Schlaug et al., 1999; Tatum et al., 2023), increasing the potential recovery.

Strategies to Modulate Cortical Reorganization

It is expected that in the future, different interventions could upregulate the production of critical trophic factors—for example, BDNF. NIBS techniques, such as TMS, have shown promise in inducing neural changes and promoting cortical reorganization in rehabilitation settings (Dayan et al., 2013). By modulating neural activity, NIBS aims to enhance functional recovery and improve outcomes for individuals with neurological disorders (Hummel & Cohen, 2005).

Understanding the functional consequences of cortical reorganization has important implications for designing effective rehabilitation strategies. Rehabilitation programs should aim to promote adaptive plasticity while minimizing maladaptive changes in neural networks. This may involve a combination of task-specific training, environmental enrichment, and NIBS techniques to optimize functional outcomes. Rehabilitation interventions should be tailored to the individual needs and characteristics of patients, taking into account factors such as age, severity of injury, and cognitive status. Multidisciplinary approaches that incorporate physical therapy, occupational therapy, speech therapy, and cognitive rehabilitation can influence the diverse range of deficits resulting from brain damage and improve the potential for functional recovery.

In summary, cortical reorganization following brain damage can relate to functional recovery or simply be an epiphenomenon. It is crucial to determine the causality of this link on a case-by-case basis to determine when interventional approaches that up- or down-regulate cortical reorganization are desirable and can improve function.

Conclusion

Cortical reorganization following brain damage encompasses an extensive variety of forms and dynamics. Determining the causal link between each form of reorganization and function remains one of the important frontiers in cognitive and clinical neuroscience. The CNS demonstrates remarkable plasticity from restoring lost functions to developing compensatory mechanisms. The translation from basic science documentation of mechanisms of disability to neuromodulation of cortical reorganization, when it plays an adaptive role, will evolve into more effective interventions than presently available. Importantly, developing individualized interventions will likely enrich the therapeutic armamentarium in neurorehabilitation.

REFERENCES

Amedi, A., Floel, A., Knecht, S., Zohary, E., & Cohen, L. G., (2004). Transcranial magnetic stimulation of the occipital pole interferes with verbal processing in blind subjects. *Nature Neuroscience, 7*, 1266–1270.

Amedi, A., Stern, W. M., Camprodon, J. A., Bermpohl, F., Merabet, L., Rotman, S., et al. (2007). Shape conveyed by visual-to-auditory sensory substitution activates the lateral occipital complex. *Nature Neuroscience, 10*, 687–689.

Bach-y-Rita, P., & Balliet, R. (1987). Recovery from stroke. In P. W. Duncan & M. B. Badke (Eds.), *Stroke rehabilitation: The recovery of motor control* (pp. 79–107). Year Book Medical.

Ball, E. L., Shah, M., Ross, E., Sutherland, R., Squires, C., Mead, G. E., et al. (2023). Predictors of post-stroke cognitive impairment using acute structural MRI neuroimaging: A systematic review and meta-analysis. *International Journal of Stroke, 18*, 543–554.

Bass, C. R., Panzer, M. B., Rafaels, K. A., Wood, G., Shridharani, J., & Capehart, B. (2012). Brain injuries from blast. *Annals of Biomedical Engineering, 40*, 185–202.

Bernhardt, J., Hayward, K. S., Kwakkel, G., Ward, N. S., Wolf, S. L., Borschmann, K., et al. (2017). Agreed definitions and a shared vision for new standards in stroke recovery research: The Stroke Recovery and Rehabilitation Roundtable taskforce. *International Journal of Stroke, 12*(5), 444–450.

Bestmann, S., Swayne, O., Blankenburg, F., Ruff, C. C., Teo, J., Weiskopf, N., et al. (2010). The role of contralesional dorsal premotor cortex after stroke as studied with concurrent TMS-fMRI. *Journal of Neuroscience, 30*, 11926–11937.

Bhembre, N., Bonthron, C., & Opazo, P. (2023). Synaptic compensatory plasticity in Alzheimer's disease. *Journal of Neuroscience, 43*, 6833–6840.

Bönstrup, M., Krawinkel, L., Schulz, R., Cheng, B., Feldheim, J., Thomalla, G., et al. (2019). Low-frequency brain oscillations track motor recovery in human stroke. *Annals of Neurology, 86*, 853–865.

Buch, E. R., Rizk, S., Nicolo, P., Cohen, L. G., Schnider, A., & Guggisberg, A. G. (2016). Predicting motor improvement after stroke with clinical assessment and diffusion tensor imaging. *Neurology, 86*, 1924–1925.

Buonomano, D. V., & Merzenich, M. M. (1998). Cortical plasticity: From synapses to maps. *Annual Review of Neuroscience, 21*, 149–186.

Carrera, E., & Tononi, G. (2014). Diaschisis: Past, present, future. *Brain, 137*, 2408–2422.

Chaves, C. J., Silver, B., Schlaug, G., Dashe, J., Caplan, L. R., & Warach, S. (2000). Diffusion- and perfusion-weighted MRI patterns in borderzone infarcts. *Stroke, 31*, 1090–1096.

Chen, R., Cohen, L. G., & Hallett, M. (2002). Nervous system reorganization following injury. *Neuroscience, 111*, 761–773.

Cheung, V. C. K., Cheung, B. M. F., Zhang, J. H., Chan, Z. Y. S., Ha, S. C. W., Chen, C.-Y., & Cheung, R. T. H. (2020). Plasticity of muscle synergies through fractionation and merging during development and training of human runners. *Nature Communications, 11*, 4356.

Chu, H.-Y., (2020). Synaptic and cellular plasticity in Parkinson's disease. *Acta Pharmacologica Sinica, 41*, 447–452.

Cohen, L. G., Celnik, P., Pascual-Leone, A., Corwell, B., Faiz, L., Dambrosia, J., et al. (1997). Functional relevance of cross-modal plasticity in blind humans. *Nature, 389*, 180–183.

Dalise, S., Ambrosio, F., & Modo, M. (2014). Brain plasticity and recovery in preclinical models of stroke. *Archives Italiennes de Biologie, 152*, 190–215.

Dayan, E., Censor, N., Buch, E. R., Sandrini, M., & Cohen, L. G. (2013). Noninvasive brain stimulation: From physiology to network dynamics and back. *Nature Neuroscience, 16*, 838–844.

Dayan, E., & Cohen, L. G. (2011). Neuroplasticity subserving motor skill learning. *Neuron, 72*, 443–454.

Di Pino, G., Pellegrino, G., Assenza, G., Capone, F., Ferreri, F., Formica, D., et al. (2014). Modulation of brain plasticity in stroke: A novel model for neurorehabilitation. *Nature Reviews Neurology, 10*, 597–608.

Dimyan, M. A., & Cohen, L. G. (2011). Neuroplasticity in the context of motor rehabilitation after stroke. *Nature Reviews Neurology, 7*, 76–85.

Duncan, P. W., & Sue Min Lai, M. L. (1997). Stroke recovery. *Topics in Stroke Rehabilitation, 4*, 51–58.

Duque, J., Hummel, F., Celnik, P., Murase, N., Mazzocchio, R., & Cohen, L. G. (2005). Transcallosal inhibition in chronic subcortical stroke. *NeuroImage, 28*, 940–946.

Duque, J., Murase, N., Celnik, P., Hummel, F., Harris-Love, M., Mazzocchio, R., et al. (2007). Intermanual differences in movement-related interhemispheric inhibition. *Journal of Cognitive Neuroscience, 19*, 204–213.

Duymuş, H., Verma, M., Güçlütürk, Y., Öztürk, M., Varol, A. B., Kurt, Ş., et al. (2024). The visual cortex in the blind but not the auditory cortex in the deaf becomes multiple-demand regions. *Brain, 187*(10), 3624–3637.

Fesharaki-Zadeh, A., & Datta, D. (2024). An overview of preclinical models of traumatic brain injury (TBI): Relevance to pathophysiological mechanisms. *Frontiers in Cellular. Neuroscience, 18*, 1371213.

Floel, A., & Cohen, L. G. (2006). Translational studies in neurorehabilitation: From bench to bedside. *Cognitive and Behavioral Neurolology, 19*(1), 1–10.

Flor, H. (2008). Maladaptive plasticity, memory for pain and phantom limb pain: Review and suggestions for new therapies. *Expert Review of Neurotherapeutics, 8*, 809–818.

Flor, H., Nikolajsen, L., & Staehelin Jensen, T. (2006). Phantom limb pain: A case of maladaptive CNS plasticity? *Nature Reviews Neuroscience, 7*, 873–881.

Gleichman, A. J., & Carmichael, S. T. (2014). Astrocytic therapies for neuronal repair in stroke. *Neuroscience Letters, 565*, 47–52.

Gulino, R. (2023). Synaptic dysfunction and plasticity in amyotrophic lateral sclerosis. *International Journal of Molecular Sciences, 24*, 4613.

Hallett, M., & Cohen, L. G. (1989). Magnetism: A new method for stimulation of nerve and brain. *JAMA, 262*, 538–541.

Hammerbeck, U., Yousif, N., Hoad, D., Greenwood, R., Diedrichsen, J., & Rothwell, J. C. (2017). Chronic stroke survivors improve reaching accuracy by reducing movement variability at the trained movement speed. *Neurorehabilitation and Neural Repair, 31*(6), 499–508.

Hebscher, M., Wing, E., Ryan, J., & Gilboa, A. (2019). Rapid cortical plasticity supports long-term memory formation. *Trends in Cognitive Science, 23*, 989–1002.

Hummel, F. C., & Cohen, L. G. (2005). Drivers of brain plasticity. *Current Opinion in Neurology, 18*, 667–674.

Jang, S. H., (2010). Prediction of motor outcome for hemiparetic stroke patients using diffusion tensor imaging: A review. *NeuroRehabilitation, 27*, 367–372.

Jang, S. H. (2011). A review of diffusion tensor imaging studies on motor recovery mechanisms in stroke patients. *NeuroRehabilitation, 28*, 345–352.

Joy, M. T., & Carmichael, S. T. (2021). Encouraging an excitable brain state: Mechanisms of brain repair in stroke. *Nature Reviews Neuroscience, 22*, 38–53.

Kaas, J. H. (2000). The reorganization of somatosensory and motor cortex after peripheral nerve or spinal cord injury in primates. In F. J. Seil (Ed.), *Progress in brain research, neural plasticity and regeneration* (pp. 173–179), Elsevier.

Kawamata, T., Dietrich, W. D., Schallert, T., Gotts, J. E., Cocke, R. R., Benowitz, L. I., & Finklestein, S. P. (1997). Intracisternal basic fibroblast growth factor enhances functional recovery and up-regulates the expression of a molecular marker of neuronal sprouting following focal cerebral infarction. *Proceedings of the National Academy of Sciences of the United States of America, 94*, 8179–8184.

Kleim, J. A., & Jones, T. A. (2008). Principles of experience-dependent neural plasticity: Implications for rehabilitation after brain damage. *Journal of Speech, Language, and Hearing Research, 51*, S225–239.

Kolb, B., Cote, S., Ribeiro-da-Silva, A., & Cuello, A. C. (1997). Nerve growth factor treatment prevents dendritic atrophy and promotes recovery of function after cortical injury. *Neuroscience, 76*, 1139–1151.

Liew, S.-L., Santarnecchi, E., Buch, E. R., & Cohen, L. G. (2014). Non-invasive brain stimulation in neurorehabilitation: Local and distant effects for motor recovery. *Frontiers in Human Neuroscience, 8*, 378.

Makin, T. R., & Krakauer, J. W. (2023). Against cortical reorganisation. *eLife, 12*, e84716.

McAllister, T. W., Flashman, L. A., McDonald, B. C., & Saykin, A. J. (2006). Mechanisms of working memory dysfunction after mild and moderate TBI: Evidence from functional MRI and neurogenetics. *Journal of Neurotrauma, 23*, 1450–1467.

Merzenich, M., Wright, B., Jenkins, W., Xerri, C., Byl, N., Miller, S., & Tallal, P. (1996). Cortical plasticity underlying perceptual, motor, and cognitive skill development: Implications for neurorehabilitation. *Cold Spring Harbor Symposia on Quantitative Biology, 61*, 1–8.

Merzenich, M. M., & Jenkins, W. M. (1993). Reorganization of cortical representations of the hand following alterations of skin inputs induced by nerve injury, skin island transfers, and experience. *Journal of Hand Therapy*, 6, 89–104.

Moisello, C., Blanco, D., Fontanesi, C., Lin, J., Biagioni, M., Kumar, P., et al. (2015). TMS enhances retention of a motor skill in Parkinson's disease. *Brain Stimulation: Basic, Translational, and Clinical Research in Neuromodulation, 8*, 224–230.

Murase, N., Duque, J., Mazzocchio, R., & Cohen, L. G. (2004). Influence of interhemispheric interactions on motor function in chronic stroke. *Annals of Neurology, 55*, 400–409.

Nielsen, J. B., & Cohen, L. G. (2008). The Olympic brain. Does corticospinal plasticity play a role in acquisition of skills required for high-performance sports? *Journal of Physiology, 586*(1), 65–70.

Nudo, R. J. (2003). Retuning the misfiring brain. *Proceedings of the National Academy of Sciences, 100*, 7425–7427.

Nudo, R. J., Wise, B. M., SiFuentes, F., & Milliken, G. W. (1996). Neural substrates for the effects of rehabilitative training on motor recovery after ischemic infarct. *Science, 272*, 1791–1794.

Penhune, V., Watanabe, D., & Savion-Lemieux, T. (2005). The effect of early musical training on adult motor performance. *Annals of the New York Academy of Sciences, 1060*, 265–268.

Penndorf, D., Witte, O. W., & Kretz, A. (2018). DNA plasticity and damage in amyotrophic lateral sclerosis. *Neural Regenerenation Research, 13*, 173–180.

Quandt, F., & Hummel, F. C. (2014). The influence of functional electrical stimulation on hand motor recovery in stroke patients: A review. *Experimental and Translational Stroke Medicine, 6*, 9.

Quentin, R., Awosika, O., & Cohen, L. G. (2019). Plasticity and recovery of function. In M. D'Esposito & J. H. Grafman (Eds.), *Handbook of clinical neurology: Vol. 163. The frontal lobes* (pp. 473–483). Elsevier.

Ramachandran, V. S., & Altschuler, E. L. (2009). The use of visual feedback, in particular mirror visual feedback, in restoring brain function. *Brain, 132*, 1693–1710.

Ransohoff, R. M. (2016). How neuroinflammation contributes to neurodegeneration. *Science, 353*, 777–783.

Schlaug, G., Benfield, A., Baird, A. E., Siewert, B., Lövblad, K. O., Parker, R. A., et al. (1999). The ischemic penumbra. *Neurology, 53*, 1528–1528.

Simons, M., Levin, J., & Dichgans, M. (2023). Tipping points in neurodegeneration. *Neuron, 111*, 2954–2968.

Soto, C., & Estrada, L. D. (2008). Protein misfolding and neurodegeneration. *Archives of Neurology, 65*, 184–189.

Staudt, M., Gerloff, C., Grodd, W., Holthausen, H., Niemann, G., & Krägeloh-Mann, I. (2004). Reorganization in congenital hemiparesis acquired at different gestational ages. *Annals of Neurolology, 56*, 854–863.

Stefanou, M.-I., Desideri, D., Belardinelli, P., Zrenner, C., & Ziemann, U. (2018). Phase synchronicity of μ-rhythm determines efficacy of interhemispheric communication between human motor cortices. *Journal of Neuroscience, 38*, 10525–10534.

Tatum, P. S., Kornbluth, J., & Soroka, A. (2023). Embolic MCA stroke treated with tPA and TICI-3 mechanical thrombectomy complicated by hemiballismus: A case study and literature review. *Military Medicine, 188*, e2738–e2740.

Tavazzi, E., Bergsland, N., Pirastru, A., Cazzoli, M., Blasi,V., & Baglio, F. (2021). MRI markers of functional connectivity and tissue microstructure in stroke-related motor rehabilitation: A systematic review. *NeuroImage: Clinical, 33*, 102931.

Tedesco Triccas, L., Meyer, S., Mantini, D., Camilleri, K., Falzon, O., Camilleri, T., & Verheyden, G. (2019). A systematic review investigating the relationship of electroencephalography and magnetoencephalography measurements with sensorimotor upper limb impairments after stroke. *Journal of Neuroscience Methods, 311*, 318–330.

Tomblin, J. B., Barker, B. A., & Hubbs, S. (2007). Developmental constraints on language development in children with cochlear implants. *International Journal of Audiology, 46*, 512–523.

Udupa, K., Bhattacharya, A., Bhardwaj, S., Pal, P. K., & Chen, R. (2022). Parkinson's disease: Alterations of motor plasticity and motor learning. In A. Quartarone, M. F. Ghilardi, & F. Boller (Eds.), *Handbook of clinical neurology: Vol. 184. Neuroplasticity from bench to bedside* (pp. 135–151) Elsevier.

VanItallie, T. B. (2019). Traumatic brain injury (TBI) in collision sports: Possible mechanisms of transformation into chronic traumatic encephalopathy (CTE). *Metabolism, 100S*, 15394.

Vargha-Khadem, F., Salmond, C. H., Watkins, K. E., Friston, K. J., Gadian, D. G., & Mishkin, M. (2003). Developmental amnesia: Effect of age at injury. *Proceedings of the National Academy of Sciences, 100*, 10055–10060.

Villamar, M. F., Portilla, A. S., Fregni, F., & Zafonte, R. (2012). Noninvasive brain stimulation to modulate neuroplasticity in traumatic brain injury. *Neuromodulation, 15*, 326–338.

Ward, N. S., & Carmichael, S. T. (2020). Blowing up neural repair for stroke recovery. *Stroke, 51*, 3169–3173.

Ward, N. S., & Cohen, L. G. (2004). Mechanisms underlying recovery of motor function after stroke. *Archives of Neurology, 61*, 1844–1848.

Werhahn, K. J., Mortensen, J., Kaelin-Lang, A., Boroojerdi, B., & Cohen, L. G. (2002). Cortical excitability changes induced by deafferentation of the contralateral hemisphere. *Brain, 125*, 1402–1413.

Werhahn, K. J., Mortensen, J., Van Boven, R. W., Zeuner, K. E., & Cohen, L. G. (2002). Enhanced tactile spatial acuity and cortical processing during acute hand deafferentation. *Nature Neuroscience, 5*, 936–938.

Wessel, M. J., Egger, P., & Hummel, F. C. (2021). Predictive models for response to non-invasive brain stimulation in stroke: A critical review of opportunities and pitfalls. *Brain Stimulation Basic Translational and Clinical Research in Neuromodulation, 14*, 1456–1466.

Xu, J., Branscheidt, M., Schambra, H., Steiner, L., Widmer, M., Diedrichsen, J., et al. (2019). Rethinking interhemispheric imbalance as a target for stroke neurorehabilitation. *Annals of Neurology, 85*, 502–513.

Yamada, K., Kinoshita, A., Kohmura, E., Sakaguchi, T., Taguchi, J., Kataoka, K., & Hayakawa, T. (1991). Basic fibroblast growth factor prevents thalamic degeneration after cortical infarction. *Journal of Cerebral Blood Flow & Metabolism, 11*, 472–478.

Zhao, Y., Zhang, X., Chen, X., & Wei, Y. (2022). Neuronal injuries in cerebral infarction and ischemic stroke: From mechanisms to treatment [Review]. *International Journal of Molecular Medicine, 49*(2), 15.

CHAPTER 9

Brain Plasticity, Cognitive Reserve, and Aging

Georgette Argiris, Christian Habeck, and Yaakov Stern

Introduction

The concept of reserve against brain damage was first introduced into the scientific community to account for the observed discrepancy between an individual's degree of brain pathology and the expected clinical manifestations of that pathology. In an early study by Katzman and colleagues (1988), 10 nursing home residents were described who, despite showing Alzheimer's disease (AD) pathology upon postmortem examination (i.e., neocortical plaques), exhibited cognitive abilities during their lifetimes that were on par with or superior to those of their healthy counterparts. It was speculated that the larger brain size and consequently greater number of neurons observed in these 10 individuals functioned as a protective factor in preserving their cognition. This was the first mention in the literature of individuals possessing greater "reserve" to mitigate cognitive decline. Katzman and colleagues asserted that "this group of patients [with incipient AD but no clinical presentation] started with more neurons and a larger brain and thus had greater reserve." However, even earlier work noticed discrepancies between the postmortem presence of senile plaques and premorbid ability (Blessed et al., 1968). The indeterminate causal relationship between senile plaques and clinical outcomes led Grünthal (1927) to conclude that there must exist qualitative and quantitative differences between dementia pathology and normal senescence.

Although these early works speculated on factors causing the observed discrepancies, formal and systematic investigation into "qualitative" and "quantitative" factors, facilitated by scientific advancements and the advent of neuroimaging, wouldn't arrive until several decades later. Through the years, the study of factors that allow some individuals to age more successfully than others has embraced more complex and nuanced research lines and methodological practices. This research expansion has also led to a system of nomenclature around observed phenomena potentially related to differential susceptibility to brain aging and disease that has often invoked disparate definitions for the same terms. To formalize operational definitions and facilitate standardized research development, a collaborative consortium recently convened to develop a consensus framework around key concepts in the resilience and reserve literature (Stern et al., 2023). These core concepts will be defined at relevant points in the chapter.

Models of Reserve

Observations from early studies, alongside observations of recovery from brain injury (Satz, 1993) and noninvasive neuroimaging of dementia patients (Stern et al., 1992), initially led researchers to hypothesize that certain individuals possess a reserve that enables them to endure the effects of cognitive aging and mitigate the cognitive impairment typically associated with brain pathology. These studies highlighted the structural properties of brain morphology—greater brain volume conferring a higher number of neurons/synapses—that could support normal cognitive functioning (Katzman, 1993; Schofield et al., 1997). In this context, reserve was conceived strictly in terms of brain reserve (BR), defined as the neurobiological status of the brain at any measured point in time, which does not involve active adaptation of functional cognitive processes in the presence of injury (Stern et al., 2023). One of the best articulated models of BR was put forth by Satz (1993), who proposed the BR capacity threshold model to explain variability in the clinical expression of brain damage severity. According to this model, once an individual exceeds a specific threshold of brain damage, clinical symptoms will appear. However, having a larger brain volume and higher neuronal count can act as a buffer against reaching this impairment threshold. Thus, two individuals with the same amount of AD brain pathology, for example, may exhibit different clinical symptoms depending on the quantity of healthy intact brain tissue. BR is considered a passive model of reserve because it only addresses the amount of damage the brain can sustain before cognitive deficits emerge. Additionally, it assumes that reserve is an additive quantity, where having more intact brain tissue provides a uniform benefit to everyone, affecting individuals in the same scalar way. While this model attempts to account for individual variability in the brain's protective benefits, it overlooks functional brain adaptability and fails to capture the intricate interplay between structure, function, and the influence of environmental and genetic factors on cognitive outcomes.

Cognitive reserve (CR) emerged from the need to better explain the observed variability in cognitive outcomes among individuals with similar levels of brain pathology, beyond a simple quantification of brain "hardware" (Stern, 2009). *Cognitive reserve* is defined as a property of the brain that allows for cognitive performance that is better than expected given the degree of life course–related brain changes and brain injury or disease (Stern et al., 2023). It is considered an active model of reserve because it describes the brain's ability to engage adaptive strategies or recruit alternative neural pathways to cope with existing brain pathology. Two individuals could possess identical BR, yet one may still be able to tolerate more pathological insult than the other before clinical impairment becomes manifest due, for example, to more efficient processing mechanisms. Thus, the critical threshold for functional impairment varies across individuals. CR encompasses a broader range of factors that include life experiences, genetics, and neural adaptability, providing a more comprehensive framework for understanding individual differences in cognitive outcomes and resilience to brain damage. Although no established indices exist to directly measure CR, it is often estimated via proxy variables that capture some of the variability in susceptibility to brain aging and disease pathology. Initial evidence for CR came from patients with probable AD, showing that among patients matched for clinical severity, those with higher education levels exhibited greater neuropathological deficits, suggesting that education may be compensating for the impact of brain pathology (Stern et al., 1992).

A longitudinal study of incident dementia revealed that individuals with higher educational and lifetime occupational attainment levels displayed lower AD risk (Stern et al., 1994). In a subsequent study, the categorization of leisure activities based on their level of social or intellectual engagement also revealed a protective effect of high engagement against developing dementia (Scarmeas et al., 2001). A systematic review examining the impact of education, occupation, premorbid IQ, and mental activities on dementia incidence found that higher CR was linked to lower dementia rates. Additionally, increased involvement in complex mental activities, even in late life, led to reduced dementia incidence in a dose-response fashion, regardless of other influencing factors (Valenzuela & Sachdev, 2006). These findings highlight the malleability of cognitive processing, indicating that accruing CR through such activities can still potentially confer protective benefits, even if initiated during late adulthood. While CR can be shaped by multiple environmental and genetic factors that can operate across the lifespan, it is essential to recognize that CR is fundamentally a property of the brain.

Neural Mechanisms of Reserve

Functional imaging studies have explored how neural networks might mediate CR. One theory for the neural implementation of CR has distinguished between the efficiency, capacity, and flexibility of existing networks (neural reserve) versus the engagement of alternative networks (neural compensation; Stern, 2009). This distinction serves to understand the different patterns of neural activity: primary networks essential for successful cognition versus secondary networks recruited when primary networks are affected by age-related inefficiency or damage.

Neural Reserve

Neural reserve refers to the preexisting brain networks that are more efficient or have a greater capacity or flexibility to resist pathological changes, best understood through those neural resources recruited in the healthy brain (Stern, 2009). These networks have developed over the lifespan through innate capacity conferred by genetics and/or life exposures, allowing for more efficient network activation or more flexible network recruitment. The instantiation of neural reserve has typically been linked to the observation of differential age-related increases in brain activation in response to task load, aligning with differences in neural efficiency and capacity. For example, a functional magnetic resonance imaging study investigating neural activation to a working memory task where task difficulty was parametrically varied found a similar pattern of activation for both younger and older adults. However, whereas younger adults expressed maximal activation of this pattern in the highest task load condition, older adults expressed similar levels of neural expression in the lowest task load, suggesting an inefficiency of neural processing (Stern et al., 2012). Moreover, these differences were not only present at the group level but were observed when tracking individual changes in expression across task load, suggesting that some individuals may display higher network efficiency or capacity when confronted with pathological change. Indeed, it has been shown that age-related atrophy modulates the relationship between engagement of identified network patterns due to age-related gray matter volume loss impacting network efficiency (Steffener et al., 2011). Additionally, network efficiency was shown to mediate the relationship between age and behavioral performance on a task of executive function (Gazes et al., 2015). Recent work has also revealed a mediation of functional network connectivity on the relationship between age and longitudinal cognitive performance on fluid intelligence, suggesting additional instantiations of neural reserve factors (Argiris et al., 2023).

Neural Compensation

Alternatively, neural compensation involves recruiting additional neural resources to "compensate" for damaged neural circuitry. An early study modeling load-related activation patterns also found that age effects on the slope of activation increase across task loads, suggesting reduced processing efficiency. However, load-related activation during the maintenance phase indicated two different processing networks that coactivated with increasing task demand, suggesting a compensatory mechanism (Zarahn et al., 2007). Importantly, both neural efficiency and compensation were conceptually grounded in behavioral performance. First, during the stimulus retention period, there was a pattern of behavior that was consistent across different age groups, showing a decrease in performance, as behavior-normalized pattern expression for load-independent processing was linked to age-related negative slopes. Second, the expression of the second pattern was near zero for young activation patterns and higher-performing older adults, suggesting greater coactivation in the face of reduced performance, and could still suggest a successful recruitment strategy relative to its theoretical absence, despite not improving cross-sectional task performance. Individual variability in the ability to compensate for the same degree of pathology, framed in the context of CR, was speculated, although not formally tested due to the lack of a brain pathology index. The identification of neural compensatory mechanisms thus does not necessarily require enhanced cognitive performance, but functions to sustain performance levels, despite aging or pathology (Stern et al., 2005).

In an early positron emission tomography (PET) study, scaled subprofile modeling was used to identify a task-related activation topography that differed maximally between younger and older adults in response to a load-related two-condition task; the correlation between change in network topography expression across these two task conditions and its relation to a CR factor was evaluated for each age group. The hypothesis was that the relationship between CR and network expression should be the same for both age groups, but a moderation effect of CR on the relationship between pattern expression and age group could shed light on potential compensatory reorganization. A directionality effect was found such that reduced network expression was observed in older adults with high CR compared with low CR and the opposite pattern observed in the younger group, suggesting that older high-CR individuals were utilizing alternative networks for optimal functioning (Stern et al., 2005).

Models of Neural Compensation

Neural compensation is a well-studied phenomenon in the literature with several models aimed at explaining how the brain adapts to age-related changes. It is important to acknowledge the contributions of these models to our understanding of the brain's coping capacities without necessarily endorsing or refuting them. The term *compensation* is often used broadly as an umbrella term to encompass various neural adaptations in response to age-related structural degeneration, including enhanced neural activation of normal pathways and alternative neural processes to maintain healthy cognition (see Bunzeck et al., 2023; Cabeza et al., 2018). It's important to note that age-related differential expression of the same neural network in younger and older adults does not align with the intended concept of neural compensation within the CR framework (Stern, 2009).

The hemispheric asymmetry reduction in older adults model first formally described the phenomenon of an age-related shift from less lateralized to more bilateral activation patterns in the prefrontal cortex to compensate for cognitive decline and/or facilitate recovery after brain damage (Cabeza, 2002). Evidence for this model has also come from studies showing that neural overrecruitment in bilateral frontoparietal regions occurs not only with aging, but also in response to increasing task demands (i.e., task load), and that this overrecruitment is linked to improved performance in tasks requiring high levels of inhibitory control (Vallesi et al., 2011). Additionally, beta-amyloid deposition, a pathological hallmark of AD, is also associated with load-dependent hyperactivation in frontoparietal regions (Oh et al., 2015). The compensation-related utilization of neural circuits hypothesis (CRUNCH) model further elaborated on these findings to focus on age-related, region-specific overactivations in addition to the "hidden" costs that result in resource depletion (Reuter-Lorenz & Mikels, 2006). It suggests that older adults recruit more neural resources at lower task demands compared with younger adults, with neural resources potentially recruited as a function of CR (Scarmeas et al., 2003). This reliance leads to quicker resource depletion, causing older adults to reach their resource limit sooner.

The arrival at this resource ceiling impacts behavioral performance, particularly at increasing levels of task demand (Reuter-Lorenz & Lustig, 2005). The CRUNCH model includes the overrecruitment of the same neural networks in both younger and older adults. This differs from the neural *compensation* framework proposed by Stern (2002) and is more aligned with neural reserve. The model suggests that different neural networks are used based on efficiency and capacity limits, serving as a generalized compensatory model.

Analogous to hemispheric "shifts" in activation via overrecruitment processes, another model has instead postulated a posterior–anterior shift in aging (PASA) that has been attributed to functional compensation to combat neurocognitive decline (Davis et al., 2008). Evidence for PASA was first found in a PET imaging study where older adults displayed weaker activity in occipitotemporal regions coupled with greater activity in frontal regions in a visual perception task (Grady et al., 1994). While several subsequent studies have reported similar findings, there has not been ubiquitous consensus for age-related frontal increases (e.g., Myrum, 2019). It has additionally been noted that age-related differences may be the result of differential age-related increases in task difficulty that exacerbate already limited cognitive resources. Davis and colleagues (2008) found what they considered pivotal compensatory validity for PASA in that, even when matching performance across age groups, they observed age-related increases in frontal activity that were both positively correlated with cognitive performance and negatively correlated with occipital activity decreases. However, more recent evidence suggests that increased prefrontal activation reflects reduced neural efficiency and/or specificity of processing, rather than compensation (Morcom & Henson, 2018). Additionally, a comparison between cross-sectional and longitudinal changes in lifespan activation patterns revealed peak increases in age-related activation in more posterior regions when examining 5-year changes (Argiris et al., 2021).

Another conceptual neural compensatory model—the scaffolding theory of aging and cognition (STAC) model—assumes that the brain naturally engages in what is termed compensatory "scaffolding" when confronted with structural alterations and consequential cognitive declines (Park & Reuter-Lorenz, 2009). This scaffolding refers to the brain's ability to utilize alternative neural circuitry to successfully perform a given task or function and is a process that is present throughout the lifespan. An increase in frontal lobe activation is considered one marker of the adaptive capacity of the brain to protect or enhance cognitive functioning. Empirical evidence has shown that task practice effects can induce remodeling of utilized brain regions and lead to longitudinal gray matter increases, even suggesting structural neuroplasticity (Ilg et al., 2008). The impetus for compensatory scaffolding is usually linked to some form of neurophysiological deterioration or neural injury. Thus, individuals with greater brain maintenance—or relative absence of changes in neural resources or neuropathological change over time as a determinant of preserved cognition in older age (Nyberg et al., 2012; Stern, 2017; Stern et al., 2023)—should require less neural reorganization. For instance, a study stratifying older adults by their ability to maintain cognitive performance over time revealed less volumetric loss in the medial temporal lobe and cingulate cortex among cognitive maintainers (Rosano et al., 2012).

With respect to brain activation, Duzel and colleagues (2011) found that a subgroup of older adults with memory performance akin to their younger counterparts had brain activation patterns akin to younger adults, indicating preserved neurobiology, rather than reliance on compensatory mechanisms. In contrast, another subgroup exhibited poorer memory and compensatory overactivation in prefrontal and parietal regions, suggesting that preserved cognition in older adults can result from either maintained neural hardware, compensatory mechanisms, or some combination of the two.

Further elaboration of STAC-r (i.e., STAC-Revised; Reuter-Lorenz & Park, 2014) integrated life course factors that could lead to the enrichment or depletion of resources relating to brain structure, function, and cognition. The original STAC model was more grounded in cross-sectional comparisons between younger and older adults, envisioned to explain intrinsic intraindividual lifespan processes that counteract structural and/or functional neural deterioration. Age was initially the primary factor of consideration, much to the exclusion of genetic, environmental, and lifestyle factors that could influence neural functioning and, consequentially, cognitive performance.

STAC-r proposes two constructs through which these factors combine to either enhance or deplete neural resources. The incorporation of lifestyle experiences into age-related cognitive ability fits well with the CR framework, where environmental factors can offset structural resource depletion via improved compensatory mechanisms, which can be further enhanced through intervention programs (Reuter-Lorenz & Park, 2014; Stern, 2013). It is important to note though that, in the CR framework, neural compensation specifically refers to the recruitment of alternative brain regions not initially engaged in successful task processing, as a response to age-related pathology. While STAC-r similarly emphasizes compensatory processes through the recruitment of additional neural circuitry, including neurogenesis, to "facilitate" compromised primary circuits, it also allows for the possibility of magnitude increases in activation and connectivity strength as a source of compensation. According to the CR framework, network efficiency would be subsumed under neural reserve.

The first construct, neural resource enrichment, highlights factors that enhance brain structure or function along two potential paths. The first pathway involves neural factors that can directly promote brain health; for example, cardiovascular fitness has been shown to have a beneficial effect on cognitive performance. This is likely due to increased blood flow that stimulates the release of brain-derived neurotrophic factor (BDNF; de Vargas et al., 2017; Erickson et al., 2013). The second pathway considers life-course enrichment factors that could indirectly promote compensatory scaffolding to offset the neural degradation and sustain healthy cognitive functioning. Support for this pathway is evident in findings that individuals with higher levels of education can tolerate greater brain pathology before cognitive decline becomes apparent compared with those with lower education (Brickman et al., 2012; Stern, 2002, 2012).

Proponents of the STAC-r model have noted that these pathways have strong parallels with the concepts of brain and CR (Barulli & Stern, 2013), respectively, where enrichment factors either sustain the underlying neural hardware or enhance the brain's "software" through adaptive strategies and coping mechanisms in the face of existing pathology. While Reuter-Lorenz and Park (2014) have also interpreted points of discrepancy with CR, it is important to note that the current formulation of CR indicates that it can be influenced by multiple genetic and environmental factors that can potentially operate at various points or continuously across the lifespan (Stern et al., 2023). Potential developmental origins (e.g., genetics) and lifelong utility are both integrated into its framework, with mechanisms of CR characterized via biological or cognitive-experimental approaches.

The second construct, neural resource depletion, refers to factors that have negative effects on the brain and cognition. For example, individuals carrying the epsilon-4 allele of the apolipoprotein E gene (ApoE4) tend to display lower cognitive performance and higher conversion rates to AD compared with noncarriers (Reitz & Mayeux, 2010). Additionally, the presence of amyloid and tau positivity, as detected by PET, has been associated with higher rates of cognitive decline, even among clinically cognitively unimpaired individuals (Ossenkoppele et al., 2022). Other factors that can contribute to cognitive decline include vascular issues, genetic predispositions, and environmental influences (see Reuter-Lorenz & Park, 2014). A recent review by Oosterhuis and colleagues (2023) aimed to delineate the overlap and divergence between the CR and STAC-r theories of cognitive aging. One major focus of proposed divergence is on the integration of adverse life effects in the engagement of compensatory strategies. One presented example is the relationship between cortical thinning and reductions in working memory (WM) performance that is moderated by the brain's capacity for dopamine synthesis (Ciampa et al., 2022). In this study, higher levels of dopamine synthesis capacity mitigated the impact of cortical atrophy on WM decline. The relationship between cortical thinning, or more generally, intraindividual differences in cortical thickness and aging, is a well-established finding in the literature and an essential element of the CR framework.

Although cortical thickness tends to decline throughout the lifespan (Fjell et al., 2015), studies have shown that preserved cortical thickness in older individuals is closely associated with better WM performance (Burzynska et al., 2012). Among older adults ages 70 to 100, better performance on WM and other executive tasks was associated with preserved regional cortical thickness, particularly in the cingulate cortex (Dominguez et al., 2021). This suggests that certain brain regions may be more susceptible to the effects of aging. Another longitudinal study found that aging is linked to accelerated changes in the temporal and occipital cortices, along with decelerating changes in the prefrontal and anterior cingulate cortices (Storsve et al., 2014). The findings from a multivariate principal component regression analysis also revealed that education is associated with regional cortical thickness, displaying a robust pattern of both negative and positive loadings across several right-sided brain regions (Habeck et al., 2020). It is a rather simple conceptual shift from emphasizing deleterious factors linked to cortical thinning and relating life course–related brain changes to protective factors that impact cognitive outcomes (Stern et al., 2023). The crux of the CR hypothesis is to identify CR measures that can moderate the relationship between brain changes, which might be more severe for some individuals and less for others, and cognitive changes over time. Additionally, adverse life events can be subsumed under risk factors that impact brain health.

Plasticity and Reserve

The CR–BR Distinction

Although CR and BR were established as distinct concepts, evidence suggests that a strict delineation between the two may at times be challenging. As CR is a brain-mediated process, the difference between these two forms of reserve necessarily lies at the level of analysis. BR involves the neurobiological status of the brain via a quantification of brain matter (e.g., neuronal count, synaptic density, etc.). CR, on the other hand, implies variability at the level of synaptic organization and brain regional recruitment as an active adaptation of functional cognitive processes to help cope with or compensate for brain changes, injury, or disease. Factors that are associated with greater CR may also confer a direct benefit on the amount of BR at a given point. Thus, it is likely a misguided endeavor to isolate variables that uniquely and strictly relate to either CR or BR.

In a randomized controlled trial, aerobic exercise training resulted in approximately 2% increases in hippocampal volume, which was linked to greater serum levels of BDNF, a key mediator of neurogenesis in the dentate gyrus; moreover, these increases were linked to improvements in spatial memory (Erickson et al., 2011). BDNF plays an important role in brain plasticity by mediating changes in cortical thickness and synaptic density. It is particularly responsive to acute physical activity and related to WM performance (Håkansson et al., 2017). Physical exercise has even been linked to enhanced hippocampal neurogenesis and learning in older mice (van Praag et al., 2005).

Evidence has also demonstrated that physical exercise boosts both BDNF and serotonin (5-hydroxytryptamine [5-HT]) systems, leading to an increase in mature hippocampal CA1 neurons and better cognitive function (Pietrelli et al., 2018). Serotonin also plays a modulatory role in stress and depression and can be a neural marker for memory deficits. The direct causal pathways between factors that exclusively contribute to brain or CR can be extremely complex if not impossible. Recent research has shown that while BR and CR are formalized as independent processes, BR can influence whether and how CR can be utilized. The relationship between CR and its associated network expression is modulated by the level of BR available (Coors et al., 2024).

In addition to aerobic physical exercise, dietary intake of omega-3 fatty acids has been positively linked to greater gray matter volume of corticolimbic regions (Conklin et al., 2007). Cross-sectional volumetric differences have been linked to intellectual stimulation (Coffey et al., 1999), with education providing a protective effect on regional gray matter volume in the presence age-related declines (Boller et al., 2017). Longitudinal changes in gray matter volume in response to training have also been observed at different time scales and developmental periods. For instance, young adults who learned to juggle over a 3-month period displayed transient bilateral expansion in gray matter in specific motor-selective regions, supporting learning-induced cortical plasticity (Draganski et al., 2004). Musical training over a 15-month period in early childhood was linked to structural brain changes in motor and auditory areas critical to instrumental training, which was also correlated with enhanced performance on musical tests (Hyde et al., 2009). In a study of London trainee taxi drivers over a 4-year learning period, qualifying as a driver was associated with volume increases in the posterior hippocampus and changes to their memory profiles (Woollett & Maguire, 2011).

Recent studies have also suggested that memory training can lead to equivalent increases in hippocampal volume in both younger and older adults (Bråthen et al., 2022). Memory training among older adults has also been linked to changes in white matter microstructures that are related to improved performance (Engvig et al., 2012). A subsequent study found that these changes in white matter microstructures and memory improvements were evident in older but not in younger groups, even when training programs were titrated to individual performance levels (de Lange et al., 2017). This suggests that white matter integrity may be a marker for cognitive plasticity, specifically in older adults (de Lange et al., 2016).

Cognitive Training and Enhancement

The notion that the brain can undergo plasticity, leading to cognitive improvements, relies on the assumption that cognitive performance is mutable throughout the lifespan. Several studies have investigated the effects of playing cognitive-engaging games on complex skill acquisition. For instance, training on a complex video game designed to explore different learning strategies led to improvements on an executive control task (Stern et al., 2011). Another study found evidence for improved memory performance after working memory training in a group of older adults (Buschkuehl et al., 2008). The extent to which cognitive training is transferable across cognitive domains may be dependent on the similarity between trained and untrained tasks, the inherent hierarchical structure within cognitive abilities, the temporal window of study, and the life stage (for a review, see Noack et al., 2014). While the benefits of memory training on a specific task were sustained among both younger and older adults over a 3-year period, only younger adults displayed transfer effects to a nontargeted memory task (Bråthen et al., 2022).

A recent meta-analysis compared the effect of single- versus multiple-component training, which targets one or multiple cognitive abilities, respectively, in both healthy aging and mild cognitive impairment (MCI; Basak et al., 2020). They found that both groups showed comparable cognitive improvements on both trained and untrained skills, which also extended to everyday functioning. Additionally, the multicomponent training condition demonstrated more generalized effects. In contrast, the impact of single-component training depended on the training domain; executive function training showed similar effects on both near and far transfer, while only processing speed training improved everyday functioning. Moreover, healthy older adults with lower educational attainment displayed greater cognitive gains from cognitive training, regardless of the training module. The authors suggest that healthy older adults with less educational attainment may be able to recover fluid abilities through cognitive training and consequentially lower the risk of conversion to MCI or AD. Previous research has demonstrated that training effects are dependent on the amount of practice and can generalize from complex working memory task demands to improvements in fluid intelligence ability (Jaeggi et al., 2008).

Theoretical Framework of Plasticity

The research described presents an intricate relationship between cognitive training and structural brain changes, which is further complicated by factors that influence individual capacities for enhancement and plasticity, at both the cognitive and functional level. This intricacy also has implications for the distinction between BR and CR, particularly in terms of their relationship with brain plasticity. Lövdén and colleagues (2010) defined a conceptual framework to address the pervasive use of the term *plasticity* as applied to any changes in brain or behavior, emphasizing the need to clarify its specific characteristics. They posit that the driving force for plasticity is not the primary changes in the system itself (e.g., brain injury, cognitive training), but the secondary reactive response of the brain's ability to compensate and restore for injury or meet changing cognitive demands. Pivotal to this reactive response is the brain's current functional supply, or the limits in its capacity for adaptation. Flexibility refers to the brain's ability to optimize its performance within the current structural and functional constraints, allowing it to dynamically represent and process different environmental stimuli by reconfiguring existing neural activity patterns. It emphasizes the brain's inherent capacity to shift between different states of activity, depending on the stimuli it encounters, thus maintaining optimal functioning, despite varying challenges. However, it is argued that this flexibility does not signify *plasticity* per se but rather constitutes the initial stage for plasticity. When cognitive and functional reactions rely on flexibility, they use existing resources. In contrast, reactions based on plasticity depend on changes to functional supply and structural alterations.

The catalyst for true plasticity is a prolonged mismatch between the functional supply of the system and the environmental demands, resulting in enduring changes to how the brain functions or processes information. Plasticity can alter mental representations themselves, or the processes that manipulate and alter those representations. Cognitive aging is attributed to negative changes in functional supply, such as declines in gray matter (Fjell et al., 2015) and white matter microstructures (Cox et al., 2016) and reductions in neurotransmitter concentrations, such as dopamine (Kaasinen & Rinne, 2002), and cerebrovascular health (Zimmerman et al., 2021) that are associated with reduced processing efficiency. This impacts both existing knowledge and the acquisition of new information. Distinguishing between knowledge- versus process-based alterations can help determine whether phenomena such as increased prefrontal activation and cognitive training gains reflect true plastic changes in the brain. For example, it is theorized that rapid changes in activation patterns are likely due to the brain's flexible engagement without any accompanying structural changes that would necessitate a longer time lag. Similarly, cognitive training-induced performance increases could reflect knowledge-based mnemonic strategies or updated response mappings that do not reflect a true change in processing and efficiency underlying the generalizability of cognitive training gains. Even if there are reported increases in gray matter volume, these effects may only be temporary, as the brain's posttraining functional capacity may not match with environmental demands, resulting in the reduction of excess functional capacity over time.

Ultimately, it is argued that plastic alterations in processing may occur only through prolonged supply–demand mismatches, such as those related to neural compensatory mechanisms, and are the result of macro- or micro-level structural brain changes. Structural changes may include processes such as neurogenesis and gliogenesis, especially in the hippocampus (Kempermann et al., 2015; Moreno-Jiménez et al., 2021), long-term potentiation between neurons (Abraham et al., 2019), synaptogenesis reflecting increases in dendritic and axonal growth (for a review, see Qi et al., 2022), and changes in myelination (for a review, see Sampaio-Baptista & Johansen-Berg, 2017). A large body of work from animal studies has shown that the morphology of neurons in the hippocampus and prefrontal cortex is particularly susceptible to age-related declines. One potential target for intervention to regulate long-term potentiation in these regions is the concentration of calcium ions (Burke & Barnes, 2006).

Additionally, it has been suggested that age-related cognitive decline is, at least in part, linked to decline and impairment of neuroglia; as the primary defense mechanism of the central nervous system, they arguably play a fundamental role in the brain's resilience and reserve capacities via multiple pathways (Verkhratsky & Zorec, 2024). Both animal and human work have demonstrated that the deleterious effects of brain aging, such as atrophy and reduced functionality of astrocytes and microglia, can potentially be reversed via environmental enrichment and dietary changes (Augusto-Oliveira & Verkhratsky, 2021).

Neural Dynamics and Plasticity

In the plasticity framework, neural compensation is viewed as a process-based mechanism of functional reorganization that may explain changes in cognitive ability (Barulli & Stern, 2013). It occurs when primary task-related networks are affected by pathology or age-related changes, prompting the recruitment of additional compensatory networks to carry out the same task. However, whether compensation is the result of neural rewiring of primary networks or simply mistaken for the flexibility of activity within preexisting networks is best clarified through longitudinal studies that employ a multimodal approach to measure both micro- and macro-level brain changes. Morphological changes in the aging brain include differential rates of regional atrophy in cortical thickness and surface area, with some studies reporting decelerating changes in the prefrontal cortex relative to the occipitotemporal regions (Strosve et al., 2014). Additionally, higher cortical thickness has been found in anterior cingulate and prefrontal regions among high-performing older adults (Harrison et al., 2018; Sun et al., 2016). Given models suggesting age-related shifts or increased prefrontal cortex activation as possible compensatory activity, it is essential to link neural activity to underlying brain structures. This link should be grounded in intra-individual differences in cognitive ability and CR mechanisms that may provide differential coping capacities to negative age-related changes.

Evidence for neural compensation has also been supported by examining the relationship between structural changes and functional connectivity from resting-state analysis (rsFC). In a study investigating age-related cortical thinning, reductions in functional amplitude of low-frequency fluctuations (fALFF), and altered rsFC, researchers found a co-localization between age-related declines in cortical thickness and fALFF, as well as a mixed pattern of association between regional atrophy and functional connectivity (FC) strength (Vieira et al., 2020). Notably, they observed an increase in connectivity in highly atrophic frontal regions, alongside a general age-related decline in connectivity magnitude, with several connections shifting from negative to positive. These findings were interpreted as reflecting compensatory scaffolding alongside dedifferentiation of processing, respectively, whereby the latter typically reflects a loss of neural specificity due to a decline in dopaminergic neuromodulation (Li et al., 2001).

Another study examined the impact of cognitive training on rsFC and reported posttraining increases in functional network integration; these changes were more similar to the pretraining patterns observed in younger adults and were further correlated with levels of educational attainment (Deng et al., 2019). Cognitive training has also been linked to increases in cerebral blood flow and rsFC, particularly within the default mode and central executive networks. This suggests enhanced neurovascular coupling that correlates with cognitive improvements (Chapman et al., 2015). In a recent review, Nguyen and colleagues (2019) examined the effect of cognitive training in three core executive functioning domains on cognitive and neural enhancements. Although functional changes varied across studies, a notable trend emerged, indicating increased subcortical activation and decreased frontoparietal activation. This suggests that training might reduce the brain's reliance on compensatory neural mechanisms. Both rsFC studies that were reviewed reported training-related increases between the right hippocampus and left superior temporal gyrus, in addition to cerebral blood flow increases within the right inferior frontal cortex (Lampit et al., 2015; Mozolic et al., 2010). Interestingly, the left inferior frontal cortex is considered a candidate region for CR given its association with more beneficial network structure and relationship with education (Franzmeier et al., 2018).

In addition to cognitive training studies, other research has investigated the neural underpinnings of cognitive flexibility using a dynamic FC approach. Dynamic FC employs specific methodologies to capture how spontaneous fluctuations in the brain change and covary over time, revealing how brain networks dynamically reconfigure to produce different brain states. Transitions between different brain states, characterized by distinct connectivity patterns, are then tracked and linked to various cognitive processes or responses to external stimuli. The brain's ability to rapidly switch between different connectivity states is considered crucial for flexible cognitive functioning and adapting to changing environmental demands (for a review, see Calhoun et al., 2014). A study of dynamic FC among older adults found that greater temporal similarity in FC and more robust switching patterns between different FC states were associated with better cognitive performance (Cabral et al., 2017). Finally, evidence suggests that neural flexibility, as measured by the number of times a network's node changes network assignment over a given time window, is more robust at predicting age-related cognitive outcomes when measured during task performance rather than rest (Varangis et al., 2022). While these latter studies do not directly relate to neural plasticity, they highlight the brain's potential for flexible network engagement.

Additionally, flexible neural engagement can also be observed in task activation patterns. For example, a "task-invariant network" whose expression relates to IQ that has been observed during disparate task performance could help preserve cognitive performance in the face of aging or disease (Stern et al., 2018). Notably though, derivations of these patterns have occurred at the group level, reflecting shared variance in neural activation, where an individual's degree of pattern expression moderates the relationship between brain status and cognitive outcome. Any pattern derived from shared variance inherently constrains the ability to capture individual variability in the flexible engagement of neural resources. However, the idea that a domain-general network may serve as a compensatory mechanism to off-load high neural demands of specific cognitive processes has been endorsed by the STAC-r model (Reuter-Lorenz & Park, 2014).

Plasticity and CR

The theoretical framework for cognitive plasticity proposed by Lövdén and colleagues (2010) aimed to discern whether the benefits of enriched lifestyle could induce enduring positive effects akin to plasticity, countering the negative effects of age and other factors on cognition. Within this framework, CR plays a crucial role in determining individual differences in the intrinsic potential for plasticity in the system. An individual's current level of flexibility, influenced by both genetic and environmental factors, will determine whether a supply–demand mismatch will occur and if it is sufficient to trigger plasticity. For example, if an individual with low functional supply is faced with a demanding working memory task outside of their capacity limits, an appropriate mismatch may not occur because the potential for change is insufficient.

Functional capacity is likely influenced by CR factors that enhance an individual's capacity to manage a wider range of environmental demands and increase the efficiency or flexibility of functional brain networks (Stern et al., 2020). A wealth of data from both observational and epidemiological studies supports the idea that various modifiable lifestyle factors such as physical activity, diet, sleep, and cognitive leisure activity may benefit cognitive function and promote higher CR. For instance, recent work has demonstrated a protective effect of high engagement in leisure activity on cognitive trajectories over a 5-year period (Simon et al., 2023). Traditionally, studies have used proxies of CR, the most common being education, general IQ, and occupational attainment to investigate the moderating role of CR on the association between brain pathology and cognitive outcomes (for a review, see Song et al., 2022). Another recent study revealed that both IQ and education moderated 5-year changes in fluid reasoning and processing speed, respectively (Gazes et al., 2023).

Another more direct measure of CR involves extracting model residuals of cognition after adjusting for structural brain and demographic factors. This residual reserve variable was associated with lower probability of dementia conversion and less decline in language abilities over a 3-year interval (Zahodne et al., 2013). In addition, unexplained variance has been associated with both education and IQ (Habeck et al., 2017). However, while this is an attractive statistical technique amenable to the CR framework, it should be approached with caution. First, it is not ideal given the typically high amount of unexplained variance in a model. Second, ordinary least squares regression models inherently create a positive correlation between the residuals and the dependent variable (in this case, cognition) due to their mathematical properties (Elman et al., 2022; Habeck et al., 2017). Given evidence suggesting positive effects of life course exposures on increased CR against age-related or disease-related pathology, cognitive intervention may be a useful tool for successful aging. However, rather than focusing on enhancing any one cognitive function, the goal should be to increase reserve, which may impart a domain-general functional supply in adapting to age- and disease-related brain change. The optimal strategy should encompass multiple lifestyle targets of intervention sustained over an extended period to enable genuine plastic change. While measurements of CR attempt to quantify the magnitude of its impact on cognitive outcomes, capturing CR in action through intervention studies is a complementary and necessary process.

Conclusion

In our current review, we have only covered the tip of the iceberg of the research related to CR, cognitive enhancement, and the brain's capacity for plasticity, with particular focus on the aging brain. For instance, we only briefly mention AD as an endpoint in the continuum from healthy to pathological aging; however, there is extensive literature on this topic (Groot et al., 2018; Menardi et al., 2018; Nelson et al., 2021). Additional work in the field of plasticity has addressed recovery from traumatic brain injury, lesion burden, and stroke patients. In cases of traumatic brain injury, the extent of recovery may depend on how well reserve factors might mitigate neuronal loss and facilitate compensation, thereby enhancing the brain's natural reparative and redundancy mechanisms (Bigler & Stern, 2015). For stroke patients, some studies have advocated for a shift in rehabilitation approaches, moving away from methods that focus on functional compensation toward those that promote neuronal regeneration and neuroplasticity via electromechanical training, virtual reality technology, and brain stimulation (Aderinto et al., 2023; Grefkes & Fink, 2020). Even in healthy adults, repetitive transcranial magnetic, electric, and deep brain stimulation, despite operating at different time scales and focal localization, have all shown indirect signs of neuroplasticity. This is evidenced by changes in brain signal amplitude and behavioral outcomes (Kricheldorff et al., 2022). Thus, enhancing alternative pathways through brain stimulation may offer a promising approach.

To effectively study plasticity, it is essential to agree on the best research practices and have clear definitions of what plasticity is and what it is not. As previously mentioned, a collaborative research consortium convened to develop a consensus framework around key concepts for studying resilience and reserve literature, aiming to set guidelines for future research (Stern et al., 2023). Lövdén and colleagues (2010) also attempted to create such a framework for plasticity, offering a critical perspective on studies claiming plastic gains and providing research principles for evaluating evidence for cognitive plasticity. However, as they point out, the issue is complex and multifaceted. To understand how an individual's cognitive abilities change over the lifespan, we need to consider the interaction of various factors, such as age-related cognitive decline, genetic and environmental factors, processing efficiency, and critically, CR factors that affect the potential for change. While greater CR may enhance an individual's current flexibility, the exact factors that trigger the shift from flexibility to plasticity remain unclear.

Evidence for neural plasticity demonstrates that it can operate at the level of BR by increasing the neurobiological status of the brain or CR by enabling the utilization of alternative networks when primary networks are challenged, as indicated by neural compensation. It is challenging to determine the order of processing to assess the independent contributions of reserve to plasticity. For instance, while CR and brain maintenance, defined as the relative absence of changes in neural resources or neuropathological change over time, are both correlated with education and IQ, they are orthogonal concepts with little relation to one another (Habeck et al., 2017). The catalyst behind gains in "hardware" is unclear. Additionally, this relationship is further complicated by the small but significant correlation between IQ, a proxy for CR, and brain volume (McDaniel, 2005).

Finally, some additional unanswered questions remain. To what extent is the accumulation of CR a finite resource, limited by physiological constraints, and how do protective and risk factors influence its development and expression? Similarly, does the use (and potential overuse) of the same neural pathways naturally lead to decay in processing over time beyond structural degeneration? Given that there is no definitive upper bound for the brain's processing capacities, predicting how multiple factors impact an individual's cognitive and neural profile is challenging. Is an individual's ability to accumulate CR constant throughout the lifespan, or does it change over time? What factors affect this ability, such as specific life experiences that may have depleted cognitive resources during critical periods? Do the factors contributing to CR produce additive benefits, or do they interact in a way that synergistically enhances CR? Future work will need to implement a common framework for the principles that constitute neural plasticity and how CR factors causally enhance the capacity for plastic change.

In the current chapter, we discussed key concepts in the resilience and reserve framework formally defined by the recent collaborative research consortium (Stern et al., 2023). Our aim was to briefly explain the possible links between CR, cognitive enhancement, and neural plasticity. A substantial body of research supports the idea that the brain can make adaptive changes throughout the lifespan, and these changes can be harnessed through targeted lifestyle interventions to reduce age-related declines in neural and cognitive functioning. While this work does not provide an exhaustive list of how CR can promote plasticity, we hope it offers a comprehensive overview of significant trends in the field.

REFERENCES

Abraham, W. C., Jones, O. D., & Glanzman, D. L. (2019). Is plasticity of synapses the mechanism of long-term memory storage? *NPJ Science of Learning, 4*(1), 9.

Aderinto, N., AbdulBasit, M. O., Olatunji, G., & Adejumo, T. (2023). Exploring the transformative influence of neuroplasticity on stroke rehabilitation: A narrative review of current evidence. *Annals of Medicine and Surgery, 85*(9), 4425–4432.

Argiris, G., Stern, Y., & Habeck, C. (2021). Quantifying age-related changes in brain and behavior: A longitudinal versus cross-sectional approach. *Eneuro, 8*(4).

Argiris, G., Stern, Y., Lee, S., Ryu, H., & Habeck, C. (2023). Simple topological task-based functional connectivity features predict longitudinal behavioral change of fluid reasoning in the RANN cohort. *NeuroImage, 277*, 120237.

Augusto-Oliveira, M., & Verkhratsky, A. (2021). Lifestyle-dependent microglial plasticity: Training the brain guardians. *Biology Direct, 16*(1), 12.

Barulli, D., & Stern, Y. (2013). Efficiency, capacity, compensation, maintenance, plasticity: Emerging concepts in cognitive reserve. *Trends in Cognitive Sciences, 17*(10), 502–509.

Basak, C., Qin, S., & O'Connell, M. A. (2020). Differential effects of cognitive training modules in healthy aging and mild cognitive impairment: A comprehensive meta-analysis of randomized controlled trials. *Psychology and Aging, 35*(2), 220.

Bigler, E. D., & Stern, Y. (2015). Traumatic brain injury and reserve. In J. Grafman & A. M. Salazar (Eds.), *Handbook of clinical neurology: Vol. 128. Traumatic brain injury, part II* (pp. 691–710). Elsevier.

Blessed, G., Tomlinson, B. E., & Roth, M. (1968). The association between quantitative measures of dementia and of senile change in the cerebral grey matter of elderly subjects. *British Journal of Psychiatry, 114*(512), 797–811.

Boller, B., Mellah, S., Ducharme-Laliberté, G., & Belleville, S. (2017). Relationships between years of education, regional grey matter volumes, and working memory-related brain activity in healthy older adults. *Brain Imaging and Behavior, 11*, 304–317.

Bråthen, A. C. S., Sørensen, Ø., De Lange, A. M. G., Mowinckel, A. M., Fjell, A. M., & Walhovd, K. B. (2022). Cognitive and hippocampal changes weeks and years after memory training. *Scientific Reports, 12*(1), 7877.

Brickman, A. M., Meier, I. B., Korgaonkar, M. S., Provenzano, F. A., Grieve, S. M., Siedlecki, K. L., et al. (2012). Testing the white matter retrogenesis hypothesis of cognitive aging. *Neurobiology of Aging, 33*(8), 1699–1715.

Bunzeck, N., Steiger, T. K., Krämer, U. M., Luedtke, K., Marshall, L., Obleser, J., & Tune, S. (2023). Trajectories and contributing factors of neural compensation in healthy and pathological aging. *Neuroscience & Biobehavioral Reviews*, 105489.

Burke, S. N., & Barnes, C. A. (2006). Neural plasticity in the ageing brain. *Nature Reviews Neuroscience, 7*(1), 30–40.

Burzynska, A. Z., Nagel, I. E., Preuschhof, C., Gluth, S., Bäckman, L., Li, S. C., et al. (2012). Cortical thickness is linked to executive functioning in adulthood and aging. *Human Brain Mapping, 33*(7), 1607–1620.

Buschkuehl, M., Jaeggi, S. M., Hutchison, S., Perrig-Chiello, P., Däpp, C., Müller, M., et al. (2008). Impact of working memory training on memory performance in old-old adults. *Psychology and Aging, 23*(4), 743.

Cabeza, R. (2002). Hemispheric asymmetry reduction in older adults: The HAROLD model. *Psychology and Aging, 17*(1), 85–100.

Cabeza, R., Albert, M., Belleville, S., Craik, F. I., Duarte, A., Grady, C. L., et al. (2018). Maintenance, reserve and compensation: The cognitive neuroscience of healthy ageing. *Nature Reviews Neuroscience, 19*(11), 701–710.

Cabral, J., Vidaurre, D., Marques, P., Magalhães, R., Silva Moreira, P., Miguel Soares, J., et al. (2017). Cognitive performance in healthy older adults relates to spontaneous switching between states of functional connectivity during rest. *Scientific Reports, 7*(1), 5135.

Calhoun, V. D., Miller, R., Pearlson, G., & Adalı, T. (2014). The chronnectome: Time-varying connectivity networks as the next frontier in fMRI data discovery. *Neuron, 84*(2), 262–274.

Chapman, S. B., Aslan, S., Spence, J. S., Hart Jr., J. J., Bartz, E. K., Didehbani, N., et al. (2015). Neural mechanisms of brain plasticity with complex cognitive training in healthy seniors. *Cerebral Cortex, 25*(2), 396–405.

Ciampa, C. J., Parent, J. H., Lapoint, M. R., Swinnerton, K. N., Taylor, M. M., Tennant, V.

R., et al. (2022). Elevated dopamine synthesis as a mechanism of cognitive resilience in aging. *Cerebral Cortex, 32*(13), 2762–2772.

Coffey, C. E., Saxton, J. A., Ratcliff, G., Bryan, R. N., & Lucke, J. F. (1999). Relation of education to brain size in normal aging: Implications for the reserve hypothesis. *Neurology, 53*(1), 189–189.

Conklin, S. M., Gianaros, P. J., Brown, S. M., Yao, J. K., Hariri, A. R., Manuck, S. B., & Muldoon, M. F. (2007). Long-chain omega-3 fatty acid intake is associated positively with corticolimbic gray matter volume in healthy adults. *Neuroscience Letters, 421*(3), 209–212.

Coors, A., Lee, S., Gazes, Y., Gacheru, M., Habeck, C., & Stern, Y. (2024). Brain reserve affects the expression of cognitive reserve networks. *Human Brain Mapping, 45*(5), e26658.

Cox, S. R., Ritchie, S. J., Tucker-Drob, E. M., Liewald, D. C., Hagenaars, S. P., Davies, G., et al. (2016). Ageing and brain white matter structure in 3,513 UK Biobank participants. *Nature Communications, 7*(1), 13629.

Davis, S. W., Dennis, N. A., Daselaar, S. M., Fleck, M. S., & Cabeza, R. (2008). Que PASA? The posterior–anterior shift in aging. *Cerebral Cortex, 18*(5), 1201–1209.

de Lange, A. M. G., Bråthen, A. C. S., Grydeland, H., Sexton, C., Johansen-Berg, H., Andersson, J. L., et al. (2016). White matter integrity as a marker for cognitive plasticity in aging. *Neurobiology of Aging, 47*, 74–82.

de Lange, A. M. G., Bråthen, A. C. S., Rohani, D. A., Grydeland, H., Fjell, A. M., & Walhovd, K. B. (2017). The effects of memory training on behavioral and microstructural plasticity in young and older adults. *Human Brain Mapping, 38*(11), 5666–5680.

Deng, L., Cheng, Y., Cao, X., Feng, W., Zhu, H., Jiang, L., et al. (2019). The effect of cognitive training on the brain's local connectivity organization in healthy older adults. *Scientific Reports, 9*(1), 9033.

de Vargas, L. D. S., das Neves, B. H. S., Roehrs, R., Izquierdo, I., & Mello-Carpes, P. (2017). One-single physical exercise session after object recognition learning promotes memory persistence through hippocampal noradrenergic mechanisms. *Behavioural Brain Research, 329*, 120–126.

Dominguez, E. N., Stark, S. M., Ren, Y., Corrada, M. M., Kawas, C. H., & Stark, C. E. (2021). Regional cortical thickness predicts top cognitive performance in the elderly. *Frontiers in Aging Neuroscience*, 758.

Draganski, B., Gaser, C., Busch, V., Schuierer, G., Bogdahn, U., & May, A. (2004). Changes in grey matter induced by training. *Nature, 427*, 311–312.

Duzel, E., Schutze, H., Yonelinas, A. P., & Heinze, H. J. (2011). Functional phenotyping of successful aging in long-term memory: Preserved performance in the absence of neural compensation. *Hippocampus, 21*(8), 803–814.

Elman, J. A., Vogel, J. W., Bocancea, D. I., Ossenkoppele, R., van Loenhoud, A. C., Tu, X. M., et al. (2022). Issues and recommendations for the residual approach to quantifying cognitive resilience and reserve. *Alzheimer's Research & Therapy, 14*(1), 102.

Engvig, A., Fjell, A. M., Westlye, L. T., Moberget, T., Sundseth, Ø., Larsen, V. A., & Walhovd, K. B. (2012). Memory training impacts short-term changes in aging white matter: A longitudinal diffusion tensor imaging study. *Human Brain Mapping, 33*(10), 2390–2406.

Erickson, K. I., Banducci, S. E., Weinstein, A. M., MacDonald III, A. W., Ferrell, R. E., Halder, I., et al. (2013). The brain-derived neurotrophic factor Val66Met polymorphism moderates an effect of physical activity on working memory performance. *Psychological Science, 24*(9), 1770–1779.

Erickson, K. I., Voss, M. W., Prakash, R. S., Basak, C., Szabo, A., Chaddock, L., et al. (2011).

Exercise training increases size of hippocampus and improves memory. *Proceedings of the National Academy of Sciences, 108*(7), 3017–3022.

Fjell, A. M., Grydeland, H., Krogsrud, S. K., Amlien, I., Rohani, D. A., Ferschmann, L., et al. (2015). Development and aging of cortical thickness correspond to genetic organization patterns. *Proceedings of the National Academy of Sciences, 112*(50), 15462–15467.

Franzmeier, N., Hartmann, J., Taylor, A. N., Araque-Caballero, M. Á., Simon-Vermot, L., Kambeitz-Ilankovic, L., et al. (2018). The left frontal cortex supports reserve in aging by enhancing functional network efficiency. *Alzheimer's Research & Therapy, 10*, 1–12.

Gazes, Y., Habeck, C., O'Shea, D, Razlighi, Q. R., Steffener, J., & Stern, Y. (2015). Functional network mediates age-related differences in reaction time: A replication and extension study. *Brain and Behavior, 5*(5), e00324.

Gazes, Y., Lee, S., Fang, Z., Mensing, A., Noofoory, D., Hidalgo Nazario, G., et al. (2023). Effects of brain maintenance and cognitive reserve on age-related decline in three cognitive abilities. *Journals of Gerontology: Series B, 78*(8), 1284–1293.

Grady, C. L., Maisog, J. M., Horwitz, B., Ungerleider, L. G., Mentis, M. J., Salerno, J. A., et al. (1994). Age-related changes in cortical blood flow activation during visual processing of faces and location. *Journal of Neuroscience, 14*(3), 1450–1462.

Grefkes, C., & Fink, G. R. (2020). Recovery from stroke: Current concepts and future perspectives. *Neurological Research and Practice, 2*(1), 17.

Groot, C., van Loenhoud, A. C., Barkhof, F., van Berckel, B. N., Koene, T., Teunissen, C. C., et al. (2018). Differential effects of cognitive reserve and brain reserve on cognition in Alzheimer disease. *Neurology, 90*(2), e149–e156.

Grünthal, E. (1927). Klinisch-anatomisch vergleichende Untersuchungen über den Greisenblödsinn. *Zeitschrift für die gesampte Neurologie und Psychiatrie, 111*, 763–818.

Habeck, C., Gazes, Y., Razlighi, Q., & Stern, Y. (2020). Cortical thickness and its associations with age, total cognition and education across the adult lifespan. *PLOS ONE, 15*(3), e0230298.

Habeck, C., Razlighi, Q., Gazes, Y., Barulli, D., Steffener, J., & Stern, Y. (2017). Cognitive reserve and brain maintenance: Orthogonal concepts in theory and practice. *Cerebral Cortex, 27*(8), 3962–3969.

Håkansson, K., Ledreux, A., Daffner, K., Terjestam, Y., Bergman, P., Carlsson, R., et al. (2017). BDNF responses in healthy older persons to 35 minutes of physical exercise, cognitive training, and mindfulness: Associations with working memory function. *Journal of Alzheimer's Disease, 55*(2), 645–657.

Harrison, T. M., Maass, A., Baker, S. L., & Jagust, W. J. (2018). Brain morphology, cognition, and μ-amyloid in older adults with superior memory performance. *Neurobiology of Aging, 67*, 162–170.

Hyde, K. L., Lerch, J., Norton, A., Forgeard, M., Winner, E., Evans, A. C., & Schlaug, G. (2009). Musical training shapes structural brain development. *Journal of Neuroscience, 29*(10), 3019–3025.

Ilg, R., Wohlschläger, A. M., Gaser, C., Liebau, Y., Dauner, R., Wöller, A., et al. (2008). Gray matter increase induced by practice correlates with task-specific activation: A combined functional and morphometric magnetic resonance imaging study. *Journal of Neuroscience, 28*(16), 4210–4215.

Jaeggi, S. M., Buschkuehl, M., Jonides, J., & Perrig, W. J. (2008). Improving fluid intelligence with training on working memory. *Proceedings of the National Academy of Sciences, 105*(19), 6829–6833.

Kaasinen, V., & Rinne, J. O. (2002). Functional imaging studies of dopamine system and cognition in normal aging and Parkinson's disease. *Neuroscience & Biobehavioral Reviews, 26*(7), 785–793.

Katzman, R. (1993). Education and the prevalence of dementia and Alzheimer's disease. *Neurology, 43*(1), 13–20.

Katzman, R., Terry, R., DeTeresa, R., Brown T., Davies P., Fuld P., et al. (1988). Clinical, pathological, and neurochemical changes in dementia: A subgroup with preserved mental status and numerous neocortical plaques. *Annals of Neurology, 23*(2), 138–144.

Kempermann, G., Song, H., & Gage, F. H. (2015). Neurogenesis in the adult hippocampus. *Cold Spring Harbor Perspectives in Biology, 7*(9), a018812.

Kricheldorff, J., Göke, K., Kiebs, M., Kasten, F. H., Herrmann, C. S., Witt, K., & Hurlemann, R. (2022). Evidence of neuroplastic changes after transcranial magnetic, electric, and deep brain stimulation. *Brain Sciences, 12*(7), 929.

Lampit, A., Hallock, H., Suo, C., Naismith, S. L., & Valenzuela, M. (2015). Cognitive training-induced short-term functional and long-term structural plastic change is related to gains in global cognition in healthy older adults: A pilot study. *Frontiers in Aging Neuroscience, 7*, 14.

Li, S. C., Lindenberger, U., & Sikström, S. (2001). Aging cognition: From neuromodulation to representation. *Trends in Cognitive Sciences, 5*(11), 479–486.

Lövdén, M., Bäckman, L., Lindenberger, U., Schaefer, S., & Schmiedek, F. (2010). A theoretical framework for the study of adult cognitive plasticity. *Psychological Bulletin, 136*(4), 659.

McDaniel, M. A. (2005). Big-brained people are smarter: A meta-analysis of the relationship between in vivo brain volume and intelligence. *Intelligence, 33*(4), 337–346.

Menardi, A., Pascual-Leone, A., Fried, P. J., & Santarnecchi, E. (2018). The role of cognitive reserve in Alzheimer's disease and aging: A multi-modal imaging review. *Journal of Alzheimer's Disease, 66*(4), 1341–1362.

Morcom, A. M., & Henson, R. N. A. (2018). Increased prefrontal activity with aging reflects nonspecific neural responses rather than compensation. *Journal of Neuroscience, 38*(33), 7303–7313.

Moreno-Jiménez, E. P., Terreros-Roncal, J., Flor-García, M., Rábano, A., & Llorens-Martín, M. (2021). Evidences for adult hippocampal neurogenesis in humans. *Journal of Neuroscience, 41*(12), 2541–2553.

Mozolic, J. L., Hayaska, S., & Laurienti, P. J. (2010). A cognitive training intervention increases resting cerebral blood flow in healthy older adults. *Frontiers in Human Neuroscience, 4*, 1080.

Myrum, C. (2019). Is PASA passé?: Rethinking compensatory mechanisms in cognitive aging. *Journal of Neuroscience, 39*(5), 786–787.

Nelson, M. E., Jester, D. J., Petkus, A. J., & Andel, R. (2021). Cognitive reserve, Alzheimer's neuropathology, and risk of dementia: A systematic review and meta-analysis. *Neuropsychology Review, 31*(2), 233–250.

Nguyen, L., Murphy, K., & Andrews, G. (2019). Cognitive and neural plasticity in old age: A systematic review of evidence from executive functions cognitive training. *Ageing Research Reviews, 53*, 100912.

Noack, H., Lövdén, M., & Schmiedek, F. (2014). On the validity and generality of transfer effects in cognitive training research. *Psychological Research, 78*, 773–789.

Nyberg, L., Lövdén, M., Riklund, K., Lindenberger, U., & Bäckman, L. (2012). Memory aging and brain maintenance. *Trends in Cognitive Sciences, 16*(5), 292–305.

Oh, H., Steffener, J., Razlighi, Q. R., Habeck, C., Liu, D., Gazes, Y., et al. (2015). A β-related hyperactivation in frontoparietal control regions in cognitively normal elderly. *Neurobiology of Aging, 36*(12), 3247–3254.

Oosterhuis, E. J., Slade, K., May, P. J. C., & Nuttall, H. E. (2023). Toward an understanding of healthy cognitive aging: The importance of lifestyle in cognitive reserve and the scaffolding theory of aging and cognition. *Journals of Gerontology: Series B, 78*(5), 777–788.

Ossenkoppele, R., Pichet Binette, A., Groot, C., Smith, R., Strandberg, O., Palmqvist, S., et al. (2022). Amyloid and tau PET-positive cognitively unimpaired individuals are at high risk for future cognitive decline. *Nature Medicine, 28*(11), 2381–2387.

Park, D. C., & Reuter-Lorenz, P. (2009). The adaptive brain: Aging and neurocognitive scaffolding. *Annual Review of Psychology, 60*(1), 173–196.

Pietrelli, A., Matković, L., Vacotto, M., Lopez-Costa, J. J., Basso, N., & Brusco, A. (2018). Aerobic exercise upregulates the BDNF-Serotonin systems and improves the cognitive function in rats. *Neurobiology of Learning and Memory, 155*, 528–542.

Qi, C., Luo, L. D., Feng, I., & Ma, S. (2022). Molecular mechanisms of synaptogenesis. *Frontiers in Synaptic Neuroscience, 14*, 939793.

Reitz, C., & Mayeux, R. (2010). Use of genetic variation as biomarkers for mild cognitive impairment and progression of mild cognitive impairment to dementia. *Journal of Alzheimer's Disease, 19*(1), 229–251.

Reuter-Lorenz, P. A., & Lustig, C. (2005). Brain aging: Reorganizing discoveries about the aging mind. *Current Opinion in Neurobiology, 15*(2), 245–251.

Reuter-Lorenz, P. A., & Mikels, J. A. (2006). The aging mind and brain: Implications of enduring plasticity for behavioral and cultural change. In P. B. Baltes, P. A. Reuter-Lorenz, & F. Rösler (Eds.), *Lifespan development and the brain: The perspective of biocultural co-constructivism* (pp. 255–276). Cambridge University Press.

Reuter-Lorenz, P. A., & Park, D. C. (2014). How does it STAC up? Revisiting the scaffolding theory of aging and cognition. *Neuropsychology Review, 24*, 355–370.

Rosano, C., Aizenstein, H. J., Newman, A. B., Venkatraman, V., Harris, T., Ding, J., et al. (2012). Neuroimaging differences between older adults with maintained versus declining cognition over a 10-year period. *Neuroimage, 62*(1), 307–313.

Sampaio-Baptista, C., & Johansen-Berg, H. (2017). White matter plasticity in the adult brain. *Neuron, 96*(6), 1239–1251.

Satz, P. (1993). Brain reserve capacity on symptom onset after brain injury: A formulation and review of evidence for threshold theory. *Neuropsychology, 7*(3), 273–295.

Scarmeas, N., Levy, G., Tang, M. X., Manly, J., & Stern, Y. (2001). Influence of leisure activity on the incidence of Alzheimer's disease. *Neurology, 57*(12), 2236–2242.

Scarmeas, N., Zarahn, E., Anderson, K. E., Hilton, J., Flynn, J., Van Heertum, R. L., et al. (2003). Cognitive reserve modulates functional brain responses during memory tasks: A PET study in healthy young and elderly subjects. *Neuroimage, 19*(3), 1215–1227.

Schofield, P. W., Logroscino, G., Andrews, H. F., Albert, S., & Stern, Y. (1997). An association between head circumference and Alzheimer's disease in a population-based study of aging and dementia. *Neurology, 49*(1), 30–37.

Simon, S. S., Lee, S., Gu, Y., Mensing, A., Noofoory, D., Nazario, G. M. H., et al. (2023). Leisure activity engagement across adulthood predicts cognitive change after five years: Do gender and age matter? *Journal of the International Neuropsychological Society, 29*(6), 529–540.

Song, S., Stern, Y., & Gu, Y. (2022). Modifiable lifestyle factors and cognitive reserve: A systematic review of current evidence. *Ageing Research Reviews, 74*, 101551.

Steffener, J., Reuben, A., Rakitin, B. C., & Stern, Y. (2011). Supporting performance in the face of age-related neural changes: Testing mechanistic roles of cognitive reserve. *Brain Imaging and Behavior, 5*, 212–221.

Stern, Y. (2002). What is cognitive reserve? Theory and research application of the reserve concept. *Journal of the International Neuropsychological Society, 8*(3), 448–460.

Stern, Y. (2009). Cognitive reserve. *Neuropsychologia, 47*(10), 2015–2028.

Stern, Y. (2012). Cognitive reserve in ageing and Alzheimer's disease. *Lancet Neurology, 11*(11), 1006–1012.

Stern, Y. (2013). Cognitive reserve: Implications for assessment and intervention. *Folia Phoniatrica et Logopaedica, 65*(2), 49–54.

Stern, Y. (2017). An approach to studying the neural correlates of reserve. *Brain Imaging and Behavior, 11*(2), 410–416.

Stern, Y., Albert, M., Barnes, C. A., Cabeza, R., Pascual-Leone, A., & Rapp, P. R. (2023). A framework for concepts of reserve and resilience in aging. *Neurobiology of Aging, 124*, 100–103.

Stern, Y., Alexander, G. E., Prohovnik, I., & Mayeux, R. (1992). Inverse relationship between education and parietotemporal perfusion deficit in Alzheimer's disease. *Annals of Neurology, 32*(3), 371–375.

Stern, Y., Arenaza-Urquijo, E. M., Bartrés-Faz, D., Belleville, S., Cantilon, M., Chetelat, G., et al., and the Reserve, Resilience and Protective Factors PIA Empirical Definitions and Conceptual Frameworks Workgroup. (2020). Whitepaper: Defining and investigating cognitive reserve, brain reserve, and brain maintenance. *Alzheimer's & Dementia, 16*(9), 1305–1311.

Stern, Y., Blumen, H. M., Rich, L. W., Richards, A., Herzberg, G., & Gopher, D. (2011). Space Fortress game training and executive control in older adults: A pilot intervention. *Aging, Neuropsychology, and Cognition, 18*(6), 653–677.

Stern, Y., Gazes, Y., Razlighi, Q., Steffener, J., & Habeck, C. (2018). A task-invariant cognitive reserve network. *Neuroimage, 178*, 36–45.

Stern, Y., Gurland, B., Tatemichi, T. K., Tang, M. X., Wilder, D., & Mayeux, R. (1994). Influence of education and occupation on the incidence of Alzheimer's disease. *Journal of the American Medical Association, 271*, 1004–1010.

Stern, Y., Habeck, C., Moeller, J., Scarmeas, N., Anderson, K. E., Hilton, H. J., et al. (2005). Brain networks associated with cognitive reserve in healthy young and old adults. *Cerebral Cortex, 15*(4), 394–402.

Stern, Y., Rakitin, B. C., Habeck, C., Gazes, Y., Steffener, J., Kumar, A., & Reuben, A. (2012). Task difficulty modulates young–old differences in network expression. *Brain Research, 1435*, 130–145.

Storsve, A. B., Fjell, A. M., Tamnes, C. K., Westlye, L. T., Overbye, K., Aasland, H. W., & Walhovd, K. B. (2014). Differential longitudinal changes in cortical thickness, surface area and volume across the adult life span: Regions of accelerating and decelerating change. *Journal of Neuroscience, 34*(25), 8488–8498.

Sun, F. W., Stepanovic, M. R., Andreano, J., Barrett, L. F., Touroutoglou, A., & Dickerson, B. C. (2016). Youthful brains in older adults: preserved neuroanatomy in the default mode and salience networks contributes to youthful memory in superaging. *Journal of Neuroscience, 36*(37), 9659–9668.

Valenzuela, M. J., & Sachdev, P. (2006). Brain reserve and dementia: A systematic review. *Psychological Medicine, 36*(4), 441–454.

Vallesi, A., McIntosh, A. R., & Stuss, D. T. (2011). Overrecruitment in the aging brain as a function of task demands: Evidence for a compensatory view. *Journal of Cognitive Neuroscience, 23*(4), 801–815.

van Praag, H., Shubert, T., Zhao, C., & Gage, F. H. (2005). Exercise enhances learning and hippocampal neurogenesis in aged mice. *Journal of Neuroscience, 25*, 8680–8685.

Varangis, E., Qi, W., Stern, Y., & Lee, S. (2022). The role of neural flexibility in cognitive aging. *NeuroImage, 247*, 118784.

Verkhratsky, A., & Zorec, R. (2024). Neuroglia in cognitive reserve. *Molecular Psychiatry, 29*, 3962–3967.

Vieira, B. H., Rondinoni, C., & Salmon, C. E. G. (2020). Evidence of regional associations between age-related inter-individual differences in resting-state functional connectivity and cortical thinning revealed through a multi-level analysis. *NeuroImage, 211*, 116662.

Woollett, K., & Maguire, E. A. (2011). Acquiring "the knowledge" of London's layout drives structural brain changes. *Current Biology, 21*(24), 2109–2114.

Zahodne, L. B., Manly, J. J., Brickman, A. M., Siedlecki, K. L., DeCarli, C., & Stern, Y. (2013). Quantifying cognitive reserve in older adults by decomposing episodic memory variance: Replication and extension. *Journal of the International Neuropsychological Society, 19*(8), 854–862.

Zarahn, E., Rakitin, B., Abela, D., Flynn, J., & Stern, Y. (2007). Age-related changes in brain activation during a delayed item recognition task. *Neurobiology of Aging, 28*(5), 784–798.

Zimmerman, B., Rypma, B., Gratton, G., & Fabiani, M. (2021). Age-related changes in cerebrovascular health and their effects on neural function and cognition: A comprehensive review. *Psychophysiology, 58*(7), e13796.

CHAPTER 10

Therapeutic Interventions for Maladaptive Neurological Disorders

Negar Nasrkhani, Nasem Raies, Rachel Chang, Nishaad Sheth, Amitabh Bhattacharya, Naaz Desai, and Robert Chen

Introduction

Brain plasticity, or neuroplasticity, refers to the brain's ability to reorganize itself by forming new neural connections throughout life. Several neurological disorders are associated with abnormal brain plasticity. In this chapter, we focus on therapeutic interventions in three disorders with maladaptive plasticity: Parkinson's disease (PD), dystonia, and chronic pain. These disorders often present complex challenges for both patients and clinicians and are associated with significant socioeconomic burdens.

PD is a neurodegenerative disease. Its clinical features include asymmetric onset of bradykinesia, rigidity, and rest tremor, in addition to nonmotor symptoms. PD causes substantial morbidity and shortened lifespan, as well as significant economic consequences, such as loss of earnings and cost of care. Current treatment options for PD include levodopa and other dopaminergic drug therapy and surgery, including pallidotomy and deep brain stimulation (DBS). However, with levodopa treatment, an increasing proportion of patients experience dyskinesia after 2–3 years of treatment (Udupa et al., 2022a).

Dystonia is a disabling movement disorder characterized by involuntary repetitive movements and abnormal postures. Current treatment options for dystonia

The first five authors contributed equally to this chapter.

include oral therapies such as anticholinergics, baclofen, benzodiazepines, and dopaminergic drugs; botulinum toxin injections; and surgeries such as peripheral denervation, intrathecal baclofen, ablative procedures (pallidotomy and thalamotomy) and DBS. However, these treatments are only moderately efficacious (Bronte-Stewart et al., 2011; Ellis, 2011).

Chronic pain is often characterized by persistent pain that can be challenging to treat. Current treatment options for chronic pain include medications such as nonsteroidal anti-inflammatory drugs, opioids, and antidepressants, as well as nonpharmacological approaches such as physical therapy, cognitive-behavioral therapy, and interventional procedures. However, these treatments may not always provide adequate relief, and invasive procedures are often risky and expensive (Hylands-White et al., 2017).

There has been growing interest in the use of neuromodulation techniques for the treatment of these neurological disorders. Neuromodulation involves the targeted delivery of stimuli such as electrical, magnetic, or sound waves to specific neural circuits to modulate their activities and restore normal function. These techniques aim to leverage brain plasticity to correct maladaptive plasticity associated with neurological disorders. They offer a promising alternative to traditional treatments, particularly for patients who do not respond well to conventional therapies.

DBS is an invasive neuromodulation technique, involving electrode implantation into selected brain regions to deliver electrical current. Although DBS is a treatment option for many disorders, it requires surgery. Conversely, noninvasive brain stimulation (NIBS) techniques are more accessible at lower cost. NIBS can be categorized into magnetic, electrical, or ultrasound stimulation modalities. Transcranial magnetic stimulation (TMS) is a noninvasive neurostimulation technique that generates magnetic pulses to stimulate the brain. TMS can be used for diagnostic (Vucic et al., 2023) as well as therapeutic indications. It can be used to assess changes in cortical excitability associated with neurological and psychiatric disorders (Rossini et al., 2015).

Focused ultrasound is another neuromodulation technique involving the convergence of ultrasound waves onto a small region of the brain. High-intensity focused ultrasound (HIFU) can raise local temperatures to greater than 55°C, causing coagulative necrosis of tissue at the focal point (Bachu et al., 2021). Magnetic resonance-guided focused ultrasound (MRgFUS) is a procedure that pairs focused ultrasound with magnetic resonance imaging to precisely set stereotactic coordinates for HIFU ablation. HIFU is usually delivered to brain tissue as a continuous wave at a spatial peak pulse average intensity exceeding 200 W/cm^2, while low-intensity focused ultrasound or transcranial focused ultrasound (TUS) is delivered intermittently at a spatial peak temporal average intensity of less than 100 W/cm^2 (Bowary & Greenberg, 2018; Davidson et al., 2024). TUS is a novel NIBS technique with greater spatial resolution and deeper penetration depths compared with existing NIBS techniques (Darmani et al., 2022; Fomenko et al., 2018; Yu et al., 2020), with the ability to reversibly induce brain plasticity.

This chapter provides an overview of the current state of neuromodulation in Parkinson's disease, dystonia, and chronic pain. It explores emerging trends and future directions in neuromodulation research in these areas.

Parkinson's Disease

PD is the second most common neurodegenerative disorder in the world and has become one of the leading causes of disability worldwide (Karikari et al., 2018). The incidence of PD globally was estimated to be about 1 million cases per year in 2019, with increasing prevalence in countries with a high sociodemographic index, such as the United States, Norway, and Germany (Ou et al., 2021). There are also ethnic variations in the prevalence and prognosis of PD; White populations reportedly have the highest prevalence, while Black patients have a higher risk of mortality compared with Hispanic and Asian patients (Ben-Joseph et al., 2020). The most significant risk factor associated with PD is age, with prevalence increasing exponentially between the ages of 60 and 80 (Pringsheim et al., 2014). Males appear to be affected more, with those over the age of 60 years being 1.6 times more affected than women (Moisan et al., 2016). Genetic risk factors also demonstrate associations with PD, particularly mutations in glucocerebrosidase, a lysosomal enzyme that shows deficiency in Gaucher's disease (Sidransky & Lopez, 2012).

Etiology and Clinical Presentation

The motor symptoms of PD are attributed to the degeneration of dopaminergic neurons in the substantia nigra pars compacta, whereas the nonmotor symptoms are linked to Lewy bodies accumulation in other brain areas and in the gut (Selikhova et al., 2009).

The cardinal motor symptoms of PD include rigidity, bradykinesia, and tremors (Baumann, 2012; Reichmann, 2010). Tremor is often the first motor symptom, predominantly affecting the hands and sometimes the lower extremities (Heusinkveld et al., 2018). Several tremor manifestations are distinguishable, including resting, action, and postural tremors (Reich & Savitt, 2019). Bradykinesia is characterized by slowness of movement, whereas rigidity typically results in the feeling of stiffness and can be assessed by resistance against passive stretching (Moustafa et al., 2016). Bradykinesia and rigidity are primarily related to basal ganglia dysfunction (DeLong & Wichmann, 2007). Other motor deficits include freezing of gait, handwriting impairment, and deficits in speech and grip force (Moustafa et al., 2016). The nonmotor symptoms of PD, such as autonomic disturbance, mood and cognitive symptoms, and sleep disorders, are also debilitating and are often overlooked in PD management (DeMaagd & Philip, 2015; Poewe, 2008; Tibar et al., 2018). Neuromodulation approaches for PD are summarized in Figure 10.1, which illustrates the main stimulation targets and mechanisms described below.

Neuromodulation Methods in PD

DBS in PD

The mechanisms behind the therapeutic effects of DBS in PD are not fully understood and go beyond local excitatory and inhibitory changes (Ashkan et al., 2017; Udupa & Chen, 2015). While some of the mechanisms may be specific to the stimulation target,

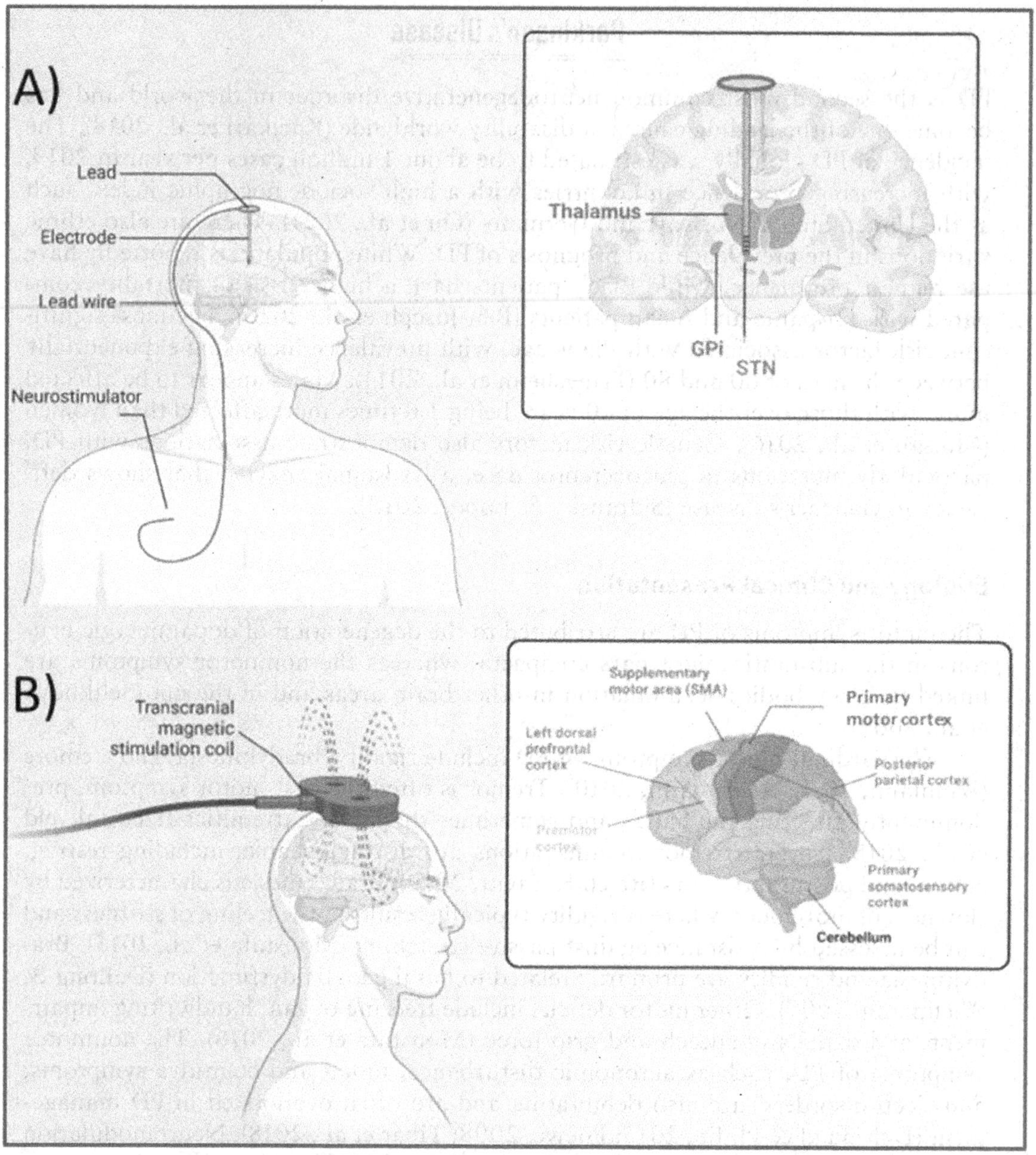

FIGURE 10.1. Neuromodulation techniques for Parkinson's disease and dystonia. (A) Deep brain stimulation (DBS) target areas. The left image shows the components of the DBS system: lead, electrode, lead wire, and neurostimulator. The right inset highlights the primary brain targets for DBS: subthalamic nucleus (STN) and globus pallidus internus (GPi), with DBS electrodes in the STN. (B) Transcranial magnetic stimulation (TMS) target areas. The left image shows placement of the TMS coil over a subject's scalp. The right inset identifies key cortical regions targeted by TMS, including the primary motor cortex, supplementary motor area (SMA), left dorsolateral prefrontal cortex, premotor cortex, posterior parietal cortex, primary somatosensory cortex, and cerebellum.

the proposed mechanisms include the inhibition of local neurons by high-frequency stimulation, excitation of axons afferent and efferent to the stimulation site, disruption of pathological oscillation, and release of endogenous opioids upon stimulation of the periaqueductal gray (Ashkan et al., 2017; Knotkova et al., 2021; Pagano et al., 2023; Sims-Williams et al., 2017). In addition, DBS may induce cortical plasticity (Kim et al., 2015; Ni et al., 2018; Udupa et al., 2016) and cellular changes such as increased neurogenesis, receptor changes, and release of gliotransmitters (Ashkan et al., 2017; Knotkova et al., 2021).

DBS surgery is a well-accepted treatment for moderate to advanced PD. A pulse generator passes electric currents to electrodes implanted in targeted deep brain areas. Several studies showed that patients treated with DBS show better improvement in motor symptoms compared with pharmacological treatment (Dharnipragada et al., 2023; Peng et al., 2018; Schuepbach et al., 2013). The subthalamic nucleus (STN) and the globus pallidus internus (GPi) are the two most common surgical targets for DBS in PD, and their efficacies have been extensively investigated (Odekerken et al., 2016; Wong et al., 2019). A meta-analysis of 38 studies of bilateral STN-DBS in PD found a 50% improvement in the Unified Parkinson's Disease Rating Scale (UPDRS) motor scores that was maintained in the 6-month to 5-year postoperative period compared with preoperative off-medication scores (Hamani et al., 2008). The motor signs with the most improvements were tremor at 81%, rigidity at 63%, bradykinesia at 52%, gait at 64%, and postural instability at 69% at the 12-month follow-up (Hamani et al., 2008).

A randomized controlled trial (RCT) investigated 299 patients treated with bilateral STN-DBS or GPi-DBS and found no significant difference in motor functions assessed by UPDRS part III scores between the two target sites (Follett et al., 2010). However, STN-DBS is superior for off-medication motor symptom reduction (Peng et al., 2018), whereas GPi-DBS yields a better reduction in dyskinesia (Williams et al., 2014). A meta-analysis of 10 RCTs confirmed similar outcomes in advanced PD and found that GPi-DBS patients experienced greater improvement in activities of daily living assessed by UPDRS part II scores (J. Zhang et al., 2021). Considering other nonmotor symptoms, GPi-DBS patients also yield better cognitive functions and mood (Rodriguez-Oroz et al., 2005; Weaver et al., 2012). However, DBS is associated with some risks. STN-DBS can lead to adverse psychiatric effects and declines in cognitive functions such as attention, working memory, processing speed, and learning (Okun et al., 2009; J.-W. Wang et al., 2016). This may be because STN has a smaller volume than the GPi, and the stimulation may affect the nonmotor regions and adjacent areas. Ultimately, the decision on the choice of DBS target between STN and GPi for patients with PD depends on the patient's clinical profile.

Other potential DBS targets include the pedunculopontine nucleus (PPN) for addressing gait disorder and postural instabilities in PD and the ventral intermediate nucleus (VIM) of the thalamus for managing tremors. Previous studies showed that unilateral PPN stimulation significantly reduced falls at 3 and 12 months after surgery (Moro et al., 2010). PPN-DBS improved gait and postural stability more than STN-DBS and showed similar effects on limb functions compared with STN-DBS (Stefani et al., 2007). Another series of 14 patients using unilateral and bilateral PPN found improvements in UPDRS part III posture and gait subscores (Mazzone et al., 2009). VIM-DBS showed improvement in off-medication motor symptoms assessed by UPDRS part III scores in the 3-month to 3-year follow-up period and therefore may be suitable for tremor-dominant PD (Mao et al., 2019).

Unlike conventional DBS, which delivers constant electrical stimulation, adaptive DBS (aDBS) uses brain signals, typically beta oscillations in local field potentials from leads in the STN or GPi to adjust the stimulation pattern and intensity according to the patient's state (Little et al., 2013; Priori et al., 2021). A study tested a brain–computer interface-controlled aDBS on the STN in eight patients with PD to assess effects on motor symptoms through blind video assessments using the UPDRS part III scores. Following aDBS, motor scores improved by over 50%, which was 27% higher than the improvement with conventional DBS (Little et al., 2013). aDBS patients also received 56% less stimulation time than conventional DBS (Little et al., 2013). In another study, bilateral aDBS was delivered to four patients, with stimulation delivered according to the amplitude of beta activity in the STN. Compared with no stimulation, the UPDRS part III scores decreased by 43% (Little et al., 2016). When delivered for over 2 hours, aDBS improved bradykinesia and dyskinesia better than conventional DBS and improved axial symptoms as effectively as traditional DBS (Beudel & Brown, 2016; Rosa et al., 2015). These advancements have provided new insights into the critical importance of selecting the appropriate DBS brain targets, devices, and stimulation parameters according to the clinical needs of patients. Future studies are expected to inform clinical trials to improve motor and nonmotor symptoms in PD patients.

NIBS Methods in PD

TMS in PD

TMS for motor physiological studies uses either single-pulse or paired-pulse stimulation. Single-pulse TMS can be used to measure the amplitude of motor-evoked potentials (MEPs) and resting and active motor thresholds (RMT/AMT). In patients with PD, most studies reported both AMT and RMT as normal (Chen et al., 2022; Chen & Rothwell, 2012). However, some studies found reduced RMT primarily on the side with greater rigidity (Spagnolo et al., 2013) and increased AMT in PD patients with bradykinesia (Ellaway et al., 1995), although these findings have not been consistently reported (Bologna et al., 2018). Another study reported reduced RMT and AMT in tremor-dominant PD patients compared with controls and akinetic-rigid patients (Khedr et al., 2021).

Paired pulse TMS delivers two magnetic pulses in close succession to the same brain region. It is commonly used in the primary motor cortex (M1) to measure cortical excitability and inhibition with parameters such as short-interval intracortical inhibition (SICI), intracortical facilitation, and short-interval intracortical facilitation (SICF; Du et al., 2014; Vucic et al., 2023). TMS can also be used to investigate changes in long-term potentiation (LTP) and long-term depression like plasticity (Bhattacharya et al., 2022; Vucic et al., 2023). Reduced SICI has been reported in PD (Ni et al., 2013) and is consistent across levodopa-naïve, nondyskinetic, and dyskinetic patients

(Ammann et al., 2020). Interestingly, SICI was also reduced on the less affected side, compared with controls, even in drug-naïve patients in whom the less affected side is minimally symptomatic (Ammann et al., 2020). Increased SICF in PD is associated with a decrease in SICI, suggesting that increased SICF could partially account for the decrease in SICI (Ni et al., 2013). A study also found that SICF is further enhanced in patients with dyskinesia (Guerra et al., 2019). These changes in cortical excitability may be used as biomarkers of disease progression (Vucic et al., 2023).

Repetitive TMS in PD

Repetitive TMS (rTMS) can be used to induce cortical plasticity. Theta burst rTMS decreases cortical excitability when applied continuously (cTBS), whereas intermittent TBS (iTBS) increases cortical excitatory (Huang et al., 2005). rTMS can induce changes in MEP amplitude for up to 60 minutes poststimulation (Hoogendam et al., 2010), and repeated sessions can lead to cumulative effects (Schulze et al., 2018; Valero-Cabré et al., 2008). Several meta-analyses and RCTs suggest that multiple sessions of high-frequency rTMS over the M1, supplementary motor area (SMA), or dorsolateral prefrontal cortex (DLPFC) elicit mild-to-moderate short- and long-term motor function improvement in areas such as gait, bradykinesia, and dyskinesia (Deng et al., 2022; Elahi et al., 2009; Li et al., 2022; Wagle Shukla et al., 2016; Zanjani et al., -2015). Notably, a systematic review suggested that high-frequency rTMS on the M1 is effective in improving motor symptoms, whereas DLPFC is effective in alleviating depression in PD patients (W. Zhang et al., 2022). A clinical trial observed a decrease in bradykinesia after 12 weeks of high-frequency rTMS at 25 Hz to the M1 (González-García et al., 2011). Some studies have also shown that high-frequency rTMS over the M1 region improves visuomotor skills and memory consolidation in PD, although systemic reviews showed conflicting results (Goodwill et al., 2017; Moisello et al., 2015). A recent meta-analysis showed that cTBS applied to the SMA improved upper limb movement functions (Cheng et al., 2021). In addition, iTBS over the DLPFC and M1 regions improved the freezing of gait. Interestingly, the changes induced by cTBS and iTBS were observed only when patients were in the *off*-medication state (Cheng et al., 2021). A consensus on the optimal rTMS protocol to improve motor symptoms in PD has not been reached (Deng et al., 2022).

Transcranial Direct Current Stimulation in PD

Transcranial direct current stimulation (tDCS) is a NIBS technique that stimulates the brain using a low-intensity direct electric current applied through electrodes on the head. Anodal tDCS has excitatory effects, as it has been proposed to induce calcium-dependent plasticity at glutamatergic synapses by stimulating glutamate transmissions and suppressing gamma-aminobutyric acid transmissions. Conversely, cathodal tDCS has the opposite effect, leading to decreased cortical excitability (Nitsche & Paulus, 2000; Pelletier & Cicchetti, 2015). Thus, tDCS has the potential to improve cognitive and motor symptoms by increasing cortical excitability with anodal tDCS and by decreasing cortical excitability with cathodal tDCS (Broeder et al., 2015). tDCS over the left DLPFC led to improvements in working memory, verbal fluency, and executive functioning, and these findings were further amplified when coupled with cognitive training in PD patients (Boggio et al., 2006; Lawrence et al., 2018; Pereira et al., 2013). Notably, remotely supervised tDCS also improved fatigue and cognitive performance when combined with cognitive training in PD patients, presenting a possible at-home rehabilitation treatment option to reduce caregiver, clinician, and patient burden (Dobbs et al., 2018).

Transcranial Alternating Current Stimulation in PD

Transcranial alternating current stimulation (tACS) is another method that can be useful for modulating motor behavior using low-intensity alternating electric current. tACS has been proposed to interact with or entrain spontaneous brain oscillations in patients with PD to reduce motor deficits (Teo et al., 2017). The advantage of tACS is that it can be applied at any frequency, leading to diverse clinical applications. For instance, 1–5 kHz of tACS can be used to induce a sustained increase in cortical excitability, and 200 kHz can stop the proliferation of cancerous cells in brain tumors (Antal & Paulus, 2013). Previous studies have demonstrated the potential use of tACS in improving bradykinesia, rest tremor, and movement variability in PD (Brittain et al., 2013; Krause et al., 2014). tACS can also boost γ oscillations when administered simultaneously with iTBS, leading to increased SICI in PD (Guerra et al., 2020). These results suggest that iTBS-tACS has therapeutic potential in restoring the LTP-like plasticity of the M1 region in PD. Another study applied tACS over the M1 to induce phase cancellation of the rest tremor, which resulted in almost a 50% reduction in the average rest tremor amplitude (Brittain et al., 2013).

MRgFUS in PD

Unlike DBS, MRgFUS is a nonsurgical procedure. The current treatment targets for MRgFUS, including VIM, STN, GPi, and pallidothalamic tract (PTT). VIM is a target for treating essential tremor and tremor-dominant PD. A study in 26 tremor-dominant PD patients found that unilateral MRgFUS VIM thalamotomy was a safe and effective treatment that provides up to 5 years of tremor relief in most patients (Sinai et al., 2022). Ablation of the STN can also ameliorate motor symptoms as abnormally sustained beta-frequency synchronization between the M1 and STN is involved in the pathophysiology of PD (Martínez-Fernández et al., 2020). Targeting the GPi with MRgFUS (pallidotomy) improved motor function and was found to be useful in the management of levodopa-induced dyskinesia (Krishna et al., 2023). The PTT is also a target for Parkinsonian tremor, akinesia, or dyskinesia. In a study of 47 patients with advanced PD, unilateral PTT MRgFUS demonstrated an improvement of 84% in tremor, 70% in rigidity, and 73% in distal bradykinesia (Gallay et al., 2019).

Adverse effects reported for MRgFUS include temporary headaches and dizziness, and most commonly, gait instability and sensory disturbances when the thalamic areas were targeted (Bretsztajn & Gedroyc, 2018). Gait ataxia and paresthesia or numbness can persist for up to 12 months following the focused ultrasound (Elias et al., 2016). Another study found constipation, anxiety, hallucinations, and one case of procedure-related nonfatal pulmonary embolism, which occurred 1 week after treatment with GPi MRgFUS. Currently, the United States Food and Drug Administration (FDA) has approved MRgFUS for the treatment of tremor-dominated PD and PD dyskinesia. Nonetheless, longer duration and larger trials are required to better determine the safety and efficacy of MRgFUS. Additionally, most studies on MRgFUS assessed unilateral focused ultrasound, which limits the treatment of tremors from dyskinesia to only one side. Further studies are needed to assess the effects of using bilateral MRgFUS in PD (Levi et al., 2024; Martínez-Fernández et al., 2024).

Low-Intensity TUS in PD

In human studies, TUS has been used primarily to investigate the primary somatosensory cortex (S1) and the M1 region, and deep brain structures such as the thalamus and caudate nuclei (P. Wang et al., 2019). TUS studies showed effectiveness in altering pain thresholds in healthy subjects (Badran et al., 2020). Depending on the sonication parameters, MEPs may be suppressed during sonication (Fomenko et al., 2020). The optimal parameters for inducing MEP suppression during TUS are a duty cycle (DC) of less than 50% and sonication durations of at least 400 milliseconds (Legon et al., 2018; Xia et al., 2021). Alternatively, high ultrasound energy with a pulse repetition frequency of 300 Hz and DC 60% may produce an online excitatory effect on the M1 (Yu et al., 2021). The same study also found these conditions to increase the amplitude of movement-related cortical potential measured with electroencephalography.

Patterned TUS protocols, such as repetitive TUS and theta-burst TUS protocols, can induce motor cortical plasticity that outlasts the stimulation period (Zeng et al., 2022; Y. Zhang et al., 2021). Trains of theta-burst patterned TUS (tbTUS) of 80–120 seconds applied to the M1 increased MEP amplitude and decreased SICI for 30–60 minutes, suggesting that the intervention reduces cortical inhibition and enhances cortical excitability (Samuel et al., 2022; Zeng et al., 2022, 2024). In PD, the tbTUS protocol led to increased M1 excitability in aged-matched healthy subjects, control, and PD patients on medication, while no plasticity was induced in the off-medication state (Grippe et al., 2024). Another study applied an accelerated tbTUS protocol with three tbTUS sessions in one day to 10 PD patients off medications and found increased M1 excitability (Samuel et al., 2023). These studies show that TUS is a feasible and promising noninvasive neuromodulation strategy in PD patients. TUS's precision, tolerability, and effectiveness in modulating brain plasticity can provide potential clinical applications in treating movement disorders. Further studies are required to investigate optimal stimulation parameters and the durability of the clinical outcomes.

Transcranial Pulse Stimulation in PD

Transcranial pulse stimulation (TPS) is a form of TUS that uses shockwave-like single pulses at lower frequencies, which minimizes brain heating (Beisteiner et al., 2020). A retrospective analysis found significant improvements in the UPDRS part III scores in 20 patients with PD after 10 sessions of TPS to the M1 region (Osou et al., 2023).

Dystonia

Dystonia is a diverse group of disorders characterized by sustained or intermittent muscle contractions, resulting in abnormal postures, repetitive movements, or both (Albanese et al., 2013). Dystonia is the third most common movement disorder after PD and essential tremor, with an estimated overall prevalence of 164 per million individuals (Steeves et al., 2012). A meta-analysis reported the prevalence of various forms of dystonia as follows: cervical dystonia (9.95 per 100,000), blepharospasm (2.82 per 100,000), laryngeal dystonia (0.40 per 100,000), upper limb dystonia (1.27 per 100,000), oromandibular dystonia (0.57 per 100,000), and all subtypes of idiopathic or inherited isolated dystonia combined (30.85 per 100,000; Medina et al., 2022). Notably, dystonia is more common in females compared with males (Medina et al., 2022). Despite these estimates, because of its wide clinical spectrum, dystonia remains underdiagnosed and is often misdiagnosed (di Biase et al., 2022). The pathophysiological changes associated with dystonia include impairment of sensorimotor integration, reduced inhibition in multiple levels of the central nervous system, and changes in synaptic plasticity. These changes may be related to the impairment of the gating mechanisms in the basal ganglia, which are involved in the "surround inhibition" process. Surround inhibition involves a balance between excitatory and inhibitory circuits, allowing appropriate movements and inhibiting undesired ones. Impairment of surround inhibition results in excessive activation of cortical areas and co-contraction of unwanted muscles (Brüggemann, 2021). There is also increasing evidence from animal, genetic, imaging, and electrophysiological studies that dystonia is a network-based disorder involving multiple brain regions, such as the cerebellum, the cerebello-thalamic connection, and the functional interplay between basal ganglia and the cerebellum (Brüggemann, 2021; Fung & Peall, 2019).

Etiology and Clinical Presentation

Dystonia can affect almost any part of the body (Brüggemann, 2021). It may be present alone or in association with other movement disorders, including chorea, myoclonus, tremor, and parkinsonism. Some dystonias are inherited, whereas others may involve both genetic predisposition and environmental factors such as repetitive practice (e.g., writer's cramp and musician's dystonia; Udupa et al., 2022b). An expert committee of the Movement Disorder Society proposed the current classification of dystonia in 2013 (Albanese et al., 2013). It proposes that dystonia can be evaluated in two main axes: a clinical axis (axis 1) and an etiological axis (axis 2). The clinical axis includes age of onset, body distribution, and temporal pattern, including disease course and variability, and other associated features. The etiological axis compromises the nervous system pathology of the disease and inheritance patterns (di Biase et al., 2022).

Dystonia is due to the exaggerated activation of muscles during the execution of certain movements. It does not, however, only appear in the context of goal-directed movements, such as focal hand dystonia or spasmodic dystonia. It may also occur at rest, such as in cervical dystonia.

Neuromodulation in Dystonia

DBS in Dystonia

Despite a growing understanding of dystonia, disease-modifying therapies do not exist for most types of dystonia, and treatment is often limited to symptomatic management. In the early 1950s, clinicians treated dystonia with functional surgeries in various target sites, such as the dentate nucleus, GPi, medial thalamus, and STN (Bledsoe et al., 2020). The symptomatic treatment of dystonia has improved significantly since the introduction of DBS. DBS offers several advantages over ablation procedures, including a more favorable side effect profile and adjustability (Bledsoe et al., 2020).

Bilateral GPi-DBS is helpful in various types of dystonia, including generalized dystonia, segmental dystonia, some forms of focal dystonia, and cervical dystonia (Coubes et al., 2000; Ni et al., 2018; Volkmann et al., 2014). A study of 40 patients with primary segmental or generalized dystonia who received bilateral GPi-DBS for 3 months showed substantial improvement in all motor symptoms (except speech and swallowing), level of disability, and quality of life compared with baseline (Kupsch et al., 2006). Another randomized, sham-controlled trial showed that 3 months of GPi-DBS was more effective than sham stimulation at reducing symptoms of cervical dystonia (Volkmann et al., 2014). However, despite the favorable outcome with pallidal DBS, there is wide variability in DBS outcomes (Bledsoe et al., 2020). Speech and swallowing abnormalities are less responsive than other dystonic symptoms. Additionally, in a few cases, there have been reports of symptom exacerbation following the initial improvement with DBS (Tagliati et al., 2011).

A less commonly used target for DBS in dystonia is the STN. In a 3-year follow-up study of 20 patients with isolated dystonia, disability, and quality of life improved with sustained benefit persisting for 3 years in 14 patients following STN stimulation (Ostrem et al., 2017). A matched retrospective cohort study comparing GPi-DBS and STN-DBS in 30 patients found that both targets produced improvement in dystonia symptoms and quality of life. However, STN stimulation produced a larger clinical improvement within 1 month of surgery, while GPi stimulation led to a greater improvement in axial symptoms compared with STN-DBS (Lin et al., 2019). STN stimulation may have some advantages over GPi stimulation, such as faster onset of symptom improvement and longer battery life, due to lower stimulation intensities needed (Lin et al., 2019). However, a drawback of STN-DBS is that it produces transient dyskinesia in a large proportion of patients (Contarino et al., 2016).

TMS in Dystonia

rTMS to specific brain areas has shown benefits in dystonia. A study using low-frequency (0.2 Hz) rTMS inhibitory stimulation led to improved handwriting ratings in patients with writer's cramp (WC) when targeting the premotor cortex (PMC) but not the M1 (Murase et al., 2005). In 20 cervical dystonia patients, 2 weeks of cerebellar cTBS led to a 15% improvement in symptoms as measured by the Toronto Western Spasmodic Torticollis Rating Scale (Koch et al., 2014). Furthermore, cTBS applied to the dorsal PMC improved writing in patients with WC (Huang et al.,

2010). The effects of cTBS and iTBS on the S1 have been investigated in patients with focal hand dystonia (FHD), but no clinical benefit was found (Conte et al., 2014).

tDCS in Dystonia

A randomized, double-blinded, sham-controlled study tested real or sham biparietal tDCS with the cathode on the left side for 2 weeks in 30 musicians with dystonia undergoing neurorehabilitation. The active tDCS group showed significantly better improvement in dystonia severity compared with the sham tDCS group (Rosset-Llobet et al., 2015). Bilateral simultaneous M1 tDCS (cathode over the affected cortex and anode over the unaffected cortex) resulted in improvement in rhythmic accuracy and sequential finger movements in 10 pianists with FHD (Furuya et al., 2014). Anodal tDCS to the cerebellum also led to improvement in handwriting in patients with FHD (Bradnam et al., 2015). However, there are also several studies with tDCS of the M1 in FHD that found no clinical benefits (Benninger et al., 2011; Buttkus et al., 2010, 2011).

HIFU in Dystonia

In a pilot study involving 10 patients with FHD, MRgFUS of ventro-oral nucleus thalamotomy led to significant improvements in the Writer's Cramp Rating Scale, Tubiana Musician's Dystonia Scale, and Arm Dystonia Disability Scale at 12 months posttreatment (Horisawa et al., 2021). These findings suggest that MRgFUS can potentially be a safe and effective treatment of focal dystonias, although studies with a larger sample size and longer follow-up periods are needed to better determine the efficacy and safety of MRgFUS for treatment of FHD (Horisawa et al., 2021).

Chronic Pain

The International Association for the Study of Pain defines chronic pain as "an unpleasant sensory and emotional experience associated with, or resembling that associated with, actual or potential tissue damage" (Raja et al., 2020). Approximately 1 in 5 adults suffer from chronic pain, a persistent condition that severely burdens patients of all ages and health care systems worldwide (Goldberg & McGee, 2011; Hadi et al., 2019; Mills et al., 2019; Phillips, 2009). Data from the Centers for Disease Control and Prevention found higher prevalence in women, individuals from lower socioeconomic backgrounds, military veterans, and people residing in rural areas (Dahlhamer et al., 2018). From an ethnicity perspective, the highest pain intensities was recorded among non-Hispanic White people, but with a higher prevalence in racial and ethnic minorities, such as African Americans and Indigenous populations (Mills et al., 2019).

Etiology and Clinical Presentation

Chronic pain is associated with unique, and sometimes disease-specific, alterations in the *peripheral* or *central nervous system* along with decreased *quality of life*

(Clauw et al., 2019). The biopsychosocial model postulates pain and disability as multidimensional, dynamic interactions among biological, psychological, and social factors that reciprocally influence each other (Meints & Edwards, 2018). Biological factors include genetics, age, sex, sleep, hormones, and the *endogenous opiate* systems (Meints & Edwards, 2018). Psychological factors include depression, anxiety, posttraumatic stress, poor coping skills, catastrophization, and many others. Sociocultural factors include low educational attainment, culture, and poor social support (Clauw et al., 2019).

There are three main categories of chronic pain: nociceptive, neuropathic, and nociplastic. Nociceptive pain is pain caused by damage to body tissue, neuropathic pain is caused by a lesion or a disease of the somatosensory nervous system, and nociplastic pain is a persistent pain that arises from altered nociception, despite no clear evidence of actual or threatened tissue. The clinical presentation varies based on the category of chronic pain and may include sensory deficits, motor deficits, hypersensitivities, autonomic dysfunction and there may be presence of other concomitant conditions (Cohen et al., 2021). Best practice guidelines advocate for mechanism-based pain treatment. However, identifying the mechanisms behind the pain can be challenging or impossible in clinical practice; therefore, treatment may be symptom-based or disease-based (Woolf et al., 1998). Current clinical practices recommend the use of alternative therapies and/or analgesics, but these interventions often fall short in their long-term efficacy, and the use of opioids poses the risk of abuse and addiction. Additionally, traditional surgical interventions are expensive and risky (Cohen et al., 2021; Hylands-White et al., 2017). Recent advances in neuromodulation have shown great promise in providing safe and effective avenues for chronic pain relief (Knotkova et al., 2021; Todd et al., 2020). Figure 10.2 provides an overview of neuromodulation techniques applied for chronic pain management, including DBS, rTMS, HIFU, and TUS.

Neuromodulation for Chronic Pain

DBS for Chronic Pain

DBS has been used to treat chronic pain for over 50 years. However, inadequate results from large multicenter studies and advances in alternative pain treatments have led to a decline in its popularity. To date, results of long-term studies on the efficacy of DBS for chronic pain have been heterogeneous. Nonetheless, specialized centers provide this surgery to patients with severe and refractory pain and have had no success with other pain therapies.

Two large multicenter trials for DBS in pain were conducted to gain FDA approval in 1976 and 1990, enrolling 196 and 50 patients, respectively. In the 1976 trial, 53% of patients reported pain relief (≥50%) at 3 months, which dropped to 18% at 24 months (Coffey, 2001; Weintraub, 1990). The 1990 trial reported even lower rates of pain relief, and the FDA retracted its approval for this application of DBS (Coffey, 2001; Weintraub, 1990). Both trials had high attrition rates (over 70%), raising concerns about the results having a high risk of bias as withdrawn patients were counted as unsuccessful treatments in efficacy calculations (Coffey, 2001). Despite the

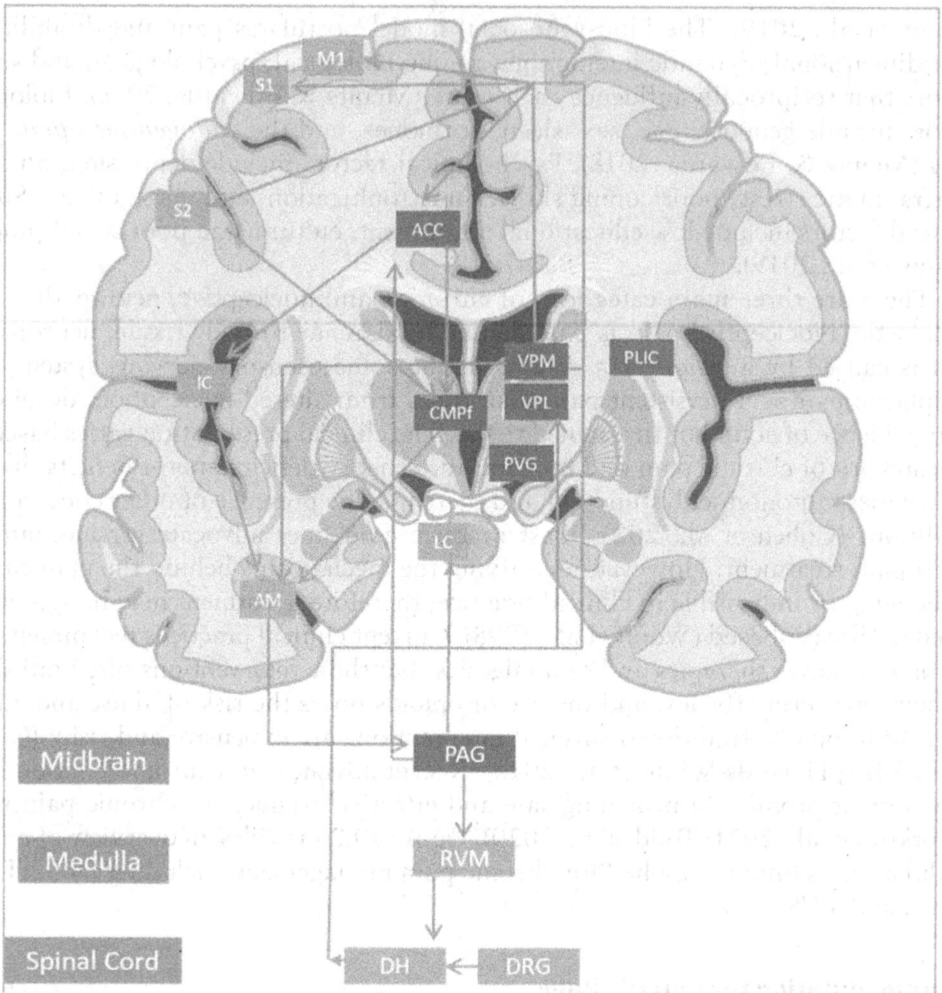

FIGURE 10.2. Pain pathways and neuromodulation targets. Primary afferent neurons, with their cell bodies in the DRG, convey nociceptive information to second-order neurons within the DH of the spinal cord. These neurons send projections to the thalamus, specifically to the VPL and VPM nuclei. Nociceptive information from the thalamus is then transmitted to the S1, S2, ACC, IC, and AM. The ascending pathways transmit nociceptive input from the DRG to the DH of the spinal cord. From the DH, projections are sent to the VPL and VPM nuclei in the thalamus. The thalamus then transmits this information to various cortical areas, including S1, S2, ACC, IC, and AM. The descending pathways originate from higher brain centers such as the ACC, IC, and AM. They project to the PAG. The PAG sends projections to the RVM. The RVM projects back to the DH of the spinal cord, modulating pain signals at the spinal level. Stimulation sites of common invasive and noninvasive neuromodulatory techniques are indicated. Specific DBS targets include the CM/Pf, PVG, and PAG. Highlighted labels mark critical nodes involved in pain pathways, some of which serve as DBS targets. ACC, anterior cingulate cortex; AM, amygdala; CM/Pf, centromedian and parafascicular nuclei; DBS, deep brain stimulation; DH, dorsal horn; DRG, dorsal root ganglion; IC, insular cortex; LC, locus coeruleus; PAG, periaqueductal gray; PFC, prefrontal cortex; PLIC, posterior limb of the internal capsule; PNS, peripheral nerve stimulation; PVG, periventricular gray; RVM, rostral ventromedial medulla; S1, primary somatosensory cortex; S2, secondary somatosensory cortex; SCS, spinal cord stimulation; VPL, ventral posterior lateral thalamus; VPM, ventral posterior medial thalamus.

off-label status of DBS for chronic pain, DBS continues to be investigated, and several studies have shown success in delivering long-term pain relief (Abreu et al., 2022; Boccard et al., 2013; Hamani et al., 2006; Levy et al., 1987; Rasche et al., 2006). A dominant theme in these studies is that careful patient selection is key in predicting effective treatment; rates of pain relief after DBS vary significantly with different characterizations of pain and stimulation targets (Bittar et al., 2005; D. Wang et al., 2024). A meta-analysis investigated the influence of chronic pain etiology and DBS target on pain relief and quality of life outcomes. The pooled mean of short-term pain reduction was 39% (n = 63) for central neuropathic pain (CNP) and 37% (n = 70) for peripheral neuropathic pain (PNP; D. Wang et al., 2024). There was a significant difference in mean long-term pain relief in CNP and PNP patients (41% vs. 61%) and initial stimulation success rate (77% vs. 93%), indicating that PNP patients may be better candidates for DBS than CNP patients (D. Wang et al., 2024).

Conventional targets of DBS for chronic pain are the ventral posterolateral/posteromedial thalamus and the periventricular/periaqueductal gray. Interest in the anterior cingulate cortex (ACC) as a DBS target has emerged in recent years, as the ACC is a critical structure for the affective component of pain (Farrell et al., 2018). However, long-term effectiveness of ACC stimulation is a concern, as ACC-DBS in CNP had significantly lower efficacy in the long term compared with stimulation of conventional targets (D. Wang et al., 2024). Further research into optimizing ACC-DBS may lead to better stimulation methods and yield better results.

While DBS has an established role in movement disorders, its use in chronic pain is considered investigational in most countries. In patients who were unsuccessful with pharmacological treatment and other conservative pain therapies, DBS can be a viable option. Other pain conditions, such as cluster headaches, phantom limb pain, and failed back surgery syndromes, may see considerable benefit from DBS (Alamri & Pereira, 2022; Falowski, 2015; Nowacki et al., 2020; Rasche et al., 2006). The invasive nature of DBS poses the risk of severe adverse events, although studies have shown relatively low complication rates (Alamri & Pereira, 2022; Farrell et al., 2018). Further research on its effects on new brain targets and advances in technology, such as closed-loop (adaptive) stimulation, may revitalize its utility in chronic pain (Shirvalkar et al., 2018).

NIBS in Chronic Pain

TMS in Chronic Pain

TMS is the most frequent noninvasive technique studied in chronic pain. The idea to use rTMS to treat chronic pain was derived from the efficacy of implanted electric stimulation for the M1 to treat refractory neuropathic pain (Tsubokawa et al., 1991). Researchers have used rTMS to predict the effects of the implanted surgical stimulation and found that a single session of rTMS could decrease the intensity of neuropathic pain for a few days (Ramger et al., 2019). rTMS has been proposed as a therapeutic option for pain relief with analgesic effects (Hamid et al., 2019; Leung et al., 2009). High-frequency rTMS (20–50 Hz) can lead to pain relief. For instance, in a study of 48 patients with trigeminal neuralgia and poststroke pain, rTMS at 20 Hz and 80% of motor threshold over the M1 for 10 minutes for 5 consecutive days led to a significant reduction in pain immediately after the treatment assessed by the visual analogue scale (VAS). This reduction in pain was maintained for 1 month (Khedr et al., 2005). According to a meta-analysis of 12 clinical trials, the target sites for stimulation with rTMS in chronic pain ranged from M1 contralateral to the painful site, DLPFC, and secondary somatosensory cortex. The study found that effective pain control could be achieved with high-frequency rTMS to M1 contralateral to pain localization (Hamid et al., 2019). rTMS has demonstrated positive effects in pain reduction in a variety of pain syndromes, including CNP and PNP, complex regional pain syndrome, trigeminal, facial, hand, phantom limb pain, postoperative pain, low back pain, central spinal cord injury, fibromyalgia, myofascial pain syndrome, and irritable bowel syndrome.

While a study on TBS alone did not lead to analgesic effects, priming with TBS has been shown to have greater analgesic effects than rTMS alone. In a study of 14 patients with chronic treatment-refractory pain, 10-Hz rTMS over M1 alone was compared with TBS priming. Compared with baseline pain levels, iTBS followed by conventional 10-Hz rTMS led to 33% pain reduction in contrast with the 28% seen after cTBS followed by rTMS and 20% after unprimed rTMS (Lefaucheur et al., 2012).

Overall, while TMS has potential utility in the management of chronic pain, contradictory results have been reported in studies partly due to the use of different stimulation parameters. Additional research, including longitudinal studies with larger sample size, is needed to standardize the optimal stimulation parameters for the management of chronic pain. An expert consensus panel provided recommendations for the optimal use of rTMS in treating neuropathic pain (NP) and post-traumatic brain injury–related headaches (PTBI-HA; Leung et al., 2020). For NP, the panel recommended 5–10 rTMS sessions at 10–20 Hz, 2000–3000 pulses per session, and a stimulation intensity of 80–90% RMT to the contralateral M1 for unilateral NP or left DLPFC for diffuse neuropathic pain conditions. For PTBI-HA, the panel recommended five rTMS sessions at 10–20 Hz, 2,000–3,000 pulses per session, and a stimulation intensity of 80–90% of RMT to either left M1 or left DLPFC (Leung et al., 2020). Another expert group on the therapeutic uses of rTMS also recommended high-frequency rTMS of M1 contralateral to pain side in patients with NP (Lefaucheur et al., 2020).

HIFU in Chronic Pain

Thalamotomy with MRgFUS for chronic neuropathic pain may be a potential treatment for patients unresponsive to pharmacological treatment. The central lateral thalamic nucleus plays an important role in neuropathic pain through a process known as thalamocortical dysrhythmia. Thus, surgical interventions for neuropathic pain are commonly focused on this brain area (Jeanmonod et al., 2005; Kinfe, 2023). In a study with nine patients, postoperative mean VAS scores improved by 42.3% at 3 months and 40.7% at 1 year, while improvement in mean global pain relief was 49.4% and 56.9% at 3 and 12 months, respectively (Jeanmonod et al., 2012). Similar results were found in a retrospective analysis of 55 patients with chronic, therapy-resistant neuropathic pain who had undergone MRgFUS of the central lateral thalamus (Gallay et al., 2023). Patients demonstrated a 41% reduction in mean VAS scores, and 49% had pain relief greater than 50% at the 1-year follow-up (Gallay et al., 2023). The treatment effects were stable over time, showing long-term efficacy, as 51% of patients experienced >50% pain relief at the last follow-up, which was at 55 months on average. Additionally, quality of life, Montreal Cognitive Assessment, and Hospital Anxiety and Depression Scale scores were significantly improved at the 1-year follow-up (Gallay et al., 2023). In these two studies, there were only two serious complications. One patient reported persistent numbness in the upper lip, and another suffered a bleed in the motor thalamus. However, the complication rate in these two studies may be less than that of stereotactic radiosurgery of the medial thalamus (Franzini et al., 2022; Gallay et al., 2023; Jeanmonod et al., 2012). HIFU is approved in Europe for thalamotomy in chronic neuropathic pain. Nonetheless, further high-quality clinical trials and research to establish standardized procedures are needed (di Biase et al., 2021).

TUS in Chronic Pain

There are only a few TUS studies in patients with chronic pain (Sarica et al., 2022). A study that applied 15 seconds of unilateral TUS to the posterior frontal cortex in chronic pain patients found that subjective reports of mood were improved at 10 and 40 minutes postintervention, although there were no significant improvements in the numeric rating scale for pain (Hameroff et al., 2013). TUS of the right anterior thalamus in healthy participants resulted in the attenuation of thermal pain sensitivity (Badran et al., 2020). A study explored the clinical potential of stimulating the anterior cingulate cortex in patients with chronic neuropathic pain. Participants underwent six sessions of TUS over 2 weeks and showed improvement in the VAS pain scores by 21% at 2 weeks and 24% at 4 weeks postintervention. Patients also reported a decrease in daily-life pain interference scores (Shin et al., 2023). TUS could be further developed as an alternative to invasive neuromodulatory procedures such as DBS.

Summary on Neuromodulation Techniques

Neuromodulation techniques present promising alternatives to existing treatments for PD, dystonia, and chronic pain. DBS, targeting the STN and GPi, is an established surgical treatment for PD. High-frequency rTMS has shown efficacy in reducing PD motor symptoms, such as gait, bradykinesia, and overall motor function, and is currently suggested for PD treatment (Lefaucheur et al., 2020). HIFU, particularly MRgFUS, is emerging as a nonsurgical alternative to DBS, showing the potential to enhance motor function and quality of life in PD. Additionally, TUS offers a novel approach capable of reversibly altering cortical excitability and inducing plasticity in the M1, with greater depth and precision compared with conventional NIBS techniques. For PD, the combination of DBS, rTMS, and HIFU provides a comprehensive set of tools to address motor symptoms and improve patients' quality of life. TUS represents a cutting-edge addition, potentially offering more targeted and reversible noninvasive interventions.

In dystonia, GPi-DBS has shown efficacy across various forms, including generalized, segmental, and cervical dystonia. Low-frequency rTMS and tDCS have demonstrated promise in improving handwriting in writer's cramp and alleviating cervical dystonia symptoms. MRgFUS also shows potential as a safe and effective treatment for focal dystonias, such as for FHD, though further studies with larger sample sizes and longer follow-up periods are necessary. For dystonia, the effectiveness of GPi-DBS is well documented, while rTMS and tDCS provide potentially valuable noninvasive alternatives. MRgFUS offers a promising new approach, but its full potential requires further validation.

Chronic pain management has yielded variable outcomes with DBS, with PNP patients experiencing greater pain relief compared with CNP patients. High-frequency rTMS targeting the M1 has shown promise as a safe analgesic tool. HIFU, specifically MRgFUS, has proven effective in treating chronic neuropathic pain by targeting the central lateral thalamic nucleus. Furthermore, TUS has demonstrated potential in clinical studies for reducing pain sensitivity and improving pain scores, providing a noninvasive alternative to invasive neuromodulatory procedures, but further studies are needed to establish TUS as a therapeutic procedure.

In PD, dystonia, and chronic pain, maladaptive plasticity manifests as pathological changes in brain circuitries that are associated with symptoms such as motor dysfunction, involuntary movements, and pain. The brain's inherent ability to adapt, reorganize, and form new neural connections is key to overcoming the maladaptive processes seen in these disorders. The therapeutic interventions discussed in this chapter, such as DBS, TMS, and focused ultrasound, all aim to tap into brain plasticity to correct imbalances in circuit functions. By targeting specific neural circuits, these interventions work to recalibrate maladaptive patterns of activity, either by inhibiting pathological activity or by promoting the formation of new, healthy connections.

Conclusion

In conclusion, this chapter illustrates how the development of neuromodulation therapies for PD, dystonia, and chronic pain are aligned with broader understanding of brain plasticity. These therapies engage the plastic potentials of the brain to restore balance and promote recovery to address the symptoms of these brain disorders. These techniques demonstrate the remarkable capacity of the brain to self-repair, and this capacity holds promise for future treatments that could further harness neuroplasticity.

Future research in DBS should prioritize identifying optimal targets to enhance therapeutic efficacy and minimize side effects. Optimizing individualized stimulation patterns through aDBS holds significant potential for developing patient-specific treatment plans. Expanding clinical trials for HIFU with larger sample sizes and extended follow-up periods is crucial to ascertain its long-term efficacy and safety, especially for bilateral treatments. Further research into TUS should explore its therapeutic effects on various brain structures and optimize sonication parameters to maximize clinical benefits. Ensuring the safety and efficacy of HIFU and TUS through rigorous research will support their broader clinical application.

Efforts should also focus on establishing a consensus on optimal rTMS protocols to effectively improve motor and pain symptoms. Additional research into tDCS and MRgFUS for dystonia is needed to provide comprehensive data on their long-term efficacy and safety. Future studies on TMS should aim to standardize optimal stimulation parameters for chronic pain management. High-quality clinical trials on HIFU are necessary to establish standardized procedures and confirm long-term safety and efficacy. Investigating the use of TUS as an alternative to invasive neuromodulatory procedures could lead to significant advancements in chronic pain treatment. Consistency in rTMS protocols will enhance its therapeutic effectiveness. Comprehensive data on tDCS, MRgFUS, and TUS will further validate their use in clinical practice.

Advancing neuromodulation techniques through targeted research will enhance treatment outcomes and ensure patient safety and well-being. Through focused research and development, these neuromodulation techniques have the potential to revolutionize treatment paradigms for various neurological as well as psychiatric disorders, including PD, dystonia, and chronic pain, improving quality of life for countless patients.

ACKNOWLEDGMENTS

This work was supported by the Canadian Institutes of Health Research (FDN 154292, PJT 198046). Amitabh Bhattacharya is supported by a Parkinson Foundation Posdoctoral Fellowship (PF-PRF-1262111).

REFERENCES

Abreu, V., Vaz, R., Chamadoira, C., Rebelo, V., Reis, C., Costa, F., et al. (2022). Thalamic deep brain stimulation for post-traumatic neuropathic limb pain: Efficacy at five years' follow-up and effective volume of activated brain tissue. *Neurochirurgie, 68*(1), 52–60.

Alamri, A., & Pereira, E. A. C. (2022). Deep brain stimulation for chronic pain. *Neurosurgery Clinics of North America, 33*(3), 311–321.

Albanese, A., Bhatia, K., Bressman, S. B., Delong, M. R., Fahn, S., Fung, V. S. C., et al. (2013). Phenomenology and classification of dystonia: A consensus update. *Movement Disorders, 28*(7), 863–873.

Ammann, C., Dileone, M., Pagge, C., Catanzaro, V., Mata-Marín, D., Hernández-Fernández, F., et al. (2020). Cortical disinhibition in Parkinson's disease. *Brain, 143*(11), 3408–3421.

Antal, A., & Paulus, W. (2013). Transcranial alternating current stimulation (tACS). *Frontiers in Human Neuroscience, 7*, 317.

Ashkan, K., Rogers, P., Bergman, H., & Ughratdar, I. (2017). Insights into the mechanisms of deep brain stimulation. *Nature Reviews Neurology, 13*(9), 548–554.

Bachu, V. S., Kedda, J., Suk, I., Green, J. J., & Tyler, B. (2021). High-intensity focused ultrasound: A review of mechanisms and clinical applications. *Annals of Biomedical Engineering, 49*(9), 1975–1991.

Badran, B. W., Caulfield, K. A., Stomberg-Firestein, S., Summers, P. M., Dowdle, L. T., Savoca, M., et al. (2020). Sonication of the anterior thalamus with MRI-guided transcranial focused ultrasound (tFUS) alters pain thresholds in healthy adults: A double-blind, sham-controlled study. *Brain Stimulation, 13*(6), 1805–1812.

Baumann, C. R. (2012). Epidemiology, diagnosis and differential diagnosis in Parkinson's disease tremor. *Parkinsonism & Related Disorders, 18*(Suppl. 1), S90–92.

Beisteiner, R., Matt, E., Fan, C., Baldysiak, H., Schönfeld, M., Philippi Novak, T., et al. (2020). Transcranial pulse stimulation with ultrasound in Alzheimer's disease: A new navigated focal brain therapy. *Advanced Science, 7*(3), 1902583.

Ben-Joseph, A., Marshall, C. R., Lees, A. J., & Noyce, A. J. (2020). Ethnic variation in the manifestation of Parkinson's disease: A narrative review. *Journal of Parkinson's Disease, 10*(1), 31–45.

Benninger, D. H., Lomarev, M., Lopez, G., Pal, N., Luckenbaugh, D. A., & Hallett, M. (2011). Transcranial direct current stimulation for the treatment of focal hand dystonia. *Movement Disorders, 26*(9), 1698–1702.

Beudel, M., & Brown, P. (2016). Adaptive deep brain stimulation in Parkinson's disease. *Parkinsonism & Related Disorders, 22*, S123–S126.

Bhattacharya, A., Mrudula, K., Sreepada, S. S., Sathyaprabha, T. N., Pal, P. K., Chen, R., et al. (2022). An overview of noninvasive brain stimulation: Basic principles and clinical applications. *Canadian Journal of Neurological Sciences, 49*(4), 479–492.

Bittar, R. G., Kar-Purkayastha, I., Owen, S. L., Bear, R. E., Green, A., Wang, S., et al. (2005). Deep brain stimulation for pain relief: A meta-analysis. *Journal of Clinical Neuroscience, 12*(5), 515–519.

Bledsoe, I. O., Viser, A. C., & San Luciano, M. (2020). Treatment of dystonia: Medications, neurotoxins, neuromodulation, and rehabilitation. *Neurotherapeutics, 17*(4), 1622–1644.

Boccard, S. G. J., Pereira, E. A. C., Moir, L., Aziz, T. Z., & Green, A. L. (2013). Long-term outcomes of deep brain stimulation for neuropathic pain. *Neurosurgery, 72*(2), 221.

Boggio, P. S., Ferrucci, R., Rigonatti, S. P., Covre, P., Nitsche, M., Pascual-Leone, A., et al. (2006). Effects of transcranial direct current stimulation on working memory in patients with Parkinson's disease. *Journal of the Neurological Sciences, 249*(1), 31–38.

Bologna, M., Guerra, A., Paparella, G., Giordo, L., Alunni Fegatelli, D., Vestri, A. R., et al. (2018). Neurophysiological correlates of bradykinesia in Parkinson's disease. *Brain, 141*(8), 2432–2444.

Bowary, P., & Greenberg, B. D. (2018). Noninvasive focused ultrasound for neuromodulation: A review. *Psychiatric Clinics of North America, 41*(3), 505–514.

Bradnam, L. V., Graetz, L. J., McDonnell, M. N., & Ridding, M. C. (2015). Anodal transcranial direct current stimulation to the cerebellum improves handwriting and cyclic drawing kinematics in focal hand dystonia. *Frontiers in Human Neuroscience, 9*, 286.

Bretsztajn, L., & Gedroyc, W. (2018). Brain-focussed ultrasound: What's the "FUS" all about?: A review of current and emerging neurological applications. *British Journal of Radiology, 91*, 20170481.

Brittain, J.-S., Probert-Smith, P., Aziz, T. Z., & Brown, P. (2013). Tremor suppression by rhythmic transcranial current stimulation. *Current Biology: CB, 23*(5), 436–440.

Broeder, S., Nackaerts, E., Heremans, E., Vervoort, G., Meesen, R., Verheyden, G., & Nieuwboer, A. (2015). Transcranial direct current stimulation in Parkinson's disease: Neurophysiological mechanisms and behavioral effects. *Neuroscience and Biobehavioral Reviews, 57*, 105–117.

Bronte-Stewart, H., Taira, T., Valldeoriola, F., Merello, M., Marks, W. J., Albanese, A., et al. (2011). Inclusion and exclusion criteria for DBS in dystonia. *Movement Disorders, 26 Suppl 1*(Suppl 1), S5–16.

Brüggemann, N. (2021). Contemporary functional neuroanatomy and pathophysiology of dystonia. *Journal of Neural Transmission, 128*(4), 499–508.

Buttkus, F., Baur, V., Jabusch, H.-C., de la Cruz Gomez-Pellin, M., Paulus, W., Nitsche, M. A., et al. (2011). Single-session tDCS-supported retraining does not improve fine motor control in musician's dystonia. *Restorative Neurology and Neuroscience, 29*(2), 85–90.

Buttkus, F., Weidenmüller, M., Schneider, S., Jabusch, H.-C., Nitsche, M. A., Paulus, W., et al. (2010). Failure of cathodal direct current stimulation to improve fine motor control in musician's dystonia. *Movement Disorders, 25*(3), 389–394.

Chen, R., Berardelli, A., Bhattacharya, A., Bologna, M., Chen, K.-H. S., Fasano, A., et al. (2022). Clinical neurophysiology of Parkinson's disease and parkinsonism. *Clinical Neurophysiology Practice, 7*, 201–227.

Chen, R., & Rothwell, J. C. (Eds.). (2012). *Cortical connectivity: Brain stimulation for assessing and modulating cortical connectivity and function.* Springer.

Cheng, B., Zhu, T., Zhao, W., Sun, L., Shen, Y., Xiao, W., & Zhang, S. (2021). Effect of theta burst stimulation-patterned rTMS on motor and nonmotor dysfunction of Parkinson's disease: A systematic review and metaanalysis. *Frontiers in Neurology, 12*, 762100.

Clauw, D. J., Essex, M. N., Pitman, V., & Jones, K. D. (2019). Reframing chronic pain as a disease, not a symptom: Rationale and implications for pain management. *Postgraduate Medicine, 131*(3), 185–198.

Coffey, R. J. (2001). Deep brain stimulation for chronic pain: Results of two multicenter trials and a structured review. *Pain Medicine, 2*(3), 183–192.

Cohen, S. P., Vase, L., & Hooten, W. M. (2021). Chronic pain: An update on burden, best practices, and new advances. *Lancet, 397*, 2082–2097.

Contarino, M. F., Smit, M., van den Dool, J., Volkmann, J., & Tijssen, M. A. J. (2016). Unmet needs in the management of cervical dystonia. *Frontiers in Neurology, 7*, 165.

Conte, A., Rocchi, L., Ferrazzano, G., Leodori, G., Bologna, M., Li Voti, P., et al. (2014). Primary somatosensory cortical plasticity and tactile temporal discrimination in focal hand dystonia. *Clinical Neurophysiology, 125*(3), 537–543.

Coubes, P., Roubertie, A., Vayssiere, N., Hemm, S., & Echenne, B. (2000). Treatment of DYT1-generalised dystonia by stimulation of the internal globus pallidus. *Lancet, 355*, 2220–2221.

Dahlhamer, J., Lucas, J., Zelaya, C., Nahin, R., Mackey, S., DeBar, L., et al. (2018). Prevalence of chronic pain and high-impact chronic pain among adults—United States, 2016. *Morbidity and Mortality Weekly Report, 67*(36), 1001–1006.

Darmani, G., Bergmann, T. O., Butts Pauly, K., Caskey, C. F., de Lecea, L., Fomenko, A., et al. (2022). Non-invasive transcranial ultrasound stimulation for neuromodulation. *Clinical Neurophysiology, 135*, 51–73.

Davidson, B., Bhattacharya, A., Sarica, C., Darmani, G., Raies, N., Chen, R., et al. (2024). Neuromodulation techniques—From non-invasive brain stimulation to deep brain stimulation. *Neurotherapeutics, 21*(3), e00330.

DeLong, M. R., & Wichmann, T. (2007). Circuits and circuit disorders of the basal ganglia. *Archives of Neurology, 64*(1), 20–24.

DeMaagd, G., & Philip, A. (2015). Parkinson's disease and its management: Part 1: Disease entity, risk factors, pathophysiology, clinical presentation, and diagnosis. *P & T: A Peer-Reviewed Journal for Formulary Management, 40*(8), 504–532.

Deng, S., Dong, Z., Pan, L., Liu, Y., Ye, Z., Qin, L., et al. (2022). Effects of repetitive transcranial magnetic stimulation on gait disorders and cognitive dysfunction in Parkinson's disease: A systematic review with meta-analysis. *Brain and Behavior, 12*(8), e2697.

Dharnipragada, R., Denduluri, L. S., Naik, A., Bertogliat, M., Awad, M., Ikramuddin, S., et al. (2023). Frequency settings of subthalamic nucleus DBS for Parkinson's disease: A systematic review and network meta-analysis. *Parkinsonism & Related Disorders, 116*, 105809.

di Biase, L., Di Santo, A., Caminiti, M. L., Pecoraro, P. M., & Di Lazzaro, V. (2022). Classification of Dystonia. *Life, 12*(2), 206.

di Biase, L., Falato, E., Caminiti, M. L., Pecoraro, P. M., Narducci, F., & Di Lazzaro, V. (2021). Focused ultrasound (FUS) for chronic pain management: Approved and potential applications. *Neurology Research International, 2021*, 8438498.

Dobbs, B., Pawlak, N., Biagioni, M., Agarwal, S., Shaw, M., Pilloni, G., et al. (2018). Generalizing remotely supervised transcranial direct current stimulation (tDCS): Feasibility and benefit in Parkinson's disease. *Journal of Neuroengineering and Rehabilitation, 15*(1), 1–8.

Du, X., Summerfelt, A., Chiappelli, J., Holcomb, H., H., & Hong, L. E. (2014). Individualized brain inhibition and excitation profile in response to paired pulse TMS. *Journal of Motor Behavior, 46*(1), 39–48.

Elahi, B., Elahi, B., & Chen, R. (2009). Effect of transcranial magnetic stimulation on Parkinson motor function—Systematic review of controlled clinical trials. *Movement Disorders, 24*(3), 357–363.

Elias, W. J., Lipsman, N., Ondo, W. G., Ghanouni, P., Kim, Y. G., Lee, W., et al. (2016). A randomized trial of focused ultrasound thalamotomy for essential tremor. *New England Journal of Medicine, 375*(8), 730–739.

Ellaway, P. H., Davey, N. J., Maskill, D. W., & Dick, J. P. R. (1995). The relation between bradykinesia and excitability of the motor cortex assessed using transcranial magnetic stimulation in normal and parkinsonian subjects. *Electroencephalography and Clinical Neurophysiology/Electromyography and Motor Control, 97*(3), 169–178.

Ellis, T. L. (2011). Dystonia and the role of deep brain stimulation. *ISRN Surgery, 2011*, 193718.

Falowski, S. M. (2015). Deep brain stimulation for chronic pain. *Current Pain and Headache Reports, 19*(7), 27.

Farrell, S. M., Green, A., & Aziz, T. (2018). The current state of deep brain stimulation for chronic pain and its context in other forms of neuromodulation. *Brain Sciences, 8*(8), 158.

Follett, K. A., Weaver, F. M., Stern, M., Hur, K., Harris, C. L., Luo, P., et al. (2010). Pallidal versus subthalamic deep-brain stimulation for Parkinson's disease. *New England Journal of Medicine, 362*(22), 2077–2091.

Fomenko, A., Chen, K.-H. S., Nankoo, J.-F., Saravanamuttu, J., Wang, Y., El-Baba, M., et al. (2020). Systematic examination of low-intensity ultrasound parameters on human motor cortex excitability and behavior. *eLife, 9*, e54497.

Fomenko, A., Neudorfer, C., Dallapiazza, R. F., Kalia, S. K., & Lozano, A. M. (2018). Low-intensity ultrasound neuromodulation: An overview of mechanisms and emerging human applications. *Brain Stimulation, 11*(6), 1209–1217.

Franzini, A., Rossini, Z., Moosa, S., Tropeano, M. P., Milani, D., Attuati, L., et al. (2022). Medial thalamotomy using stereotactic radiosurgery for intractable pain: A systematic review. *Neurosurgical Review, 45*(1), 71–80.

Fung, W. K. W., & Peall, K. J. (2019). What is the role of the cerebellum in the pathophysiology of dystonia? *Journal of Neurology, 266*(6), 1549–1551.

Furuya, S., Nitsche, M. A., Paulus, W., & Altenmüller, E. (2014). Surmounting retraining limits in musicians' dystonia by transcranial stimulation. *Annals of Neurology, 75*(5), 700–707.

Gallay, M. N., Magara, A. E., Moser, D., Kowalski, M., Kaeser, M., & Jeanmonod, D. (2023). Magnetic resonance–guided focused ultrasound central lateral thalamotomy against chronic and therapy-resistant neuropathic pain: Retrospective long-term follow-up analysis of 63 interventions. *Journal of Neurosurgery, 139*(3), 615–624.

Gallay, M. N., Moser, D., Rossi, F., Magara, A. E., Strasser, M., Bühler, R., et al. (2019). MRgFUS pallidothalamic tractotomy for chronic therapy-resistant Parkinson's disease in 51 consecutive patients: Single center experience. *Frontiers in Surgery, 6*, 76.

Goldberg, D. S., & McGee, S. J. (2011). Pain as a global public health priority. *BMC Public Health, 11*, 770.

González-García, N., Armony, J. L., Soto, J., Trejo, D., Alegría, M. A., & Drucker-Colín, R. (2011). Effects of rTMS on Parkinson's disease: A longitudinal fMRI study. *Journal of Neurology, 258*(7), 1268–1280.

Goodwill, A. M., Lum, J. A. G., Hendy, A. M., Muthalib, M., Johnson, L., Albein-Urios, N., et al. (2017). Using non-invasive transcranial stimulation to improve motor and cognitive function in Parkinson's disease: A systematic review and meta-analysis. *Scientific Reports, 7*(1), 14840.

Grippe, T., Shamli-Oghli, Y., Darmani, G., Nankoo, J.-F., Raies, N., Sarica, C., et al. (2024). Plasticity-induced effects of theta burst transcranial ultrasound stimulation in Parkinson's disease. *Movement Disorders, 39*(8), 1364–1374.

Guerra, A., Asci, F., D'Onofrio, V., Sveva, V., Bologna, M., Fabbrini, G., et al. (2020). Enhancing gamma oscillations restores primary motor cortex plasticity in Parkinson's disease. *Journal of Neuroscience, 40*(24), 4788–4796.

Guerra, A., Suppa, A., D'Onofrio, V., Di Stasio, F., Asci, F., Fabbrini, G., et al. (2019). Abnormal cortical facilitation and L-dopa-induced dyskinesia in Parkinson's disease. *Brain Stimulation, 12*(6), 1517–1525.

Hadi, M. A., McHugh, G. A., & Closs, S. J. (2019). Impact of chronic pain on patients' quality of life: A comparative mixed-methods study. *Journal of Patient Experience, 6*(2), 133–141.

Hamani, C., Richter, E., Schwalb, J. M., & Lozano, A. M. (2008). Bilateral subthalamic nucleus stimulation for Parkinson's disease: A systematic review of the clinical literature. *Neurosurgery, 62*, SHC-863.

Hamani, C., Schwalb, J. M., Rezai, A. R., Dostrovsky, J. O., Davis, K. D., & Lozano, A. M. (2006). Deep brain stimulation for chronic neuropathic pain: Long-term outcome and the incidence of insertional effect. *Pain, 125*(1), 188.

Hameroff, S., Trakas, M., Duffield, C., Annabi, E., Gerace, M. B., Boyle, P., et al. (2013). Transcranial ultrasound (TUS) effects on mental states: A pilot study. *Brain Stimulation, 6*(3), 409–415.

Hamid, P., Malik, B. H., & Hussain, M. L. (2019). Noninvasive transcranial magnetic stimulation (TMS) in chronic refractory pain: A systematic review. *Cureus, 11*(10), e6019.

Heusinkveld, L. E., Hacker, M. L., Turchan, M., Davis, T. L., & Charles, D. (2018). Impact of tremor on patients with early stage Parkinson's disease. *Frontiers in Neurology, 9*, 628.

Hoogendam, J. M., Ramakers, G. M. J., & Lazzaro, V. D. (2010). Physiology of repetitive transcranial magnetic stimulation of the human brain. *Brain Stimulation, 3*(2), 95–118.

Horisawa, S., Yamaguchi, T., Abe, K., Hori, H., Fukui, A., Iijima, M., et al. (2021). Magnetic resonance-guided focused ultrasound thalamotomy for focal hand dystonia: A pilot study. *Movement Disorders, 36*(8), 1955–1959.

Huang, Y.-Z., Edwards, M. J., Rounis, E., Bhatia, K. P., & Rothwell, J. C. (2005). Theta burst stimulation of the human motor cortex. *Neuron, 45*(2), 201–206.

Huang, Y.-Z., Rothwell, J. C., Lu, C.-S., Wang, J., & Chen, R.-S. (2010). Restoration of motor inhibition through an abnormal premotor–motor connection in dystonia. *Movement Disorders, 25*(6), 696–703.

Hylands-White, N., Duarte, R. V., & Raphael, J. H. (2017). An overview of treatment approaches for chronic pain management. *Rheumatology International, 37*(1), 29–42.

Jeanmonod, D., Sarnthein, J., Magnin, M., Stern, J., Lebzelter, C., Aufenberg, C., et al. (2005). Chronic neurogenic pain: Thalamocortical dysrhythmic mechanisms and their surgical treatment. *Thalamus and Related Systems, 3*(1), 63.

Jeanmonod, D., Werner, B., Morel, A., Michels, L., Zadicario, E., Schiff, G., & Martin, E. (2012). Transcranial magnetic resonance imaging-guided focused ultrasound: Noninvasive central lateral thalamotomy for chronic neuropathic pain. *Neurosurgical Focus, 32*(1), E1.

Karikari, T. K., Charway-Felli, A., Höglund, K., Blennow, K., & Zetterberg, H. (2018). Commentary: Global, regional, and national burden of neurological disorders during 1990–2015: A systematic analysis for the Global Burden of Disease Study 2015. *Frontiers in Neurology, 9*, 201.

Khedr, E. M., Kotb, H., Kamel, N. F., Ahmed, M. A., Sadek, R., & Rothwell, J. C. (2005). Longlasting antalgic effects of daily sessions of repetitive transcranial magnetic stimulation in central and peripheral neuropathic pain. *Journal of Neurology, Neurosurgery, and Psychiatry, 76*(6), 833–838.

Khedr, E. M., Lefaucheur, J.-P., Hasan, A. M., & Osama, K. (2021). Are there differences in cortical excitability between akinetic-rigid and tremor-dominant subtypes of Parkinson's disease? *Neurophysiologie Clinique, 51*(5), 443–453.

Kim, S. J., Udupa, K., Ni, Z., Moro, E., Gunraj, C., Mazzella, F., et al. (2015). Effects of subthalamic nucleus stimulation on motor cortex plasticity in Parkinson disease. *Neurology, 85*(5), 425–432.

Kinfe, T. (2023). MR-guided high-intensity focused ultrasound for chronic pain: Where do we stand? *Expert Review of Neurotherapeutics, 23*(9), 757–761.

Knotkova, H., Hamani, C., Sivanesan, E., Le Beuffe, M. F. E., Moon, J. Y., Cohen, S. P., et al. (2021). Neuromodulation for chronic pain. *Lancet, 397*, 2111–2124.

Koch, G., Porcacchia, P., Ponzo, V., Carrillo, F., Cáceres-Redondo, M. T., Brusa, L., et al. (2014). Effects of two weeks of cerebellar theta burst stimulation in cervical dystonia patients. *Brain Stimulation: Basic, Translational, and Clinical Research in Neuromodulation, 7*(4), 564–572.

Krause, V., Wach, C., Südmeyer, M., Ferrea, S., Schnitzler, A., & Pollok, B. (2014). Corticomuscular coupling and motor performance are modulated by 20 Hz transcranial alternating current stimulation (tACS) in Parkinson's disease. *Frontiers in Human Neuroscience, 7*, 928.

Krishna, V., Fishman, P. S., Eisenberg, H. M., Kaplitt, M., Baltuch, G., Chang, J. W., et al. (2023). Trial of globus pallidus focused ultrasound ablation in Parkinson's disease. *New England Journal of Medicine, 388*(8), 683–693.

Kupsch, A., Benecke, R., Müller, J., Trottenberg, T., Schneider, G.-H., Poewe, W., et al. (2006). Pallidal deep-brain stimulation in primary generalized or segmental dystonia. *New England Journal of Medicine, 355*(19), 1978–1990.

Lawrence, B. J., Gasson, N., Johnson, A. R., Booth, L., & Loftus, A. M. (2018). Cognitive training and transcranial direct current stimulation for mild cognitive impairment in Parkinson's disease: A randomized controlled trial. *Parkinson's Disease, 2018*, 4318475.

Lefaucheur, J.-P., Aleman, A., Baeken, C., Benninger, D. H., Brunelin, J., Di Lazzaro, V., et al. (2020). Evidence-based guidelines on the therapeutic use of repetitive transcranial magnetic stimulation (rTMS): An update (2014–2018). *Clinical Neurophysiology, 131*(2), 474–528.

Lefaucheur, J.-P., Ayache, S. S., Sorel, M., Farhat, W. H., Zouari, H. G., Ciampi de Andrade, D., et al. (2012). Analgesic effects of repetitive transcranial magnetic stimulation of the motor cortex in neuropathic pain: Influence of theta burst stimulation priming. *European Journal of Pain, 16*(10), 1403–1413.

Legon, W., Bansal, P., Tyshynsky, R., Ai, L., & Mueller, J. K. (2018). Transcranial focused ultrasound neuromodulation of the human primary motor cortex. *Scientific Reports, 8*(1), 10017.

Leung, A., Donohue, M., Xu, R., Lee, R., Lefaucheur, J.-P., Khedr, E. M., et al. (2009). rTMS for suppressing neuropathic pain: A meta-analysis. *Journal of Pain, 10*(12), 1205–1216.

Leung, A., Shirvalkar, P., Chen, R., Kuluva, J., Vaninetti, M., Bermudes, R., et al. (2020). Transcranial magnetic stimulation for pain, headache, and comorbid depression: INS-NANS Expert Consensus Panel review and recommendation. *Neuromodulation, 23*(3), 267–290.

Levi, V., Stanziano, M., Pinto, C., Zibordi, F., Fedeli, D., Caldiera, V., et al. (2024). Bilateral simultaneous magnetic resonance-guided focused ultrasound pallidotomy for life-threatening status dystonicus. *Movement Disorders, 39*(8), 1408–1412.

Levy, R. M., Lamb, S., & Adams, J. E. (1987). Treatment of chronic pain by deep brain stimulation: Long term follow-up and review of the literature. *Neurosurgery, 21*(6), 885.

Li, R., He, Y., Qin, W., Zhang, Z., Su, J., Guan, Q., et al. (2022). Effects of repetitive transcranial magnetic stimulation on motor symptoms in Parkinson's disease: A meta-analysis. *Neurorehabilitation and Neural Repair, 36*(7), 395–404.

Lin, S., Wu, Y., Li, H., Zhang, C., Wang, T., Pan, Y., et al. (2019). Deep brain stimulation of the globus pallidus internus versus the subthalamic nucleus in isolated dystonia. *Journal of Neurosurgery, 132*(3), 721–732.

Little, S., Beudel, M., Zrinzo, L., Foltynie, T., Limousin, P., Hariz, M., et al. (2016). Bilateral adaptive deep brain stimulation is effective in Parkinson's disease. *Journal of Neurology, Neurosurgery, and Psychiatry, 87*(7), 717–721.

Little, S., Pogosyan, A., Neal, S., Zavala, B., Zrinzo, L., Hariz, M., et al. (2013). Adaptive deep brain stimulation in advanced Parkinson disease. *Annals of Neurology, 74*(3), 449–457.

Mao, Z., Ling, Z., Pan, L., Xu, X., Cui, Z., Liang, S., et al. (2019). Comparison of efficacy of deep brain stimulation of different targets in Parkinson's disease: A network meta-analysis. *Frontiers in Aging Neuroscience, 11*, 23.

Martínez-Fernández, R., Máñez-Miró, J. U., Rodríguez-Rojas, R., Del Álamo, M., Shah, B. B., Hernández-Fernández, F., et al. (2020). Randomized trial of focused ultrasound subthalamotomy for Parkinson's disease. *New England Journal of Medicine, 383*(26), 2501–2513.

Martínez-Fernández, R., Natera-Villalba, E., Rodríguez-Rojas, R., Del Álamo, M., Pineda-Pardo, J. A., Obeso, I., et al. (2024). Staged bilateral MRI-guided focused ultrasound subthalamotomy for Parkinson disease. *JAMA Neurology, 81*(6), 638–644.

Mazzone, P., Insola, A., Sposato, S., & Scarnati, E. (2009). The deep brain stimulation of the pedunculopontine tegmental nucleus. *Neuromodulation: Technology at the Neural Interface, 12*(3), 191–204.

Medina, A., Nilles, C., Martino, D., Pelletier, C., & Pringsheim, T. (2022). The prevalence of idiopathic or inherited isolated dystonia: A systematic review and meta-analysis. *Movement Disorders Clinical Practice, 9*(7), 860–868.

Meints, S. M., & Edwards, R. R. (2018). Evaluating psychosocial contributions to chronic pain outcomes. *Progress in Neuro-Psychopharmacology & Biological Psychiatry, 87*(Pt. B), 168–182.

Mills, S. E. E., Nicolson, K. P., & Smith, B. H. (2019). Chronic pain: A review of its epidemiology and associated factors in population-based studies. *British Journal of Anaesthesia, 123*(2), e273–e283.

Moisan, F., Kab, S., Mohamed, F., Canonico, M., Le Guern, M., Quintin, C., et al. (2016). Parkinson disease male-to-female ratios increase with age: French nationwide study and meta-analysis. *Journal of Neurology, Neurosurgery, and Psychiatry, 87*(9), 952–957.

Moisello, C., Blanco, D., Fontanesi, C., Lin, J., Biagioni, M., Kumar, P., et al. (2015). TMS enhances retention of a motor skill in Parkinson's disease. *Brain Stimulation, 8*(2), 224–230.

Moro, E., Hamani, C., Poon, Y.-Y., Al-Khairallah, T., Dostrovsky, J. O., Hutchison, W. D., et al. (2010). Unilateral pedunculopontine stimulation improves falls in Parkinson's disease. *Brain, 133*(Pt. 1), 215–224.

Moustafa, A. A., Chakravarthy, S., Phillips, J. R., Gupta, A., Keri, S., Polner, B., et al. (2016). Motor symptoms in Parkinson's disease: A unified framework. *Neuroscience and Biobehavioral Reviews, 68*, 727–740.

Murase, N., Rothwell, J. C., Kaji, R., Urushihara, R., Nakamura, K., Murayama, N., et al. (2005). Subthreshold low-frequency repetitive transcranial magnetic stimulation over the premotor cortex modulates writer's cramp. *Brain, 128*(1), 104–115.

Ni, Z., Bahl, N., Gunraj, C. A., Mazzella, F., & Chen, R. (2013). Increased motor cortical facilitation and decreased inhibition in Parkinson disease. *Neurology, 80*(19), 1746–1753.

Ni, Z., Kim, S. J., Phielipp, N., Ghosh, S., Udupa, K., Gunraj, C. A., et al. (2018). Pallidal deep brain stimulation modulates cortical excitability and plasticity. *Annals of Neurology, 83*(2), 352–362.

Nitsche, M. A., & Paulus, W. (2000). Excitability changes induced in the human motor cortex by weak transcranial direct current stimulation. *Journal of Physiology, 527*(3), 633–639.

Nowacki, A., Schober, M., Nader, L., Saryyeva, A., Nguyen, T.-A. K., Green, A. L., et al. (2020). Deep brain stimulation for chronic cluster headache: Meta-analysis of individual patient data. *Annals of Neurology, 88*(5), 956–969.

Odekerken, V. J. J., Boel, J. A., Schmand, B. A., de Haan, R. J., Figee, M., van den Munckhof, P., et al. (2016). GPi vs STN deep brain stimulation for Parkinson disease: Three-year follow-up. *Neurology, 86*(8), 755–761.

Okun, M. S., Fernandez, H. H., Wu, S. S., Kirsch-Darrow, L., Bowers, D., Bova, F., et al. (2009). Cognition and mood in Parkinson's disease in subthalamic nucleus versus globus pallidus interna deep brain stimulation: The COMPARE trial. *Annals of Neurology, 65*(5), 586–595.

Osou, S., Radjenovic, S., Bender, L., Gaal, M., Zettl, A., Dörl, G., et al. (2023). Novel ultrasound neuromodulation therapy with transcranial pulse stimulation (TPS) in Parkinson's disease: A first retrospective analysis. *Journal of Neurology, 271*(3), 1462–1468.

Ostrem, J. L., San Luciano, M., Dodenhoff, K. A., Ziman, N., Markun, L. C., Racine, C. A., et al. (2017). Subthalamic nucleus deep brain stimulation in isolated dystonia. *Neurology, 88*(1), 25–35.

Ou, Z., Pan, J., Tang, S., Duan, D., Yu, D., Nong, H., et al. (2021). Global trends in the incidence, prevalence, and years lived with disability of Parkinson's disease in 204 countries/territories from 1990 to 2019. *Frontiers in Public Health, 9*, 776847.

Pagano, R. L., Dale, C. S., Campos, A. C. P., & Hamani, C. (2023). Translational aspects of deep brain stimulation for chronic pain. *Frontiers in Pain Research, 3*, 1084701.

Pelletier, S. J., & Cicchetti, F. (2015). Cellular and molecular mechanisms of action of transcranial direct current stimulation: Evidence from in vitro and in vivo models. *International Journal of Neuropsychopharmacology, 18*(2), p.pyu047.

Peng, L., Fu, J., Ming, Y., Zeng, S., He, H., & Chen, L. (2018). The long-term efficacy of STN vs GPi deep brain stimulation for Parkinson disease. *Medicine, 97*(35), e12153.

Pereira, J. B., Junqué, C., Bartrés-Faz, D., Martí, M. J., Sala-Llonch, R., Compta, Y., et al. (2013). Modulation of verbal fluency networks by transcranial direct current stimulation (tDCS) in Parkinson's disease. *Brain Stimulation, 6*(1), 16–24.

Phillips, C. J. (2009). The cost and burden of chronic pain. *Reviews in Pain, 3*(1), 2–5.

Poewe, W. (2008). Non-motor symptoms in Parkinson's disease. *European Journal of Neurology, 15*(Suppl. 1), 14–20.

Pringsheim, T., Jette, N., Frolkis, A., & Steeves, T. D. L. (2014). The prevalence of Parkinson's disease: A systematic review and meta-analysis. *Movement Disorders, 29*(13), 1583–1590.

Priori, A., Maiorana, N., Dini, M., Guidetti, M., Marceglia, S., & Ferrucci, R. (2021). Adaptive deep brain stimulation (aDBS). *International Review of Neurobiology, 159*, 111–127.

Raja, S. N., Carr, D. B., Cohen, M., Finnerup, N. B., Flor, H., Gibson, S., et al. (2020). The revised International Association for the Study of Pain definition of pain: Concepts, challenges, and compromises. *Pain, 161*(9), 1976–1982.

Ramger, B. C., Bader, K. A., Davies, S. P., Stewart, D. A., Ledbetter, L. S., Simon, C. B., et al. (2019). Effects of non-invasive brain stimulation on clinical pain intensity and experimental pain sensitivity among individuals with central post-stroke pain: A systematic review. *Journal of Pain Research, 12*, 3319–3329.

Rasche, D., Rinaldi, P. C., Young, R. F., & Tronnier, V. M. (2006). Deep brain stimulation for the treatment of various chronic pain syndromes. *Neurosurgical Focus, 21*(6), 1–8.

Reich, S. G., & Savitt, J. M. (2019). Parkinson's disease. *Medical Clinics of North America, 103*(2), 337–350.

Reichmann, H. (2010). Clinical criteria for the diagnosis of Parkinson's disease. *Neuro-Degenerative Diseases, 7*(5), 284–290.

Rodriguez-Oroz, M. C., Obeso, J. A., Lang, A. E., Houeto, J.-L., Pollak, P., Rehncrona, S., et al. (2005). Bilateral deep brain stimulation in Parkinson's disease: A multicentre study with 4 years follow-up. *Brain, 128*(Pt. 10), 2240–2249.

Rosa, M., Arlotti, M., Ardolino, G., Cogiamanian, F., Marceglia, S., Di Fonzo, A., et al. (2015). Adaptive deep brain stimulation in a freely moving parkinsonian patient. *Movement Disorders, 30*(7), 1003–1005.

Rosset-Llobet, J., Fàbregas-Molas, S., & Pascual-Leone, Á. (2015). Effect of Transcranial Direct Current stimulation on neurorehabilitation of task-specific dystonia: A double-blind, randomized clinical trial. *Medical Problems of Performing Artists, 30*(3), 178–184.

Rossini, P. M., Burke, D., Chen, R., Cohen, L. G., Daskalakis, Z., Di Iorio, R., et al. (2015). Non-invasive electrical and magnetic stimulation of the brain, spinal cord, roots and peripheral nerves: Basic principles and procedures for routine clinical and research application. An updated report from an I.F.C.N. Committee. *Clinical Neurophysiology, 126*(6), 1071–1107.

Samuel, N., Ding, M. Y. R., Sarica, C., Darmani, G., Harmsen, I. E., Grippe, T., et al. (2023). Accelerated transcranial ultrasound neuromodulation in Parkinson's disease: A pilot study. *Movement Disorders, 38*(12), 2209–2216.

Samuel, N., Zeng, K., Harmsen, I. E., Ding, M. Y. R., Darmani, G., Sarica, C., et al. (2022). Multi-modal investigation of transcranial ultrasound-induced neuroplasticity of the human motor cortex. *Brain Stimulation, 15*(6), 1337–1347.

Sarica, C., Nankoo, J.-F., Fomenko, A., Grippe, T. C., Yamamoto, K., Samuel, N., et al. (2022). Human studies of transcranial ultrasound neuromodulation: A systematic review of effectiveness and safety. *Brain Stimulation, 15*(3), 737–746.

Schuepbach, W. M. M., Rau, J., Knudsen, K., Volkmann, J., Krack, P., Timmermann, L., et al. (2013). Neurostimulation for Parkinson's disease with early motor complications. *New England Journal of Medicine, 368*(7), 610–622.

Schulze, L., Feffer, K., Lozano, C., Giacobbe, P., Daskalakis, Z. J., Blumberger, D. M., et al. (2018). Number of pulses or number of sessions?: An open-label study of trajectories of improvement for once-vs. twice-daily dorsomedial prefrontal rTMS in major depression. *Brain Stimulation, 11*(2), 327–336.

Selikhova, M., Williams, D. R., Kempster, P. A., Holton, J. L., Revesz, T., & Lees, A. J. (2009). A clinico-pathological study of subtypes in Parkinson's disease. *Brain, 132*(Pt. 11), 2947–2957.

Shin, D. H., Son, S., & Kim, E. Y. (2023). Low-energy transcranial navigation-guided focused ultrasound for neuropathic pain: An exploratory study. *Brain Sciences, 13*(10), 1433.

Shirvalkar, P., Veuthey, T. L., Dawes, H. E., & Chang, E. F. (2018). Closed-loop deep brain stimulation for refractory chronic pain. *Frontiers in Computational Neuroscience, 12*, 18.

Sidransky, E., & Lopez, G. (2012). The link between the GBA gene and parkinsonism. *Lancet. Neurology, 11*(11), 986–998.

Sims-Williams, H., Matthews, J. C., Talbot, P. S., Love-Jones, S., Brooks, J. C., Patel, N. K., et al. (2017). Deep brain stimulation of the periaqueductal gray releases endogenous opioids in humans. *Neuroimage, 146*, 833–842.

Sinai, A., Nassar, M., Sprecher, E., Constantinescu, M., Zaaroor, M., & Schlesinger, I. (2022). Focused ultrasound thalamotomy in tremor dominant Parkinson's disease: Long-term results. *Journal of Parkinson's Disease, 12*(1), 199–206.

Spagnolo, F., Coppi, E., Chieffo, R., Straffi, L., Fichera, M., Nuara, A., et al. (2013). Interhemispheric balance in Parkinson's disease: A transcranial magnetic stimulation study. *Brain Stimulation, 6*(6), 892–897.

Steeves, T. D., Day, L., Dykeman, J., Jette, N., & Pringsheim, T. (2012). The prevalence of primary dystonia: A systematic review and meta-analysis. *Movement Disorders, 27*(14), 1789–1796.

Stefani, A., Lozano, A. M., Peppe, A., Stanzione, P., Galati, S., Tropepi, D., et al. (2007). Bilateral deep brain stimulation of the pedunculopontine and subthalamic nuclei in severe Parkinson's disease. *Brain, 130*(6), 1596–1607.

Tagliati, M., Krack, P., Volkmann, J., Aziz, T., Krauss, J. K., Kupsch, A., et al. (2011). Long-term management of DBS in dystonia: Response to stimulation, adverse events, battery changes, and special considerations. *Movement Disorders, 26*(Suppl. 1), S54–S62.

Teo, W.-P., Hendy, A. M., Goodwill, A. M., & Loftus, A. M. (2017). Transcranial alternating current stimulation: A potential modulator for pathological oscillations in Parkinson's disease? *Frontiers in Neurology, 8*, 185.

Tibar, H., El Bayad, K., Bouhouche, A., Ait Ben Haddou, E. H., Benomar, A., Yahyaoui, M., et al. (2018). Non-motor symptoms of Parkinson's disease and their impact on quality of life in a cohort of Moroccan patients. *Frontiers in Neurology, 9*, 170.

Todd, N., McDannold, N., & Borsook, D. (2020). Targeted manipulation of pain neural networks: The potential of focused ultrasound for treatment of chronic pain. *Neuroscience and Biobehavioral Reviews, 115*, 238–250.

Tsubokawa, T., Katayama, Y., Yamamoto, T., Hirayama, T., & Koyama, S. (1991). Treatment of thalamic pain by chronic motor cortex stimulation. *Pacing and Clinical Electrophysiology: PACE, 14*(1), 131–134.

Udupa, K., Bahl, N., Ni, Z., Gunraj, C., Mazzella, F., Moro, E., et al. (2016). Cortical Plasticity Induction by pairing subthalamic nucleus deep-brain stimulation and primary motor cortical transcranial magnetic stimulation in Parkinson's disease. *Journal of Neuroscience, 36*(2), 396–404.

Udupa, K., Bhattacharya, A., Bhardwaj, S., Pal, P. K., & Chen, R. (2022a). Parkinson's disease: Alterations of motor plasticity and motor learning. In A. Quartarone, M. F. Ghilardi, & F. Boller (Eds.), *Handbook of clinical neurology: Vol. 184. Neuroplasticity* (pp. 135–151). Elsevier.

Udupa, K., Bhattacharya, A., & Chen, R. (2022b). Exploring the connections between basal ganglia and cortex revealed by transcranial magnetic stimulation, evoked potential and deep brain stimulation in dystonia. *European Journal of Paediatric Neurology, 36*, 69–77.

Udupa, K., & Chen, R. (2015). The mechanisms of action of deep brain stimulation and ideas for the future development. *Progress in Neurobiology, 133*, 27–49.

Valero-Cabré, A., Pascual-Leone, A., & Rushmore, R. J. (2008). Cumulative sessions of repetitive transcranial magnetic stimulation (rTMS) build up facilitation to subsequent TMS-mediated behavioural disruptions. *European Journal of Neuroscience, 27*(3), 765–774.

Volkmann, J., Mueller, J., Deuschl, G., Kühn, A. A., Krauss, J. K., Poewe, W., et al. (2014). Pallidal neurostimulation in patients with medication-refractory cervical dystonia: A randomised, sham-controlled trial. *Lancet Neurology, 13*(9), 875–884.

Vucic, S., Stanley Chen, K.-H., Kiernan, M. C., Hallett, M., Benninger, D. H., Di Lazzaro, V., et al. (2023). Clinical diagnostic utility of transcranial magnetic stimulation in neurological disorders. Updated report of an IFCN committee. *Clinical Neurophysiology, 150*, 131–175.

Wagle Shukla, A., Shuster, J. J., Chung, J. W., Vaillancourt, D. E., Patten, C., Ostrem, J., et al. (2016). Repetitive transcranial magnetic stimulation (rTMS) therapy in Parkinson disease: A meta-analysis. *PM&R, 8*(4), 356–366.

Wang, D., Lu, Y., Han, Y., Zhang, X., Dong, S., Zhang, H., et al. (2024). The influence of etiology and stimulation target on the outcome of deep brain stimulation for chronic neuropathic pain: A systematic review and meta-analysis. *Neuromodulation, 27*(1), 83–94.

Wang, J.-W., Zhang, Y.-Q., Zhang, X.-H., Wang, Y.-P., Li, J.-P., & Li, Y.-J. (2016). Cognitive and psychiatric effects of STN versus GPi deep brain stimulation in Parkinson's disease: A meta-analysis of randomized controlled trials. *PLOS ONE, 11*(6), e0156721.

Wang, P., Zhang, J., Yu, J., Smith, C., & Feng, W. (2019). Brain modulatory effects by low-intensity transcranial ultrasound stimulation (TUS): A systematic review on both animal and human studies. *Frontiers in Neuroscience, 13*, 696.

Weaver, F. M., Follett, K. A., Stern, M., Luo, P., Harris, C. L., Hur, K., et al. (2012). Randomized trial of deep brain stimulation for Parkinson disease: Thirty-six-month outcomes. *Neurology, 79*(1), 55–65.

Weintraub, M. (1990). How to evaluate reports of clinical trials. *Pharmacy and Therapeutics, 14*, 1463–1476.

Williams, N. R., Foote, K. D., & Okun, M. S. (2014). STN vs. GPi deep brain stimulation: Translating the rematch into clinical practice. *Movement Disorders Clinical Practice, 1*(1), 24–35.

Wong, J. K., Cauraugh, J. H., Ho, K. W. D., Broderick, M., Ramirez-Zamora, A., Almeida, L., et al. (2019). STN vs. GPi deep brain stimulation for tremor suppression in Parkinson disease: A systematic review and meta-analysis. *Parkinsonism & Related Disorders, 58*, 56–62.

Woolf, C. J., Bennett, G. J., Doherty, M., Dubner, R., Kidd, B., Koltzenburg, M., et al. (1998). Towards a mechanism-based classification of pain? *Pain, 77*(3), 227–229.

Xia, X., Fomenko, A., Nankoo, J.-F., Zeng, K., Wang, Y., Zhang, J., et al. (2021). Time course of the effects of low-intensity transcranial ultrasound on the excitability of ipsilateral and contralateral human primary motor cortex. *NeuroImage, 243*, 118557.

Yu, K., Liu, C., Niu, X., & He, B. (2021). Transcranial focused ultrasound neuromodulation of voluntary movement-related cortical activity in humans. *IEEE Transactions on Bio-Medical Engineering, 68*(6), 1923–1931.

Yu, K., Niu, X., & He, B. (2020). Neuromodulation management of chronic neuropathic pain in the central nervous system. *Advanced Functional Materials, 30*(37), 1908999.

Zanjani, A., Zakzanis, K. K., Daskalakis, Z. J., & Chen, R. (2015). Repetitive transcranial magnetic stimulation of the primary motor cortex in the treatment of motor signs in Parkinson's disease: A quantitative review of the literature. *Movement Disorders, 30*(6), 750–758.

Zeng, K., Darmani, G., Fomenko, A., Xia, X., Tran, S., Nankoo, J.-F., et al. (2022). Induction of human motor cortex plasticity by theta burst transcranial ultrasound stimulation. *Annals of Neurology, 91*(2), 238–252.

Zeng, K., Li, Z., Xia, X., Wang, Z., Darmani, G., Li, X., & Chen, R. (2024). Effects of different sonication parameters of theta burst transcranial ultrasound stimulation on human motor cortex. *Brain Stimulation, 17*(2), 258–268.

Zhang, J., Li, J., Chen, F., Liu, X., Jiang, C., Hu, X., et al. (2021). STN versus GPi deep brain stimulation for dyskinesia improvement in advanced Parkinson's disease: A meta-analysis of randomized controlled trials. *Clinical Neurology and Neurosurgery, 201*, 106450.

Zhang, W., Deng, B., Xie, F., Zhou, H., Guo, J.-F., Jiang, H., et al. (2022). Efficacy of repetitive transcranial magnetic stimulation in Parkinson's disease: A systematic review and meta-analysis of randomised controlled trials. *EClinicalMedicine, 52*, 101589.

Zhang, Y., Ren, L., Liu, K., Tong, S., Yuan, T.-F., & Sun, J. (2021). Transcranial ultrasound stimulation of the human motor cortex. *iScience, 24*(12), 103429.

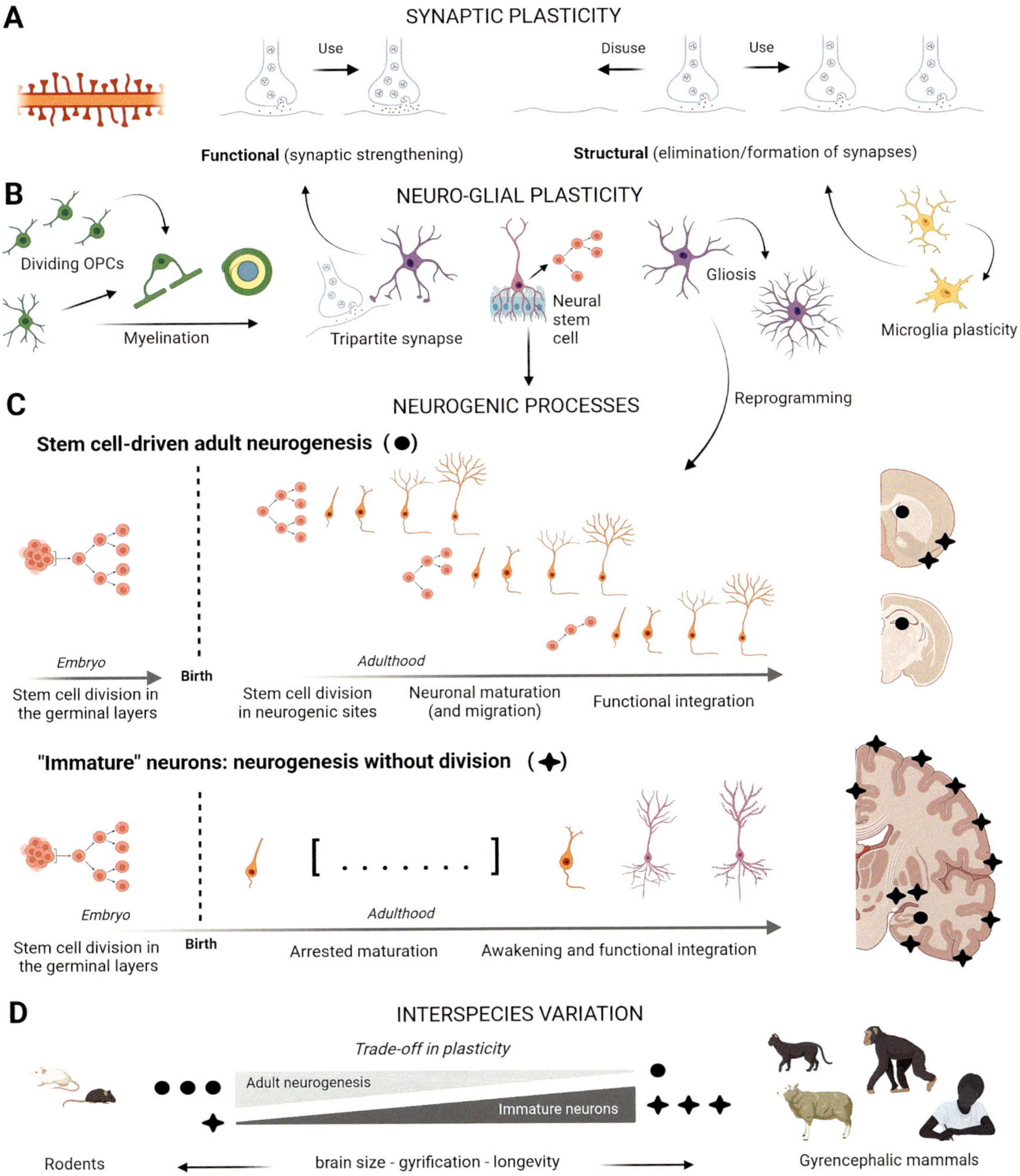

FIGURE 4.1. Heterogeneity of neural plasticity. (A–C) Different types of structural changes; (D) interspecies variation from mice to humans. (A) Functional and structural synaptic plasticity. (B) Different aspects of neuroglial plasticity, involving oligodendrocyte progenitor cells (OPCs), astrocytes, and microglia. (C) Neurogenic plasticity, in which new functional neurons can originate either from stem cell division (hosted and regulated within canonical neurogenic niches; top) or after awakening and full maturation of "dormant" neurons arrested in a state of immaturity (bottom). (D) Unlike synaptic plasticity (generally widespread in the entire nervous system and present across the animal world), neurogenic processes are restricted in mammals, showing an evolutionary "tradeoff" with a prevalence of stem cell–driven adult neurogenesis in some animal groups (small-brained, lissencephalic species, e.g., rodents) and a preference for nondividing "immature" neurons in others (large-brained, gyrencephalic species, e.g., cats, sheep, and primates), these latter including long-living species such as humans. Created with *https://app.biorender.com*.

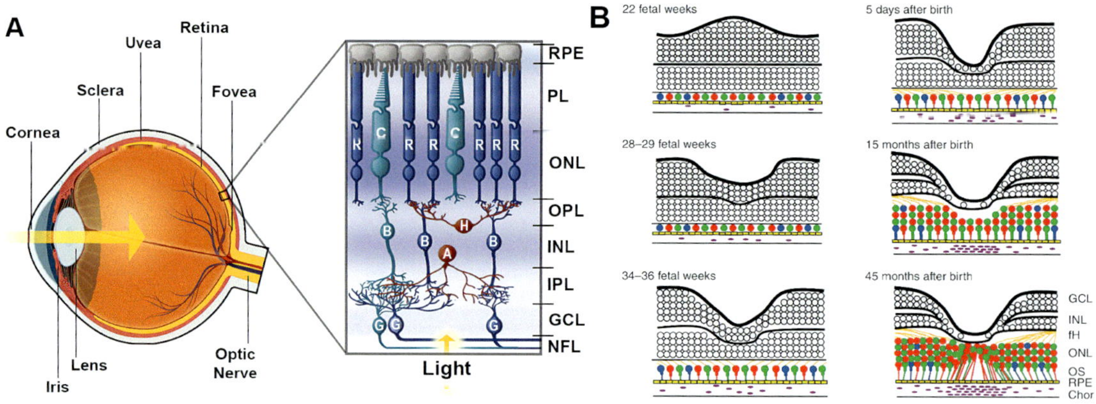

FIGURE 6.1. Maturation of the human retina. (A) The eye and the different layers of the retina. From Ptito, Bleau, and Bouskila (2021); available at *https://doi.org/10.3390/cells10123269* under a CC-BY4.0 license. (B) Pre- and postnatal maturation of the retina, viewed at the level of the fovea. From Gregory-Evans and Gregory-Evans (2011); with permission from Taylor & Francis Ltd., *www.tandfonline.com*. R, rod; C, cone; H, horizontal cells; B, bipolar cells; A, amacrine cells; G, retinal ganglion cells; RPE, retinal pigment epithelium; PL, photoreceptor layer; ONL, outer nuclear layer; OPL, outer plexiform layer; INL, inner nuclear layer; IPL, inner plexiform layer; GCL, ganglion cell layer; NFL, nerve fiber layer; Chor, choroid; fH, fibers of Henle; OS, outer segment.

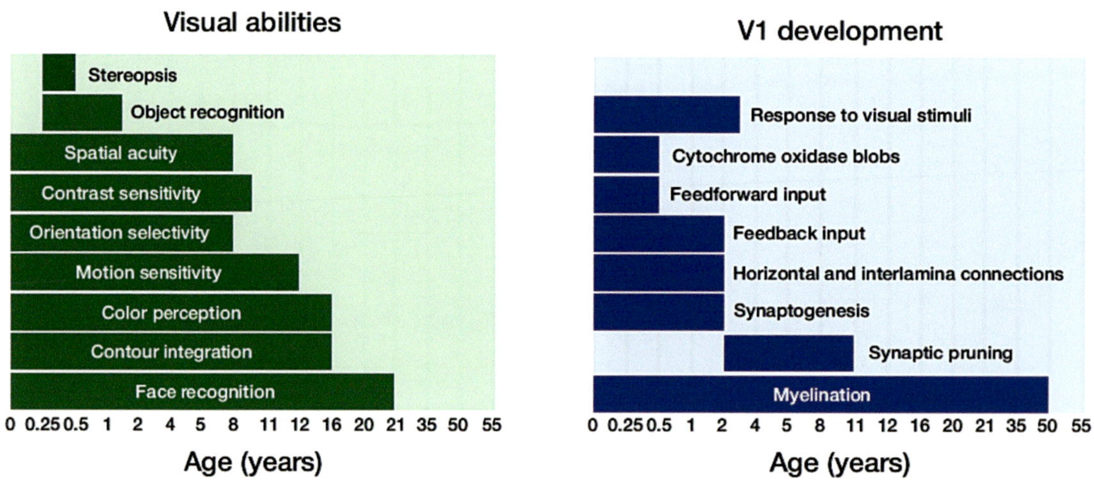

FIGURE 6.2. Postnatal development of visual functions in humans parallels the maturation of the visual cortex. Based on reviews from Danka Mohammed and Khalil (2020) and Siu and Murphy (2018).

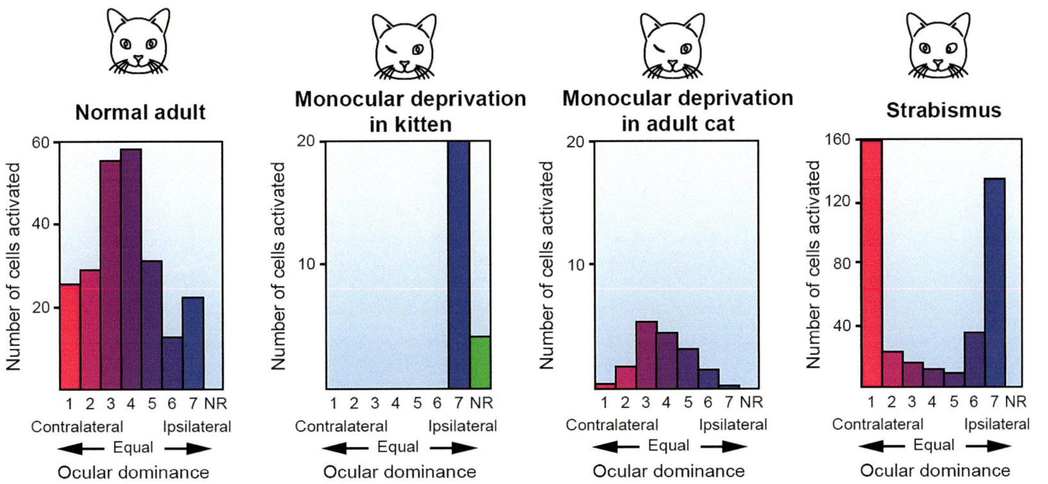

FIGURE 6.3. Monocular deprivation and unilateral strabismus in the kitten significantly affect ocular dominance in V1. Based on results from Hubel and Wiesel (1965, 1970); cat images generated by AI emoji generator. NR, not responding.

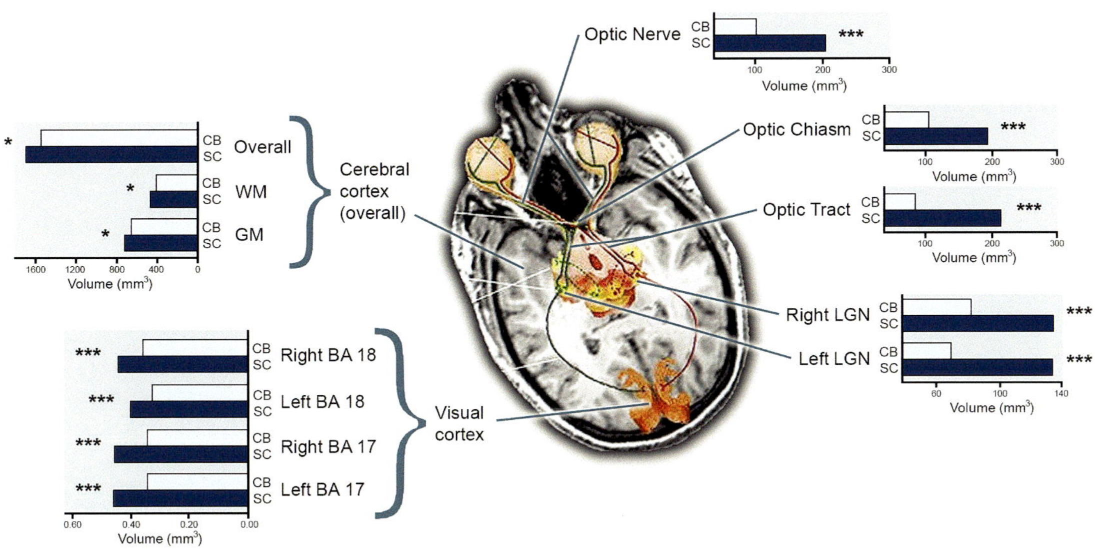

FIGURE 6.4. Anatomical changes along the visual pathway in blind individuals from the optic nerve to the visual cortex. Early, or congenitally, blind (CB) individuals show atrophy in the components of the visual system compared with controls (SC). Adapted with permission from Ptito, Schneider, et al. (2008); bar graphs based on results from Cecchetti et al. (2016), Ptito, Schneider, et al. (2008), and Ptito, Paré, et al. (2021). $^{*}p < .05$; $^{***}p < .001$.

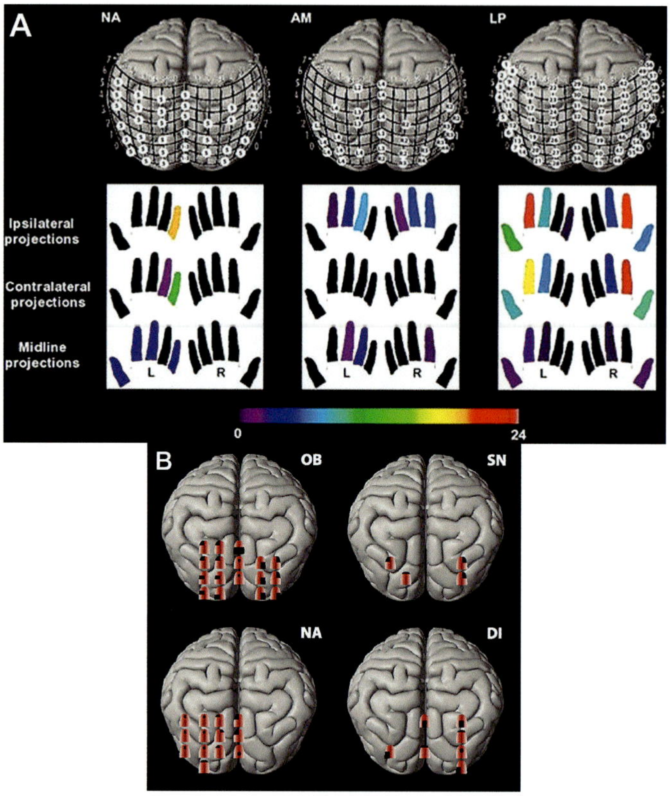

FIGURE 6.5. TMS of the visual cortex induces paresthesia in fingers of Braille readers (from Ptito, Fumal, et al., 2008) and on the tongue of individuals trained with the TDU (from Kupers et al., 2006; Copyright © 2006 Springer Nature and National Academy of Sciences, U.S.A.).

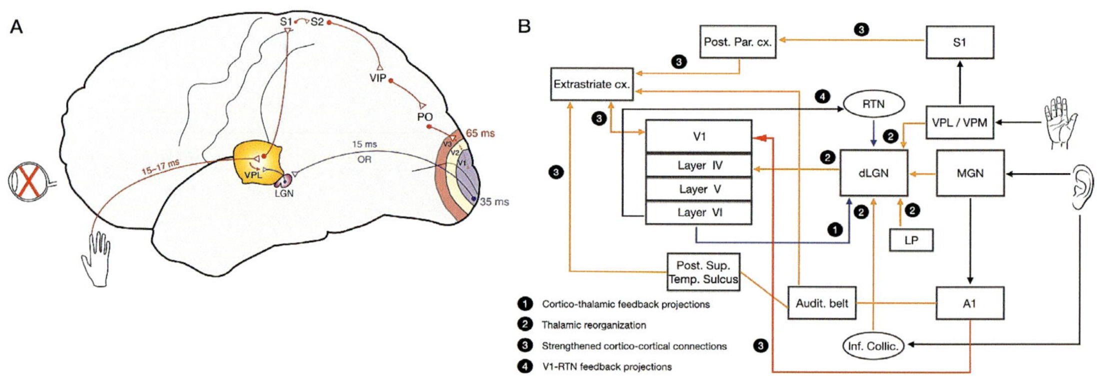

FIGURE 6.6. Anatomo-functional reorganization of the human blind brain leading to cross-modal recruitment of the visual cortex. (A) MEG results highlighting the fast thalamo-cortical pathway using a short connection between VPL and LGN and reaching V1 via the optic radiations. From Müller et al. (2019), available *at https://doi.org/10.1038/s41467-019-13173-7* under a CC-BY4.0 license. (B) Diffusion tensor imaging cartoon showing how tactile and auditory information reach the visual cortex. Note that, in both cases, the dLGN receives an ectopic projection from the somatosensory (VPL) and the auditory (MGN) thalamic nuclei en route to the visual cortex. From Ptito, Paré, et al. (2021), available at *https://doi.org/10.3389/fnhum.2021.638887* under a CC-BY4.0 license.

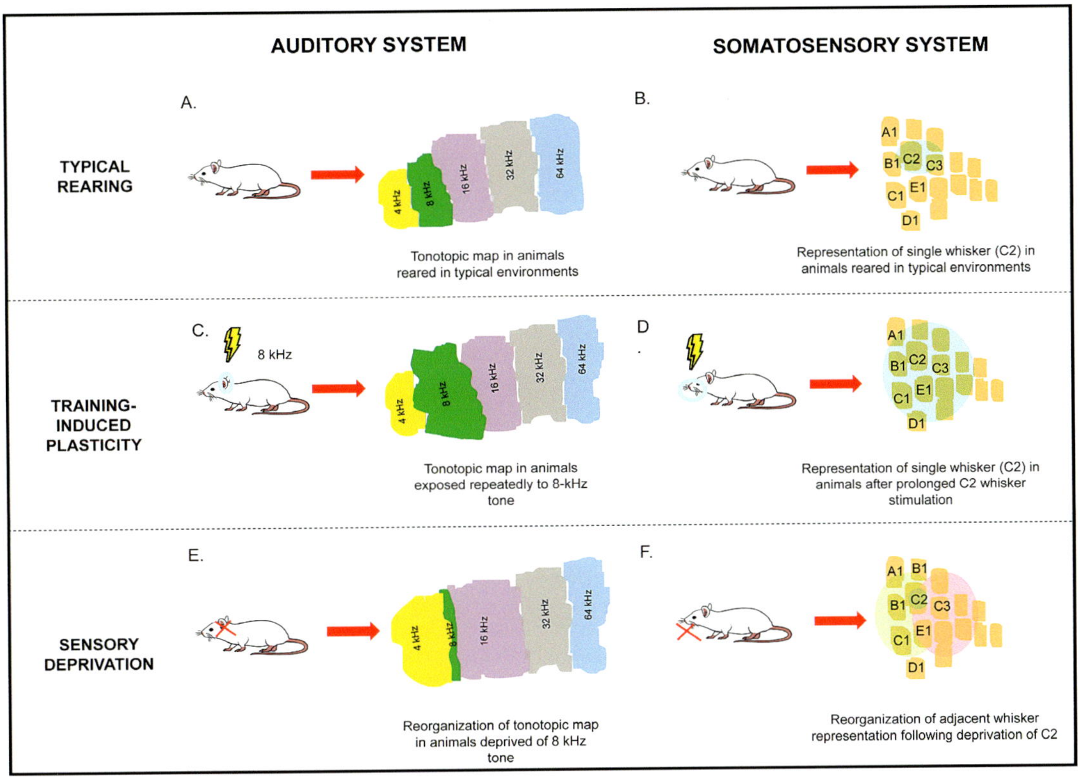

FIGURE 7.1. Summary of adaptive plastic mechanisms observed in the auditory and somatosensory cortex. Panels A and B display the cortical maps in the auditory (A) and somatosensory (B) cortex when the animal is exposed to a typical sensory experience. Panels C and D display the plastic changes observed in the tonotopic (C) and somatosensory (D) map following intense training, consisting of exposing the animal either to one single frequency or stimulation of a single whisker. Note that in both cortices, what is observed is the expansion of selective frequency and whisker representation. Finally, Panels E and F show plastic changes observed following selective deprivation of one single frequency (E) or whisker. Note that in both cases, adjacent cortical map representations expand at the expense of the deprived representation.

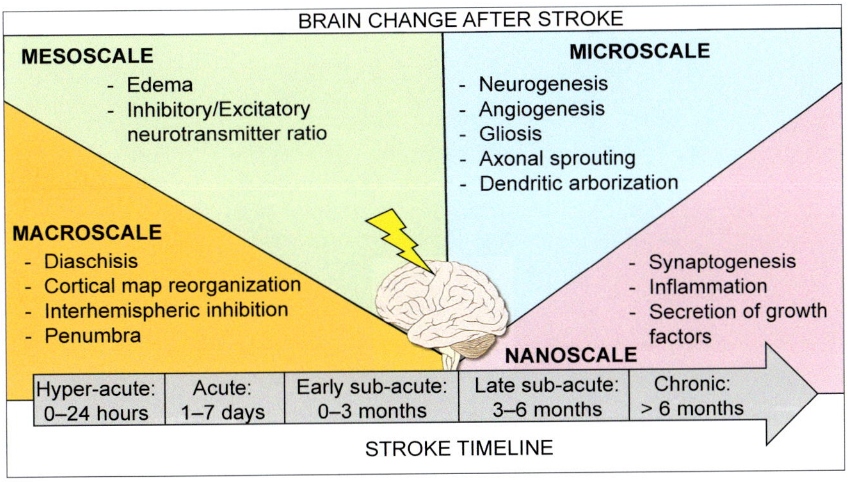

FIGURE 8.1. The main changes occurring in the brain after an injury, such as a stroke, can be visualized at different dimensional scales (Dalise et al., 2014). These changes occur during various phases of the disease, with their magnitude modulated by disease characteristics, stage of recovery, and external interventions (Bernhardt et al., 2017). This figure has been designed using assets from *Freepik.com*.

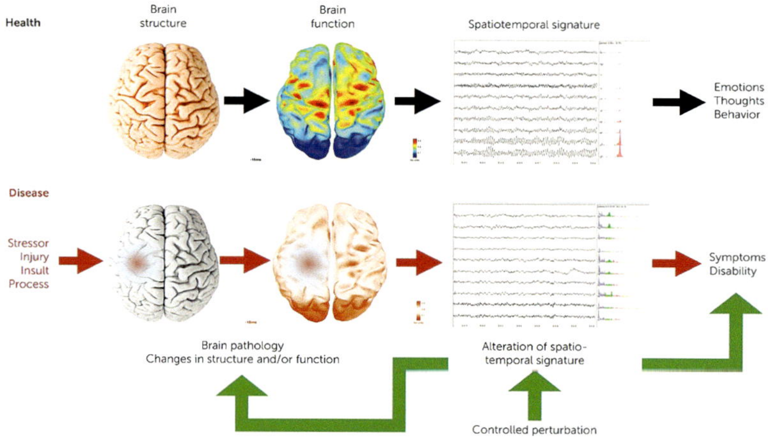

FIGURE 11.1. Conceptualization of brain–behavior relationships as manifestations of activity patterns in specific brain circuits giving rise to spatiotemporal signatures of brain function. In the context of brain diseases, these patterns can become altered, leading to specific symptoms or disabilities. This framework introduces the concept of brain-related disabilities as brain circuit disorders, or circuitopathies. Within this model, controlled perturbations of these altered spatiotemporal signatures—using techniques like repetitive transcranial magnetic stimulation (rTMS) or transcranial electrical stimulation (tES; including tDCS or tACS)—can lead to symptomatic improvement and potentially modify both the structural and functional components of the underlying brain pathology. Adapted with permission from Cappon and Pascual-Leone (2024).

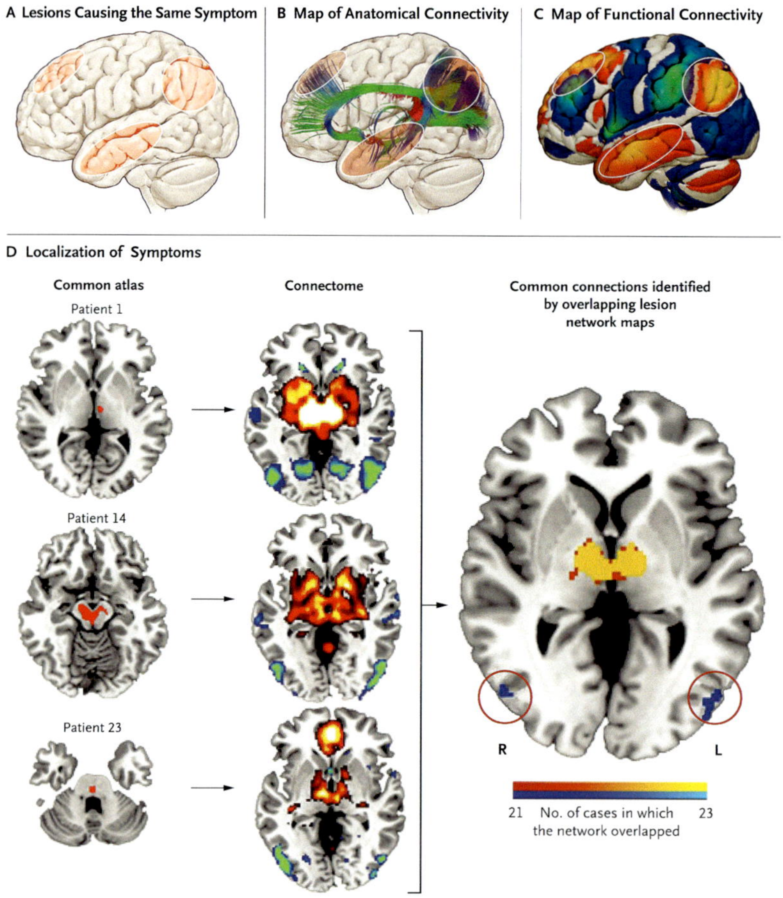

FIGURE 11.2. Conceptualization of lesion network localization involves understanding how lesions in different brain locations can lead to the same symptom. As shown in Panel A, lesions causing identical symptoms but located in different parts of the brain can be analyzed by overlaying them on maps of anatomical connectivity (Panel B) or functional connectivity (Panel C) to determine whether they are part of the same interconnected brain network. Through lesion network mapping, lesion sites from various patients with the same symptom are traced onto a common brain atlas (Panel D, left column). Using the human connectome, the functional connectivity between each lesion site and the rest of the brain is calculated (Panel D, middle column). These lesion network maps can then be superimposed to identify shared connections (Panel D, right column). In this example, lesions associated with visual hallucinations are functionally connected to a brain region involved in visual imagery (highlighted by red circles). Adapted with permission from Fox (2018).

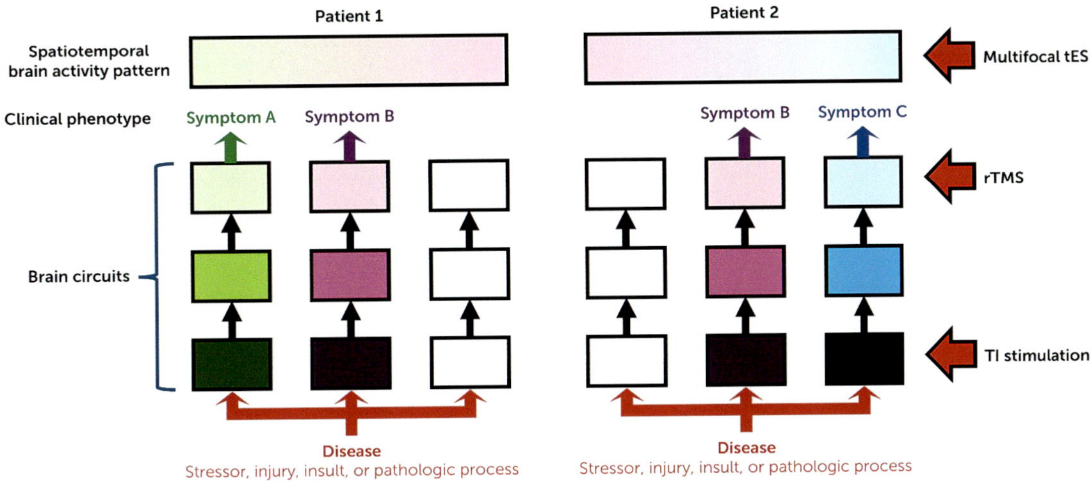

FIGURE 11.3. Approaches to brain circuit therapeutics using noninvasive electromagnetic neuromodulation techniques. Individuals experience varied impacts on their brain circuits due to factors such as illness, stress, injury, or pathological processes. This variability contributes to the diverse phenotypic and symptomatic presentations observed across patients. By identifying the altered brain circuits, targeted neuromodulation techniques like rTMS or tES can be employed to modulate specific circuits. Multifocal neuromodulation approaches allow for the targeting of multiple circuits simultaneously, while TI stimulation enables selective modulation of deep brain structures. These methods use the targeted brain regions as "windows" to influence broader brain circuits. Additionally, multifocal tES can modulate the overall disruption in the spatiotemporal patterns of brain activity associated with a patient's clinical phenotype, and multifocal tACS can even target specific frequencies of altered oscillatory activity within the brain. Adapted with permission from Cappon and Pascual-Leone (2024).

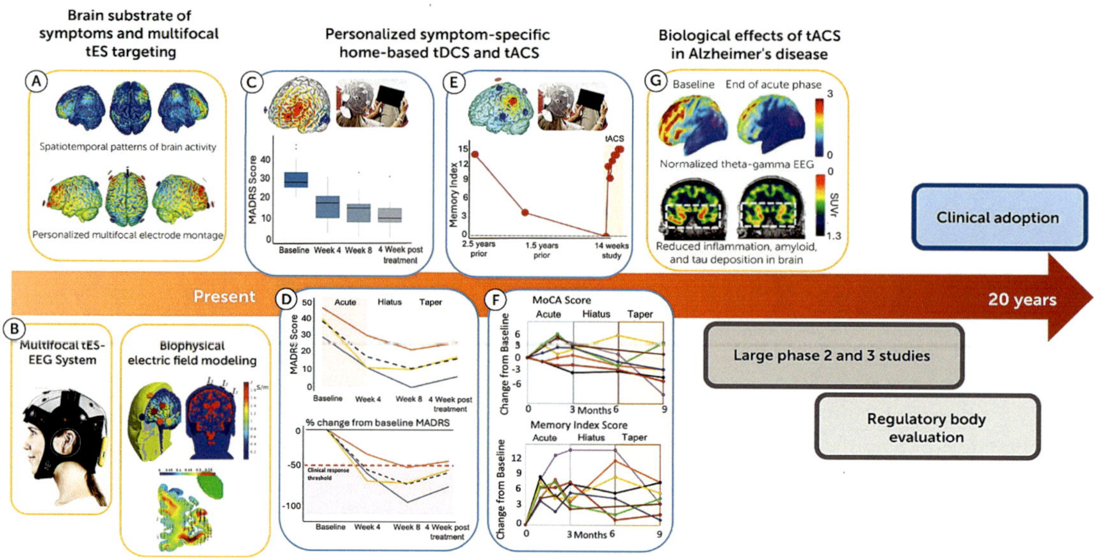

FIGURE 11.4. Recent advancements in precision tES have introduced several innovative approaches aimed at improving the efficacy of noninvasive brain stimulation. (A) (top) One such advancement is the development of AI algorithms to define multifocal electrode montages tailored to target altered spatiotemporal brain activity patterns identified through MRI and EEG (e.g., Stimweaver®). (bottom) By capturing the brain substrates of symptoms using neuroimaging techniques like EEG and fMRI, personalized tES can be applied based on each individual's unique spatiotemporal signatures. (B) Left: Another significant development is the creation of systems for multifocal recording and modulation of brain activity, such as Neuroelectrics® Enobio & Starstim, which allow for more precise interventions. Right: Additionally, advanced biophysical mathematical models have been developed to predict the distribution of induced electric currents in the brain during tDCS and tACS (Miranda et al., 2006, 2018; Ruffini et al., 2014). These models have demonstrated that the E-field can explain changes in cortical excitability (Laakso et al., 2015; Miranda et al., 2018) and that anatomical variations in the brain significantly influence the E-field generated by noninvasive stimulation methods (Antonenko et al., 2021; Laakso et al., 2019; Miranda et al., 2018; Nummenmaa et al., 2013; Thielscher et al., 2011). (C) Proof-of-concept studies have shown that tDCS targeting the DLPFC can improve depression severity. (top) Left: DLPFC targeting optimization using Stimweaver® algorithm (Ruffini et al., 2014). The color scale represents En, the normal component of the E-field induced by the optimized montage in the cortical surface (in V/m). Right: Neuroelectrics® Starstim Home system. (bottom) In a study involving 35 patients with major depressive disorder (MDD), remotely supervised tDCS resulted in an average improvement of 19.8 points after 4 weeks of daily home-based tDCS (HB-tDCS). (D) A separate proof-of-concept study investigated a novel protocol where multichannel tDCS was administered at home for older adults with MDD, supported by caregivers. The study involved five participants, with three completing the trial and showing an average 59% reduction in Montgomery–Åsberg Depression Rating Scale (MADRS) scores between baseline and 1-month follow-up. This protocol utilized a multichannel electric field–informed montage and a remotely hosted training program for caregivers, eliminating the need for lab visits (Cappon et al., 2022). (E) Initial proof of concept studies of tACS in patients with amnestic mild cognitive impairment due to AD. (top) The multichannel home-based tACS (HB-tACS) targeting the left angular gyrus. (bottom) Pilot data of one participant completing open-label 14 weeks tACS intervention showed improvement in episodic memory compared with the same participant 2.5 and 1.5 years before the study (Brechet et al., 2021). (F) A subsequent study enrolled eight participants diagnosed with mild AD who underwent multiple consecutive sessions (70–98) of multifocal HB-tACS (40 Hz, 20 minutes) targeting the left angular gyrus (AG) over 4 weeks (Cappon et al., 2023). All eight participants demonstrated memory improvements during the trial. The acute phase showed the greatest enhancement, with a 7.38-point increase in the Memory Index Score (MIS), which was maintained at 7.00 points 3 months later in the hiatus phase, and at 4.63 points 6 months later in the taper phase. Notably, despite the rise in MIS values, Montreal Cognitive Assessment (MoCA) scores remained stable, suggesting that targeting specific cognitive domains with noninvasive brain stimulation might represent a net zero-sum effect (Brem et al., 2014). (G) Additionally, tACS in AD showed initial biological effects: (top) restored theta-gamma EEG activity (Cappon et al., 2023) and (bottom) reduced inflammation, amyloid, and tau deposition on PET scans (Sprugnoli et al., 2021). All this work is progressing toward large-scale phase 2 and 3 trials, regulatory reviews, and eventual clinical adoption. Adapted with permission from Cappon and Pascual-Leone (2024).

CHAPTER 11

Therapeutic Interventions for Modulation of Brain Plasticity in Neurological and Psychiatric Diseases

Ali Jannati, Joyce Gomes-Osman, Davide B. Cappon, and Alvaro Pascual-Leone

Introduction

The World Health Organization (WHO; 2019) launched the UN Decade of Healthy Aging 2021–2030 initiative to "add life to years" and enhance the quality of life for individuals, their families, and communities. A key component of achieving this vision is addressing the growing burden of neurological and psychiatric diseases, which are leading contributors to disability worldwide. While advancements in public health, health care, and education have significantly increased global life expectancy, evidence shows that many individuals spend these additional years in illness and disability, rather than enjoying a higher quality of life (Feigin et al., 2019).

Brain diseases are now the leading cause of disability, particularly in older adults. Currently, approximately 320 million children globally have brain developmental disorders, 366 million people suffer from attention deficit disorders, 50 million experience epilepsy, 310 million live with anxiety disorders, 250 million are affected by depression, and over 100 million have dementia. Additionally, migraine is the top cause of disability for women under 50, stroke is the primary cause of disability in older men, and dementia is one of the most feared health conditions in developed nations. Overall, one in two people worldwide is impacted by brain-related disabilities—whether through direct illness or as a caregiver for someone affected.

In 2021 alone, neurological and psychiatric conditions accounted for 406 million disability-adjusted life years (DALYs)—a measure combining years lost due to premature death and years lived with disability. This figure is nearly double the DALYs attributed to cancer (260 million) and exceeds those from cardiovascular disease (402 million; Feigin et al., 2019). The burden of brain-related disabilities continues to rise, and the WHO projects that by 2030, such disabilities will account for half of the global economic impact of disability, surpassing 15% of the world's gross domestic product—more than cancer, diabetes, and respiratory diseases combined.

Despite extensive research and substantial investments, progress in treating brain-related disabilities remains limited, largely because of our incomplete understanding of the underlying biology, the complexity of their clinical presentations, and the frequent overlap of symptoms across disorders. A new approach is necessary—one that addresses individual patient disabilities while continuing to search for key pathophysiological processes that could repair core disease mechanisms and resolve all associated clinical symptoms. This shift requires a focus on disease prevention and the promotion of brain health and resilience, enhancing each individual's nervous system's ability to cope with and minimize the functional consequences of stressors, injuries, or diseases.

Strategies to promote brain health must be grounded in a deeper understanding of what constitutes a healthy brain. It is reasonable to assume that brain health and mental well-being are shaped by both genetic and environmental factors and that maintaining them depends on developing and preserving structural brain integrity and optimal function appropriate to one's age. Several principles can be used to define brain health (Gomes-Osman & Pascual-Leone, 2024), but perhaps the most fundamental is that "a healthy brain is one with the right amount of efficacy in its mechanisms of plasticity" (Pascual-Leone & Taylor, 2011).

Neuroplasticity forms the biological basis for learning, skill acquisition, and creativity, yet it also contributes to the emergence of symptoms in brain diseases and disabilities (Kloos et al., 2020). Importantly, neuroplastic changes are neither inherently beneficial nor detrimental—the key lies in directing them toward adaptive and functional outcomes (Pascual-Leone et al., 2005). Evidence suggests that the effectiveness of plasticity mechanisms declines with age (Freitas et al., 2013; Gomes-Osman et al., 2018), and alterations in plasticity are associated with conditions such as Alzheimer's disease (AD), depression, schizophrenia, and autism spectrum disorder (Jannati et al., 2023).

A healthy brain maintains optimal plasticity mechanisms that adapt to an individual's age, sex, life circumstances, and medical conditions. It also sustains a "state of brain functioning across cognitive, sensory, social-emotional, behavioral, and motor domains," enabling individuals to realize their full potential throughout life, regardless of the presence of any disorders (WHO, 2022).

Plastic ensembles of neurons—organized into dynamic brain circuits—represent the fundamental units of brain function and, consequently, the key substrates of brain health. Mounting evidence indicates that every human emotion, thought, and behavior correspond to specific patterns of activity within these neuronal ensembles or networks, each defined by distinctive spatiotemporal signatures of brain activity. These networks are continuously reshaped through experience and adaptation, and their evolving activity patterns give rise to the full spectrum of human cognition, emotion, and behavior. Conversely, the symptoms of neurological or psychiatric disorders often reflect disruptions in these patterns—altered spatiotemporal dynamics within specific neural circuits—suggesting that many such conditions may best be understood as *circuitopathies* (Figure 11.1*).

Identifying alterations in spatiotemporal signatures of brain activity that correspond to specific symptoms and disabilities provides a novel framework for understanding disease pathophysiology and guiding precise therapeutics. This paradigm addresses a major limitation of the current neuropsychiatric diagnostic system, which tends to assign broad categorical labels to syndromes arising from dysfunction across multiple, overlapping neural processes. By leveraging advanced tools that map brain activity and connectivity—such as functional magnetic resonance imaging (fMRI) and electroencephalography (EEG)—clinicians can delineate the distributed networks underlying particular symptoms and target the plastic brain circuits most amenable to intervention.

For example, building on von Monakow's framework for localizing brain dysfunction and associated disabilities (Wiesendanger, 2006), *lesion network localization* provides powerful insights into the neural basis of neurological and psychiatric symptoms. By examining how focal lesions, pathologies, or injuries alter activity across distributed brain networks, this approach reveals how network-level disruptions give rise to specific symptom profiles (Boes et al., 2015; Fox, 2018; Joutsa & Fox, 2022; Figure 11.2). Moreover, lesion network mapping enables the identification of precise neural circuits that may serve as optimal targets for neuromodulatory or therapeutic interventions (Fox et al., 2014; Ozdemir et al., 2020). By mapping the altered spatiotemporal signatures that emerge from these network disruptions and underlie an individual's symptoms or disabilities, this approach opens a complementary therapeutic pathway—one that targets dysfunctional neural dynamics directly. In doing so, it not only supports efforts to address the root cause of disease but also offers direct functional benefits to the patient.

In this chapter, we examine noninvasive brain stimulation through the lens of this conceptual framework. Rather than functioning as a direct treatment for a specific disease, noninvasive brain stimulation—and brain stimulation more broadly—acts as a means of modulating the neural substrates that give rise to symptoms and disabilities associated with brain dysfunction. By influencing plasticity and activity within targeted neural networks or circuits, it enables the adjustment of the very mechanisms that underlie these impairments, thereby offering a pathway to functional recovery and restoration (Cappon & Pascual-Leone, 2024).

Tools for Modulation of Plasticity and Circuit-Based Therapeutics

In the rapidly advancing field of neuroscience, we are approaching a pivotal moment in which emerging discoveries are poised to revolutionize our understanding of the brain's complexity. A new generation of innovative methods and technologies is enabling researchers to decode the spatiotemporal patterns of human brain activity and uncover their deep relationships with behavior, disease symptoms, and disabilities.

---

* All figures appear on the separate color insert.

These technologies offer a concrete means of modulating altered brain activity and leveraging the brain's intrinsic plasticity to restore or enhance function. An expanding body of evidence demonstrates that brain function can be precisely influenced through noninvasive methods, yielding measurable improvements in cognitive performance, mental health, and overall neurological resilience.

These neurotechnologies span a broad spectrum of approaches—both invasive and noninvasive—ranging from genetic and molecular interventions to diverse stimulation and neuromodulation techniques. In this chapter, we focus on noninvasive brain stimulation, a subset of neurotechnologies that modulate brain activity transcranially without requiring surgical procedures. Among these methods, electromagnetic approaches, particularly *transcranial magnetic stimulation* (TMS) and *transcranial electrical stimulation* (tES), have been the most extensively investigated and form the central focus of our discussion. Both TMS and tES trace their origins to the pioneering discoveries of Michael Faraday (1791–1867; Wagner et al., 2007). TMS functions as an electrode-free method of brain stimulation based on the principle of electromagnetic induction, in which the brain effectively serves as a set of "pick-up" coils that respond to a magnetic field generated by an external coil positioned over the scalp. When delivered in a series of repetitive pulses—known as repetitive TMS (rTMS)—this technique can induce lasting modulation of brain activity. The physiological effects of rTMS depend on multiple stimulation parameters, including frequency, intensity, and pattern of delivery, and can extend well beyond the stimulation period. Depending on these factors, rTMS may either enhance or suppress activity in the targeted brain region and influence connected networks through transsynaptic effects (Wagner et al., 2007). tES involves applying a low-intensity electrical current to the brain via one or more anodes and cathodes, creating an electric field that modulates neuronal excitability. Depending on the polarity and configuration of the electrodes, this current can either increase or decrease the likelihood of neuronal firing, thereby influencing patterns of brain activity and facilitating neuroplasticity through activity-dependent neuromodulation. The term *tES* encompasses several distinct techniques, including transcranial direct current stimulation (tDCS), transcranial alternating current stimulation (tACS), transcranial random noise stimulation, and temporal interference (TI) stimulation—each offering unique capabilities for noninvasively tuning neural dynamics.

Present Therapeutic Applications of TMS and tES

The use of rTMS in the treatment of depression has evolved considerably, reflecting both significant scientific progress and untapped therapeutic potential. This section highlights the key milestones that culminated in the regulatory approval of TMS for depression and its subsequent expansion into other clinical applications (Cappon & Pascual-Leone, 2024). Building on brain imaging studies that revealed functional abnormalities in the left prefrontal cortex (PFC) of individuals with major depression, George and colleagues (1994, 1995) conducted pioneering research demonstrating that applying rTMS to this region produced significant mood improvements in patients resistant to pharmacological treatment. These antidepressant effects were accompanied by widespread alterations in brain activity, showing that focal stimulation of the left PFC modulates interconnected neural circuits extending well beyond the site of stimulation. This pioneering work laid the groundwork for subsequent controlled trials and fueled the rapid growth of the field. It also underscored the importance of neurobiology-guided stimulation protocols and revealed that brain stimulation influences not only the targeted region but also interconnected neural networks. Subsequent studies have demonstrated that these distributed effects can be more precisely characterized through real-time integration of TMS with neuroimaging and EEG (Farzan et al., 2016; Fox et al., 2014; Shafi et al., 2012), offering deeper insight into how localized stimulation reshapes large-scale brain dynamics.

In one of the first controlled clinical trials, Conca and colleagues (1996) demonstrated that combining rTMS with standard antidepressant medication produced significantly greater reductions in depressive symptoms than medication alone. These findings were reinforced by Pascual-Leone and colleagues (1996), who showed that high-frequency stimulation of the left PFC consistently elicited robust antidepressant benefits. Building on these foundational studies, a landmark multicenter, randomized, sham-controlled trial involving 301 patients with major depression who had not responded to at least one adequate antidepressant treatment provided the decisive evidence leading to U.S. Food and Drug Administration (FDA) approval for the NeuroStar rTMS system in 2008 (Horvath et al., 2010; O'Reardon et al., 2007).

Since that milestone, numerous TMS devices and stimulation protocols have received FDA clearance—not only for treatment-resistant depression but also for a widening range of diagnostic and therapeutic indications (Cohen et al., 2022). In parallel, an expanding body of clinical research has provided compelling evidence for the efficacy and safety of tES across diverse neuropsychiatric conditions, including depression (Kang et al., 2024).

Currently, rTMS provides substantial therapeutic benefits for patients with medication-resistant depression, with approximately 60% achieving a clinically meaningful response and about 30% reaching full remission after a standard 6-week course of daily sessions. Accelerated rTMS protocols—delivering multiple sessions per day over 5 consecutive days—have demonstrated the potential to induce remission within just 1 week (Cole et al., 2019, 2020; van Rooij et al., 2024). With more than 600 rTMS systems in operation across the United States, it is estimated that rTMS therapy enables remission in roughly 25 patients with treatment-resistant depression every day. However, it's important to recognize that approximately 40% of patients do not achieve the desired therapeutic response, highlighting a critical challenge for the field: the need to develop personalized, precise interventions that target each individual's unique patterns of brain dysfunction to optimize symptom relief.

Recent meta-analyses indicate that tDCS effectively alleviates depressive symptoms, demonstrating moderate effect sizes and outperforming sham stimulation (Moffa et al., 2020; Razza et al., 2020). Other applications of TMS and tES have produced comparable therapeutic outcomes, though with substantial variability across individuals. Kang and colleagues (2024) have further underscored the promise of tES for treating schizophrenia and obsessive–compulsive disorder (OCD); however, larger and more rigorous randomized controlled trials are needed to confirm these emerging results. Notably, administering tDCS and tACS in home settings has proven both feasible and effective, demonstrating promising therapeutic outcomes (Cappon et al., 2022; Ruffini et al., 2024). These supervised home-based tES (HB-tES) applications have the potential to greatly expand access to care by enabling treatment independent of geographic constraints. In addition to improving accessibility, HB-tES can help reduce geographic and socioeconomic selection biases in research, enhance diversity within study populations, and support large-scale clinical trials and extended treatment protocols. Continued efforts to standardize HB-tES methodologies will be critical to fully realizing its potential across a wide range of patient groups (Cappon et al., 2024). Despite these promising developments, evidence-based guidelines from the International Federation of Clinical Neurophysiology indicate that no clinical application of tES has yet achieved a level A recommendation (definite efficacy). The strongest evidence to date supports its use in treating depression, which currently holds a level B recommendation (probable efficacy; Lefaucheur et al., 2017). To fully harness the potential of noninvasive brain stimulation within a precision medicine framework, future progress will depend on achieving far greater spatial, temporal, and contextual precision in both stimulation delivery and individual characterization (Cappon & Pascual-Leone, 2024; Jannati et al., 2023).

1. Focusing on specific symptoms and complaints, rather than relying solely on diagnostic categories, requires identifying the underlying brain mechanisms that give rise to these manifestations, while simultaneously emphasizing patient-centered goals and meaningful clinical outcomes.
2. Assessing and guiding interventions based on their neurophysiological effects, which entails monitoring the brain's physiological responses to stimulation—using real-time integration with techniques such as fMRI or EEG—to ensure accurate targeting and adaptive modulation.
3. Utilizing *state-dependent* effects to enhance the precision and efficacy of brain stimulation outcomes, that is, timing stimulation to the brain's current physiological or oscillatory state in order to align intervention with maximal responsiveness.
4. Monitoring behavioral responses in real time and dynamically adjusting stimulation parameters and targeting through closed-loop systems to optimize therapeutic efficacy and individualize treatment.

Realizing the Promise of Therapeutic Neuromodulation: Shifting Focus to Individual Symptomatology and Neurobiological Substrates and Markers

As discussed earlier, growing evidence indicates that specific symptoms within a given disorder are linked to disruptions or maladaptive modulation of distinct neural circuits governing plasticity (Cappon & Pascual-Leone, 2024). Consequently, disease symptoms may be more accurately understood as alteration of spatiotemporal patterns of brain activity that constitute the immediate substrates of human cognition, emotion, behavior, and other functional capacities (Figure 11.1). The objective, therefore, is to identify the spatiotemporal signatures, physiological biotypes, and biomarkers that correspond to individual symptom profiles. Such characterization could enable more precise, circuit-specific interventions tailored to each patient's unique neurobiological pattern. Within this framework, TMS and tES treatments can be optimized to enhance efficacy, reduce the proportion of nonresponders, and minimize the risk of adverse effects (Siddiqi et al., 2020). The following section illustrates these principles through recent advances in the use of rTMS for the treatment of depression.

Neurobiological Targets in rTMS for Depression

Early therapeutic applications of rTMS focused primarily on the left dorsolateral prefrontal cortex (DLPFC), given its established involvement in the neurobiology of depression (George et al., 1995; Pascual-Leone et al., 1996). Structural and functional imaging studies had shown that patients with left-hemisphere lesions—particularly those affecting the DLPFC—were significantly more likely to develop depressive symptoms than individuals with right-hemisphere lesions (Gainotti, 1972; Robinson et al., 1984; Robinson & Downhill, 1995). Furthermore, functional imaging studies consistently demonstrated reduced metabolic activity in the PFC in both primary and secondary forms of depression, with symptom severity closely correlating with the extent of frontal inactivity (George et al., 1994). Early rTMS investigations highlighted this hemispheric asymmetry in emotional regulation, showing that high-frequency stimulation of the left DLPFC enhanced cortical excitability and produced significant clinical improvement in depressed patients (George et al., 1995; Pascual-Leone et al., 1996). In contrast, low-frequency rTMS—which reduces cortical excitability—was found to be therapeutically beneficial when applied to the right DLPFC (Feinsod et al., 1998; Menkes et al., 1999). The differential roles of the left and right PFC in processing positive and negative emotions were further supported by electrophysiological studies in healthy individuals exposed to emotion-inducing stimuli (Davidson, 1992).

This body of evidence underscored the role of prefrontal dysfunction—particularly its regulatory influence over limbic activity—as a central factor in the emergence of depressive symptoms. Consequently, targeting the DLPFC with TMS became a logical therapeutic strategy. However, subsequent neuroimaging studies revealed an inverse relationship between prefrontal and subgenual activity, suggesting that effective treatment must account for interactions within broader, interconnected brain circuits rather than focusing solely on the DLPFC.

Recent advances in connectivity analysis have refined the identification of optimal rTMS targets within the DLPFC for achieving maximal antidepressant effects. Building on the foundational work by Mayberg and colleagues (2005; Mayberg, 2001), Fox and colleagues (2012) employed resting-state functional connectivity MRI (rs-fcMRI) to demonstrate that the most effective stimulation sites within DLPFC are those exhibiting the strongest negative functional connectivity with the subgenual cingulate cortex (sgCC). This discovery has driven increasingly sophisticated approaches to TMS targeting guided by brain connectivity profiles, consistently demonstrating that the most effective stimulation sites for depression are those exhibiting stronger negative functional connectivity with the sgCC (Cash et al., 2019; Kong et al., 2022; Weigand et al., 2018). Conceptually, the DLPFC serves as a strategic *entry point* for modulating cortico-subcortical networks that govern mood regulation and depression severity. Furthermore, the integration of rs-fcMRI now enables the identification of individualized rTMS targets within the prefrontal cortex, advancing the field toward truly personalized and precision-guided neuromodulation (Cash et al., 2021; Siddiqi et al., 2023).

Identifying Circuit-Based Biotypes

Defining circuit-level dysfunction and understanding its influence on individual patterns of brain activity remains a formidable challenge. Compounding this difficulty, the current diagnostic framework for neuropsychiatric disorders often reduces complex, heterogeneous syndromes to singular diagnostic labels. For example, what is commonly referred to as "Parkinson's disease" may, in reality, represent multiple distinct subtypes—or *Parkinson's diseases*—distinguished by differing dominant symptoms, underlying neural dysfunctions, and primary disabilities. Likewise, "major depression" likely comprises several neurobiological subtypes, each defined by distinct patterns of brain activity and disruptions within neural circuits. Given this phenotypic heterogeneity, it is plausible that the therapeutic efficacy of TMS could be enhanced by identifying and targeting specific biotypes—distinct neurobiological subgroups characterized by unique patterns of circuit dysfunction and symptom expression.

Recent research has advanced the concept of circuit-based "biotypes" that are associated with specific clinical features, underscoring the inherent heterogeneity of neuropsychiatric disorders. For instance, Drysdale and colleagues identified four depression biotypes via fMRI, each defined by unique connectivity patterns and symptom profiles, and demonstrated that these biotypes could predict response to rTMS treatment (Drysdale et al., 2017). However, subsequent machine-learning studies have highlighted challenges such as model overfitting, which can limit the reproducibility and generalizability of these findings across diverse patient populations (Dinga et al., 2019).

Liang and colleagues (2020) employed rs-fcMRI to identify two subgroups of patients with depression based on connectivity patterns within the default mode network (DMN): one marked by hyperconnectivity and the other by hypoconnectivity. Notably, individuals in the hypoconnectivity subgroup exhibited more severe anxiety symptoms than those in the hyperconnectivity group (Liang et al., 2020). Similarly, Fatt and colleagues (2023) delineated three distinct depression subgroups defined by connectivity patterns across the DMN, executive control network (ECN), and dorsal attention networks, further highlighting the complexity and network-level heterogeneity of depressive disorders. Notably, the subgroup demonstrating the highest remission rates following sertraline treatment showed markedly reduced connectivity between the DMN and the ECN (Fatt et al., 2023).

Building on these findings, Tozzi and colleagues (2024) combined resting-state and task-evoked fMRI modalities to delineate biotypes of depression and anxiety, identifying six distinct profiles characterized by unique connectivity patterns within the DMN, salience, and frontoparietal attention networks. These biotypes exhibited differential patterns of neural communication both at rest and during emotional or cognitive engagement. Importantly, they correlated with symptom severity, cognitive performance, and treatment responsiveness to both pharmacological and behavioral interventions. Collectively, these findings lay the groundwork for more precisely targeted neuromodulation strategies informed by biotype-specific neural characteristics.

Biotype-Guided Neuromodulation

Siddiqi and colleagues (2020) adopted a complementary approach by directly linking therapeutic outcomes to anatomically defined stimulation targets. In contrast to earlier biotyping methods that classified patients prior to assessing treatment relevance, their framework began with observed rTMS treatment responses to identify underlying symptom–circuit relationships. They distinguished two primary symptom clusters—dysphoric and anxio-somatic—that exhibited differential responses to stimulation of specific prefrontal regions. Notably, rTMS applied to the dorsomedial PFC produced greater reductions in anxiety symptoms, whereas stimulation of the DLPFC more effectively alleviated dysphoric symptoms. These not only predicted individual treatment outcomes across multiple studies but also provided a compelling neurobiological explanation for the variability in rTMS efficacy observed in previous clinical trials. Looking ahead, prospective experimental validation of these findings will be essential to fully personalize rTMS interventions according to each patient's unique symptom profile and functional priorities. This approach underscores the importance of a patient-centered framework, in which individuals actively participate in defining their treatment goals and therapeutic outcomes.

Collectively, these findings underscore the intricate ways in which distinct brain circuits contribute to the wide range of symptoms and disabilities observed in patients (Figure 11.3). Emerging evidence suggests that stimulating multiple interconnected brain regions through noninvasive brain stimulation may yield superior therapeutic outcomes. For example, Wei and colleagues (2023) found that a sequential bilateral stimulation protocol targeting the DLPFC, orbitofrontal cortex, and supplementary motor area led to significant symptom improvement in individuals with OCD. These results highlight the critical role of distributed neural networks in OCD and suggest that multifocal stimulation strategies may more effectively address the disorder's complex and heterogeneous symptomatology.

Moreover, rather than targeting a single neural circuit, addressing the widespread disruptions in brain activity across multiple interconnected networks may yield broader and more durable therapeutic effects. Such an approach can be advantageous even when precise knowledge of the specific circuits involved is limited. For instance, multifocal tES can be individualized by employing computational algorithms that design electrode montages to generate targeted electric fields (E-fields) aligned with each person's measured brain activity patterns, derived from EEG or neuroimaging data (Figure 11.3; Ruffini et al., 2014).

This approach employs biophysical mathematical modeling to predict how electric currents distribute throughout the brain during stimulation (Miranda et al., 2006, 2018; Ruffini et al., 2014). Research indicates that E-field strength and orientation are key determinants of cortical excitability changes, while individual anatomical variability—such as cortical folding, skull thickness, and tissue conductivity—significantly shapes the resulting E-field (Antonenko et al., 2021; Laakso et al., 2014,

2015; Nummenmaa et al., 2013; Thielscher et al., 2011). Accurate E-field simulations enable researchers to model how factors like coil or electrode placement, current intensity, and frequency influence neuronal activation, using sophisticated algorithms that account for each individual's unique brain anatomy and biophysical properties (Opitz et al., 2015; Ruffini et al., 2014; Zhao et al., 2024).

By integrating neuroanatomical data with functional neuroimaging, these computational models can predict both the spatial and temporal characteristics of the induced E-fields. This integration provides a powerful framework for optimizing stimulation precision and identifying the most effective therapeutic targets. Such individualized modeling not only enhances the safety and efficacy of noninvasive brain stimulation but also paves the way toward truly personalized, precision-guided treatment strategies.

In addition to techniques that target specific nodes within individual brain circuits (e.g., rTMS) or approaches that modulate widespread disruptions in spatiotemporal brain activity across multiple networks (as with multifocal tES), emerging methods now enable selective, noninvasive modulation of deep brain structures at specific oscillatory frequencies. One such innovation is *temporal interference* (TI) stimulation, developed by Grossman and colleagues (2017), which uses intersecting high-frequency electric fields to noninvasively and selectively activate neurons located in deep brain regions without affecting overlying cortical tissue. This technique operates by delivering two or more high-frequency E-fields that, individually, oscillate too rapidly to elicit neural firing. When these fields are applied in antiphase with a slight frequency offset—within the physiological range of neuronal firing—their interaction creates an interference pattern. Neurons located at the interference zone experience modulation at the difference frequency, allowing for targeted stimulation of deep brain regions without directly affecting surrounding tissue.

The potential of TI stimulation was first demonstrated in mice, where it enabled the selective activation of hippocampal neurons without affecting overlying cortical regions. More recently, this approach has been successfully translated to humans (Violante et al., 2023). Collectively, these advances highlight the growing suite of noninvasive neuromodulation techniques capable of precisely and personally modulating brain circuits. Together, they open new avenues for targeted interventions across diverse brain regions and oscillatory frequency bands (Figure 11.3).

While imaging and neurophysiology-based biotypes and biomarkers have propelled the field of precision neuromodulation forward, molecular markers hold the promise of achieving an even higher level of specificity and individualized care. The progress made in oncology provides a compelling paradigm for developing precision neuropsychiatry, capable of fully realizing the therapeutic potential of noninvasive brain stimulation. This vision rests on two foundational steps: (1) identifying neurobiological and molecular substrates linked to patient-defined priority symptoms or disabilities and elucidating their neurophysiological consequences, and (2) measuring the physiological impact of interventions to determine their neural and behavioral effects, then correlating these changes with clinical, cognitive, emotional, and functional outcomes. Integrating these processes within a closed-loop system would enable real-time, data-driven adjustments to stimulation parameters, continuously refining treatment for maximal efficacy and personalization.

Combining Behavioral Phenotyping and Physiological Biomarkers for Personalized Neuromodulation

Tailoring neuromodulation strategies to specific biotypes and symptom profiles represents a major advancement. However, its effectiveness relies on precise monitoring of behavioral changes and accurate characterization of behavioral phenotypes and symptom clusters. We propose that integrating neurophysiological measures with behavioral assessments is essential to advancing our understanding of psychopathology (Cappon & Pascual-Leone, 2024). Traditionally, behavioral phenotypes—distinct patterns of behavior observed in neurological and psychiatric disorders—have been assessed primarily through clinical interviews and observations, methods that are inherently subjective and susceptible to variability. However, recent technological innovations have transformed this landscape, enabling the objective, quantitative, and continuous measurement of behavior in real-world and laboratory settings. Today, smart sensors and wearable technologies enable the continuous and objective monitoring of behavioral patterns, capturing data on movement, activity levels, sleep, and social interactions to create a rich, ecologically valid picture of real-world behaviors. For example, voice-analysis algorithms can detect subtle shifts in speech patterns, tone, and prosody, providing sensitive indicators of mood and cognitive state. Together, these innovations yield digital biomarkers that deepen our understanding of behavioral phenotypes (Insel, 2018). Such biomarkers not only facilitate early detection of emerging symptoms and ongoing monitoring of disease progression but also offer objective, quantifiable measures for evaluating treatment outcomes.

While behavioral phenotyping elucidates the outward manifestations of neurological and psychiatric disorders, integrating it with physiological biomarkers provides a more complete picture of the underlying neurobiological mechanisms. The convergence of behavioral phenotypes and individual neurobiology is essential for advancing personalized approaches to noninvasive neuromodulation. For instance, digital phenotyping enables real-time monitoring of patient responses to TMS and tES by continuously capturing behavioral and physiological data through digital devices. This continuous feedback can be used to dynamically optimize stimulation parameters and improve treatment outcomes (Kelkar et al., 2023).

Precision Neuromodulation Using Closed-Loop Strategies

Closed-loop neuromodulation represents a frontier in precision medicine, utilizing real-time feedback to continuously monitor brain activity and dynamically adjust stimulation parameters for optimal effect (Soleimani et al., 2023). These systems rely on spatiotemporal brain signatures—such as blood-oxygenation-level–dependent (BOLD) signals from fMRI or electrophysiological markers from EEG—to assess the brain's current functional state relative to an individualized "normal" baseline. By integrating behavioral, cognitive, and emotional metrics with these physiological measures, adaptive algorithms can quantify deviations from an "optimal" brain state and automatically fine-tune stimulation parameters to restore functional balance and promote adaptive neuroplasticity.

The value of a closed-loop approach is illustrated by studies demonstrating that TMS can modulate oscillatory dynamics across distributed brain networks, including deep structures beyond the direct site of stimulation. For instance, using intracranial EEG recordings, Solomon and colleagues (2024) found that stimulation of DLPFC induced widespread increases in low-frequency oscillations (3–8 Hz) within frontolimbic cortices, accompanied by reductions in high-frequency oscillations (30–110 Hz) across frontotemporal regions, including the hippocampus. These findings highlight the network-level reach of TMS and underscore the potential of closed-loop systems to harness and regulate such complex oscillatory effects in real time. Another compelling example of closed-loop neuromodulation is phase-locked tACS, in which stimulation is precisely synchronized with the phase of ongoing brain oscillations detected via EEG. Early implementations employed autoregressive models to predict future EEG signals from preceding activity, allowing stimulation parameters to be continuously updated in real time. However, accurately modeling the full complexity of EEG dynamics in real time remains a significant technical challenge, as it requires rapid computation and adaptation to highly variable neural signals (Chen et al., 2013). Consequently, subsequent studies have explored alternative strategies to deliver tACS precisely at EEG frequencies aligned with specific sleep-related rhythms, such as spindles (Lustenberger et al., 2016) or slow oscillations (Ketz et al., 2018). For instance, Ketz and colleagues (2018) developed a closed-loop algorithm designed to enhance slow-wave oscillations during sleep, resulting in increased power in both slow-wave and spindle activity. These enhancements were associated with improved long-term memory performance, providing empirical support for theories of systems-level memory consolidation driven by coordinated oscillatory activity during sleep (Ketz et al., 2018).

Similarly, Gordon and colleagues (2022) demonstrated that real-time EEG-triggered rTMS, synchronized to the phase of ongoing theta oscillations, can modulate prefrontal excitability and enhance working memory (WM) performance. Specifically, rTMS delivered at the negative peak of theta oscillations increased prefrontal theta power and strengthened theta-gamma phase-amplitude coupling, resulting in faster WM response times. In contrast, stimulation at the positive peak reduced theta power without improving performance, and random-phase rTMS produced no measurable effects. These findings underscore the therapeutic promise of phase-specific, EEG-triggered rTMS for selectively enhancing cognitive control and WM-related neural networks.

Additionally, Sun and colleagues (2023) developed a closed-loop rTMS system that delivered stimulation at specific phases of each patient's prefrontal EEG alpha rhythm to enhance antidepressant efficacy. In a 6-week study involving 24 patients with major depressive disorder, they compared outcomes between phase-synchronized and unsynchronized rTMS protocols. Changes in global cortical excitability—measured via alpha-band global mean field power (6–13 Hz)—were correlated with treatment response in both groups. Notably, the synchronized group exhibited greater reductions in cortical excitability after each session compared with the unsynchronized group. Moreover, within the synchronized group, weeks showing the largest improvements in Hamilton Rating Scale for Depression scores coincided with the most pronounced posttreatment decreases in cortical excitability, underscoring the clinical potential of EEG-guided, phase-locked rTMS for depression.

Despite the promise of closed-loop systems, several challenges remain, chief among them the need for more robust real-time algorithms, reproducibility across diverse populations, and the high costs associated with integrating neuroimaging and stimulation technologies. Overcoming these barriers will require sustained interdisciplinary collaboration among neuroscientists, engineers, clinicians, and data scientists. Such efforts are essential to fully unlock the therapeutic potential of closed-loop neuromodulation for patients with neurological and psychiatric disorders.

Expanding Access with Home-Based Neuromodulation

Frequent clinic visits for neuromodulation treatments can be burdensome for patients, particularly those facing mobility limitations, socioeconomic barriers, or other logical challenges. Home-based neuromodulation offers a practical and accessible alternative, allowing treatments to be administered in familiar environments while improving adherence and convenience. For example, HB-tES enables patients or caregivers to deliver therapy under remote clinical supervision, effectively removing geographical barriers and expanding access to care.

Recent advancements in portable tDCS systems have made it possible to extend treatment durations and conduct remote, clinician-supervised sessions. These systems support optimized multichannel protocols capable of safely and effectively targeting specific brain circuits from home (Figure 11.4). Proof-of-concept studies have demonstrated the feasibility and promise of such home-based neuromodulation approaches. For instance, tACS administered at home by trained caregivers to patients with mild dementia due to AD successfully restored theta-gamma EEG activity and produced significant improvements in memory performance (Cappon et al., 2023; Figure 11.4). Other early studies have also shown similarly positive effects when targeting dysphoric symptoms in patients with major depressive disorder (Cappon et al., 2022; Ruffini et al., 2024). Larger, well-controlled trials are currently underway to confirm these findings and refine home-based treatment protocols.

Significant progress has also been made in developing comprehensive training and supervision programs for HB-tES. These initiatives aim to enhance methodological rigor and ensure consistency both within individual studies and across multicenter clinical trials implementing tES in the home environment (Cappon et al., 2024). By addressing these practical and methodological challenges, home-based neuromodulation stands to greatly expand access to safe and effective treatments, improving outcomes for individuals with a wide range of neurological and psychiatric conditions.

Conclusion

The future of neurology and psychiatry is moving toward highly personalized, multidimensional care—approaches precisely tailored to each individual's unique neurobiological profile, clinical presentation, and therapeutic needs. This integrated model will combine pharmacological treatments, neuromodulation technologies, psychotherapeutic interventions, and supportive care systems to optimize outcomes for individuals with brain circuit disorders. Within this framework, noninvasive neuromodulation techniques such as TMS and tES hold tremendous promise. However, realizing their full therapeutic potential will depend on continued advances in precision neuromodulation, enabling truly individualized and adaptive treatment strategies.

Current neuromodulation protocols typically target broad brain regions associated with specific disorders. However, the future of the field lies in achieving far greater precision. Research efforts should prioritize developing advanced targeting methods grounded in each individual's spatiotemporal neural signatures, identifiable through state-of-the-art neuroimaging and digital behavioral phenotyping. By integrating individualized brain maps with sophisticated biophysical modeling to tailor stimulation parameters, clinicians can more effectively address the unique circuitry disruptions underlying each patient's condition. This paradigm shift holds the potential to markedly enhance both treatment efficacy and overall patient outcomes.

In addition, the field must place a greater emphasis on understanding the long-term effects of neuromodulation. Longitudinal studies are essential for evaluating the durability and sustained impact of these therapies over time. Extended monitoring can yield critical insights into individual variability in treatment response and the persistence of therapeutic benefits. A deeper understanding of these long-term dynamics will enable refinement of intervention strategies, ensuring that neuromodulation not only alleviates immediate symptoms but also promotes enduring, adaptive neuroplastic changes.

Another key frontier for future progress is the integration of digital phenotyping into real-time data collection. By continuously monitoring behavioral patterns and physiological biomarkers, researchers can build predictive models that accurately forecast individual treatment responses. These digital biomarkers will enable dynamically adaptive, data-driven interventions—allowing therapies to be continuously personalized and fine-tuned based on each patient's evolving neurophysiological and behavioral state.

Together, these innovations are poised to usher neuromodulation into a new era of precision medicine. By integrating real-time monitoring of behavioral and physiological markers with advanced biophysical modeling and personalized, home-based protocols, the next generation of noninvasive brain stimulation will deliver therapies that are more effective, sustainable, and individually tailored. This evolution marks a pivotal step toward truly personalized care for disorders of brain circuitry.

ACKNOWLEDGMENTS AND DISCLOSURES

Dr. Pascual-Leone was partly supported by the National Institutes of Health (R01AG076708, R24AG06142, R01AG059089), the Jack Satter Foundation, and the Bright Focus Foundation. He is a cofounder of Linus Health and TI Solutions AG; serves on the scientific advisory boards for Neuroelectrics, Welcony-Magstim, MedRhythms, TetraNeuron, and Skin2Neuron; and is listed as an inventor on several issued and pending patents on methods for noninvasive brain stimulation and combination of noninvasive brain stimulation with EEG and fMRI, applications of noninvasive brain stimulation in various neurological disorders, as well as digital biomarkers of cognition, function, and biomarker status, and digital assessments for early diagnosis of dementia. Dr. Cappon was partly supported by the National Institutes of Health (R01AG076708), the NARSAD-Brain and Behavior Research Foundation (30772), and the Bright Focus Foundation (A2024027S). Dr. Jannati is an employee of Linus Health and is listed as an inventor on pending patents on digital biomarkers of cognition, function, and biomarker status.

REFERENCES

Antonenko, D., Grittner, U., Saturnino, G., Nierhaus, T., Thielscher, A., & Flöel, A. (2021). Inter-individual and age-dependent variability in simulated electric fields induced by conventional transcranial electrical stimulation. *NeuroImage, 224*, 1–9.

Boes, A. D., Prasad, S., Liu, H., Liu, Q., Pascual-Leone, A., Caviness Jr., V. S., et al. (2015). Network localization of neurological symptoms from focal brain lesions. *Brain, 138*(10), 3061–3075.

Brechet, L., Yu, W., & Biagi, M. C. (2021). Patient-tailored, home-based non-invasive brain stimulation for memory deficits in dementia due to Alzheimer's disease. *Frontiers in Neurology, 12*, 598135.

Brem, A.-K., Fried, P. J., Horvath, J. C., Robertson, E. M., & Pascual-Leone, A. (2014). Is neuroenhancement by noninvasive brain stimulation a net zero-sum proposition? *NeuroImage, 85*, 1058–1068.

Cappon, D., den Boer, T., Jordan, C., Yu, W., Lo, A., LaGanke, N., et al. (2022). Safety and feasibility of tele-supervised home-based transcranial direct current stimulation for major depressive disorder. *Frontiers in Aging Neuroscience, 13*, 765370.

Cappon, D., den Boer, T., Yu, W., LaGanke, N., Fox, R., Brozgol, M., et al. (2024). An educational program for remote training and supervision of home-based transcranial electrical stimulation: Feasibility and preliminary effectiveness. *Neuromodulation: Journal of the International Neuromodulation Society, 27*(4), 636–644.

Cappon, D., Fox, R., den Boer, T., Yu, W., LaGanke, N., Cattaneo, G., et al. (2023). Tele-supervised home-based transcranial alternating current stimulation (tACS) for Alzheimer's disease: A pilot study. *Frontiers in Human Neuroscience, 17*, 1168673.

Cappon, D., & Pascual-Leone, A. (2024). Toward precision noninvasive brain stimulation. *American Journal of Psychiatry, 181*(9), 795–805.

Cash, R. F. H., Weigand, A., Zalesky, A., Siddiqi, S. H., Downar, J., Fitzgerald, P. B., et al. (2021). Using brain imaging to improve spatial targeting of transcranial magnetic stimulation for depression. *Biological Psychiatry, 90*(10), 689–700.

Cash, R. F. H., Zalesky, A., Thomson, R. H., Tian, Y., Cocchi, L., & Fitzgerald, P. B. (2019). Subgenual functional connectivity predicts antidepressant treatment response to transcranial magnetic stimulation: Independent validation and evaluation of personalization. *Biological Psychiatry, 86*(2), e5–e7.

Chen, L. L., Madhavan, R., Rapoport, B. I., & Anderson, W. S. (2013). Real-time brain oscillation detection and phase-locked stimulation using autoregressive spectral estimation and time-series forward prediction. *IEEE Transactions on Bio-Medical Engineering, 60*(3), 753–762.

Cohen, S. L., Bikson, M., Badran, B. W., & George, M. S. (2022). A visual and narrative timeline of US FDA milestones for transcranial magnetic stimulation (TMS) devices. *Brain Stimulation, 15*(1), 73–75.

Cole, E. J., Gulser, M., Stimpson, K., Bentzley, B., Hawkins, J., Xiao, X., et al. (2019). Stanford accelerated intelligent neuromodulation therapy for treatment-resistant depression

(SAINT-TRD). *Brain Stimulation: Basic, Translational, and Clinical Research in Neuromodulation, 12*(2), 402.

Cole, E. J., Stimpson, K. H., Bentzley, B. S., Gulser, M., Cherian, K., Tischler, C., et al. (2020). Stanford accelerated intelligent neuromodulation therapy for treatment-resistant depression. *American Journal of Psychiatry, 177*(8), 716–726.

Conca, A., Koppi, S., König, P., Swoboda, E., & Krecke, N. (1996). Transcranial magnetic stimulation: A novel antidepressive strategy? *Neuropsychobiology, 34*(4), 204–207.

Davidson, R. J. (1992). Emotion and affective style: Hemispheric substrates. *Psychological Science, 3*(1), 39–43.

Dinga, R., Schmaal, L., Penninx, B. W. J. H., van Tol, M. J., Veltman, D. J., van Velzen, L., et al. (2019). Evaluating the evidence for biotypes of depression: Methodological replication and extension of Drysdale et al. (2017). *NeuroImage: Clinical, 22*, 101796.

Drysdale, A. T., Grosenick, L., Downar, J., Dunlop, K., Mansouri, F., Meng, Y., et al. (2017). Resting-state connectivity biomarkers define neurophysiological subtypes of depression. *Nature Medicine, 23*(1), 28–38.

Farzan, F., Vernet, M., Shafi, M. M. D., Rotenberg, A., Daskalakis, Z. J., & Pascual-Leone, A. (2016). Characterizing and modulating brain circuitry through transcranial magnetic stimulation combined with electroencephalography. *Frontiers in Neural Circuits, 10*, 73.

Fatt, C. R. C., Minhajuddin, A., Jha, M. K., Mayes, T., Rush, A. J., & Trivedi, M. H. (2023). Data driven clusters derived from resting state functional connectivity: Findings from the EMBARC study. *Journal of Psychiatric Research, 158*, 150–156.

Feigin, V. L., Nichols, E., Alam, T., Bannick, M. S., Beghi, E., Blake, N., et al. (2019). Global, regional, and national burden of neurological disorders, 1990–2016: A systematic analysis for the Global Burden of Disease Study 2016. *Lancet Neurology, 18*(5), 459–480.

Feinsod, M., Kreinin, B., Chistyakov, A., & Klein, E. (1998). Preliminary evidence for a beneficial effect of low-frequency, repetitive transcranial magnetic stimulation in patients with major depression and schizophrenia. *Depression and Anxiety, 7*(2), 65–68.

Fox, M. D. (2018). Mapping symptoms to brain networks with the human connectome. *New England Journal of Medicine, 379*(23), 2237–2245.

Fox, M. D., Buckner, R. L., Liu, H., Chakravarty, M. M., Lozano, A. M., & Pascual-Leone, A. (2014). Resting-state networks link invasive and noninvasive brain stimulation across diverse psychiatric and neurological diseases. *Proceedings of the National Academy of Sciences, 111*(41), E4367–4375.

Fox, M. D., Buckner, R. L., White, M. P., Greicius, M. D., & Pascual-Leone, A. (2012). Efficacy of TMS targets for depression is related to intrinsic functional connectivity with the subgenual cingulate. *Biological Psychiatry, 72*(7), 595–603.

Freitas, C., Farzan, F., & Pascual-Leone, A. (2013). Assessing brain plasticity across the lifespan with transcranial magnetic stimulation: Why, how, and what is the ultimate goal? *Frontiers in Neuroscience, 7*, 42.

Gainotti, G. (1972). Emotional behavior and hemispheric side of the lesion. *Cortex, 8*(1), 41–55.

George, M. S., Ketter, T. A., & Post, R. M. (1994). Prefrontal cortex dysfunction in clinical depression. *Depression, 2*(2), 59–72.

George, M. S., Wassermann, E. M., Williams, W. A., Callahan, A., Ketter, T. A., Basser, P., et al. (1995). Daily repetitive transcranial magnetic stimulation (rTMS) improves mood in depression. *Neuroreport, 6*(14), 1853–1856.

Gomes-Osman, J., Indahlastari, A., Fried, P. J., Cabral, D. L. F., Rice, J., Nissim, N. R., et al. (2018). Non-invasive brain stimulation: Probing Intracortical circuits and improving cognition in the aging brain. *Frontiers in Aging Neuroscience, 10*, 177.

Gomes-Osman, J., & Pascual-Leone, A. (2024). The 10 tenets of brain health for clinical practice in the era of technology. *Medical Research Archives, 12*(9), 1–21.

Gordon, P. C., Belardinelli, P., Stenroos, M., Ziemann, U., & Zrenner, C. (2022). Prefrontal theta phase-dependent rTMS-induced plasticity of cortical and behavioral responses in human cortex. *Brain Stimulation, 15*(2), 391–402.

Grossman, N., Bono, D., Dedic, N., Kodandaramaiah, S. B., Rudenko, A., Suk, H.-J., et al. (2017). Noninvasive deep brain stimulation via temporally interfering electric fields. *Cell, 169*(6), 1029–1041.

Horvath, J. C., Mathews, J., Demitrack, M. A., & Pascual-Leone, A. (2010). The NeuroStar TMS device: Conducting the FDA approved protocol for treatment of depression. *Journal of Visualized Experiments, 45*, 2345.

Insel, T. R. (2018). Digital phenotyping: A global tool for psychiatry. *World Psychiatry, 17*(3), 276–277.

Jannati, A., Oberman, L. M., Rotenberg, A., & Pascual-Leone, A. (2023). Assessing the mechanisms of brain plasticity by transcranial magnetic stimulation. *Neuropsychopharmacology, 48*(1), 191–208.

Joutsa, J., & Fox, M. D. (2022). Lesion network mapping for symptom localization: Recent developments and future directions. *Current Opinion in Neurology, 35*(4), 453–459.

Kang, J., Lee, H., Yu, S., Lee, M., Kim, H. J., Kwon, R., et al. (2024). Effects and safety of transcranial direct current stimulation on multiple health outcomes: An umbrella review of randomized clinical trials. *Molecular Psychiatry, 29*, 3789–3801.

Kelkar, R. S., Currey, D., Nagendra, S., Mehta, U. M., Sreeraj, V. S., Torous, J., et al. (2023). Utility of smartphone-based digital phenotyping biomarkers in assessing treatment response to transcranial magnetic stimulation in depression: Proof-of-concept study. *JMIR Formative Research, 7*, e40197.

Ketz, N., Jones, A. P., Bryant, N. B., Clark, V. P., & Pilly, P. K. (2018). Closed-loop slow-wave tACS improves sleep-dependent long-term memory generalization by modulating endogenous oscillations. *Journal of Neuroscience, 38*(33), 7314–7326.

Kloos, A., Gomes-Osman, J., & Boyd, L. (2020). Harnessing neuroplasticity for functional recovery. *Journal of Neurologic Physical Therapy, 44*(2), 119–120.

Kong, G., Wei, L., Wang, J., Zhu, C., & Tang, Y. (2022). The therapeutic potential of personalized connectivity-guided transcranial magnetic stimulation target over group-average target for depression. *Brain Stimulation, 15*(5), 1063–1064.

Laakso, I., Hirata, A., & Ugawa, Y. (2014). Effects of coil orientation on the electric field induced by TMS over the hand motor area. *Physics in Medicine and Biology, 59*(1), 203–218.

Laakso, I., Tanaka, S., Koyama, S., De Santis, V., & Hirata, A. (2015). Inter-subject variability in electric fields of motor cortical tDCS. *Brain Stimulation, 8*(5), 906–913.

Lefaucheur, J.-P., Antal, A., Ayache, S. S., Benninger, D. H., Brunelin, J., Cogiamanian, F., et al. (2017). Evidence-based guidelines on the therapeutic use of transcranial direct current stimulation (tDCS). *Clinical Neurophysiology, 128*(1), 56–92.

Liang, S., Deng, W., Li, X., Greenshaw, A. J., Wang, Q., Li, M., et al. (2020). Biotypes of major depressive disorder: Neuroimaging evidence from resting-state default mode network patterns. *NeuroImage Clinical, 28*, 102514.

Lustenberger, C., Boyle, M. R., Alagapan, S., Mellin, J. M., Vaughn, B. V., & Fröhlich, F. (2016). Feedback-controlled transcranial alternating current stimulation reveals a functional role of sleep spindles in motor memory consolidation. *Current Biology, 26*(16), 2127–2136.

Mayberg, H. S. (2001). Depression and frontal-subcortical circuits: Focus on prefrontal-limbic interactions. In D. G. Lichter & J. L. Cummings (Eds.), *Frontal-subcortical circuits in psychiatric and neurological disorders* (pp. 177–206). Guilford Press.

Mayberg, H. S., Lozano, A. M., Voon, V., McNeely, H. E., Seminowicz, D., Hamani, C., et al. (2005). Deep brain stimulation for treatment-resistant depression. *Neuron, 45*(5), 651–660.

Menkes, D. L., Bodnar, P., Ballesteros, R. A., & Swenson, M. R. (1999). Right frontal lobe slow frequency repetitive transcranial magnetic stimulation (SF r-TMS) is an effective treatment for depression: A case-control pilot study of safety and efficacy. *Journal of Neurology, Neurosurgery, and Psychiatry, 67*(1), 113–115.

Miranda, P. C., Callejón-Leblic, M. A., Salvador, R., & Ruffini, G. (2018). Realistic modeling of transcranial current stimulation: The electric field in the brain. *Current Opinion in Biomedical Engineering, 8*, 20–27.

Miranda, P. C., Lomarev, M., & Hallett, M. (2006). Modeling the current distribution during transcranial direct current stimulation. *Clinical Neurophysiology, 117*(7), 1623–1629.

Moffa, A. H., Martin, D., Alonzo, A., Bennabi, D., Blumberger, D. M., Benseñor, I. M., et al. (2020). Efficacy and acceptability of transcranial direct current stimulation (tDCS) for major depressive disorder: An individual patient data meta-analysis. *Progress in Neuro-Psychopharmacology and Biological Psychiatry, 99*, 109836.

Nummenmaa, A., Stenroos, M., Ilmoniemi, R. J., Okada, Y. C., Hämäläinen, M. S., & Raij, T. (2013). Comparison of spherical and realistically shaped boundary element head models for transcranial magnetic stimulation navigation. *Clinical Neurophysiology, 124*(10), 1995–2007.

Opitz, A., Paulus, W., Will, S., Antunes, A., & Thielscher, A. (2015). Determinants of the electric field during transcranial direct current stimulation. *NeuroImage, 109*, 140–150.

O'Reardon, J. P., Solvason, H. B., Janicak, P. G., Sampson, S., Isenberg, K. E., Nahas, Z., et al. (2007). Efficacy and safety of transcranial magnetic stimulation in the acute treatment of major depression: A multisite randomized controlled trial. *Biological Psychiatry, 62*(11), 1208–1216.

Ozdemir, R. A., Tadayon, E., Boucher, P., Momi, D., Karakhanyan, K. A., Fox, M. D., et al. (2020). Individualized perturbation of the human connectome reveals reproducible biomarkers of network dynamics relevant to cognition. *Proceedings of the National Academy of Sciences, 117*(14), 8115–8125.

Pascual-Leone, A., Amedi, A., Fregni, F., & Merabet, L. B. (2005). The plastic human brain cortex. *Annual Review of Neuroscience, 28*(1), 377–401.

Pascual-Leone, A., Rubio, B., Pallardó, F., & Catalá, M. D. (1996). Rapid-rate transcranial magnetic stimulation of left dorsolateral prefrontal cortex in drug-resistant depression. *Lancet, 348*, 233–237.

Pascual-Leone, A., & Taylor, M. J. (2011). A developmental framework of brain and cognition from infancy to old age. *Brain Topography, 24*(3–4), 183–186.

Razza, L. B., Palumbo, P., Moffa, A. H., Carvalho, A. F., Solmi, M., Loo, C. K., et al. (2020). A systematic review and meta-analysis on the effects of transcranial direct current stimulation in depressive episodes. *Depression and Anxiety, 37*(7), 594–608.

Robinson, R. G., & Downhill, J. E. (1995). *Lateralization of psychopathology in response to focal brain injury.* In R. J. Davidson & K. Hugdahl (Eds.), *Brain asymmetry* (pp. 693–711). MIT Press.

Robinson, R. G., Kubos, K. L., Starr, L. B., Rao, K., & Price, T. R. (1984). Mood disorders in stroke patients: Importance of location of lesion. *Brain: A Journal of Neurology, 107*(Pt. 1), 81–93.

Ruffini, G., Fox, M. D., Ripolles, O., Miranda, P. C., & Pascual-Leone, A. (2014).

Optimization of multifocal transcranial current stimulation for weighted cortical pattern targeting from realistic modeling of electric fields. *Neuroimage, 89*, 216–225.

Ruffini, G., Salvador, R., Castaldo, F., Baleeiro, T., Camprodon, J. A., Chopra, M., et al. (2024). Multichannel tDCS with advanced targeting for major depressive disorder: A tele-supervised at-home pilot study. *medRxiv*.

Shafi, M. M., Westover, M. B., Fox, M. D., & Pascual-Leone, A. (2012). Exploration and modulation of brain network interactions with noninvasive brain stimulation in combination with neuroimaging. *European Journal of Neuroscience, 35*(6), 805–825.

Siddiqi, S. H., Kandala, S., Hacker, C. D., Trapp, N. T., Leuthardt, E. C., Carter, A. R., et al. (2023). Individualized precision targeting of dorsal attention and default mode networks with rTMS in traumatic brain injury-associated depression. *Scientific Reports, 13*(1), 4052.

Siddiqi, S. H., Taylor, S. F., Cooke, D., Pascual-Leone, A., George, M. S., & Fox, M. D. (2020). Distinct symptom-specific treatment targets for circuit-based neuromodulation. *American Journal of Psychiatry, 177*(5), 435–446.

Soleimani, G., Nitsche, M. A., Bergmann, T. O., Towhidkhah, F., Violante, I. R., Lorenz, R., et al. (2023). Closing the loop between brain and electrical stimulation: Towards precision neuromodulation treatments. *Translational Psychiatry, 13*(1), 1–17.

Solomon, E. A., Wang, J. B., Oya, H., Howard, M. A., Trapp, N. T., Uitermarkt, B. D., et al. (2024). TMS provokes target-dependent intracranial rhythms across human cortical and subcortical sites. *Brain Stimulation: Basic, Translational, and Clinical Research in Neuromodulation, 17*(3), 698–712.

Sprugnoli, G., Munsch, F., Cappon, D., Paciorek, R., Macone, J., Connor, A., et al. (2021). Impact of multisession 40Hz tACS on hippocampal perfusion in patients with Alzheimer's disease. *Alzheimer's Research & Therapy, 13*(1), 1–14.

Sun, X., Doose, J., Faller, J., McIntosh, J., Saber, G., Lin, Y., et al. (2023). Closed-loop phase-locked rTMS treatment decreases global cortical excitability in major depressive disorder patients. *Brain Stimulation: Basic, Translational, and Clinical Research in Neuromodulation, 16*(1), 397.

Thielscher, A., Opitz, A., & Windhoff, M. (2011). Impact of the gyral geometry on the electric field induced by transcranial magnetic stimulation. *NeuroImage, 54*(1), 234–243.

Tozzi, L., Zhang, X., Pines, A., Olmsted, A. M., Zhai, E. S., Anene, E. T., et al. (2024). Personalized brain circuit scores identify clinically distinct biotypes in depression and anxiety. *Nature Medicine, 30*(7), 2076–2087.

van Rooij, S. J. H., Arulpragasam, A. R., McDonald, W. M., & Philip, N. S. (2024). Accelerated TMS—moving quickly into the future of depression treatment. *Neuropsychopharmacology, 49*(1), 128–137.

Violante, I. R., Alania, K., Cassarà, A. M., Neufeld, E., Acerbo, E., Carron, R., et al. (2023). Non-invasive temporal interference electrical stimulation of the human hippocampus. *Nature Neuroscience, 26*(11), 1994–2004.

Wagner, T., Valero-Cabre, A., & Pascual-Leone, A. (2007). Noninvasive human brain stimulation. *Annual Review of Biomedical Engineering, 9*, 527–565.

Wei, K., Luo, Y., Bai, Y., Chen, T., & Bi, B. (2023). Toward a neurocircuit-based sequential bilateral transcranial magnetic stimulation for treatment of obsessive-compulsive disorder. *Brain Stimulation: Basic, Translational, and Clinical Research in Neuromodulation, 16*(6), 1585–1587.

Weigand, A., Horn, A., Caballero, R., Cooke, D., Stern, A. P., Taylor, S. F., et al. (2018). Prospective validation that subgenual connectivity predicts antidepressant efficacy of transcranial magnetic stimulation sites. *Biological Psychiatry, 84*(1), 28–37.

Wiesendanger, M. (2006). Constantin von Monakow (1853–1930): A pioneer in interdisciplinary brain research and a humanist. *Comptes Rendus Biologies, 329*(5–6), 406–418.

World Health Organization. (2019). *Risk reduction of cognitive decline and dementia: WHO guidelines.* www.who.int/publications/i/item/9789241550543.

World Health Organization. (2022). *Optimizing brain health across the life course: WHO position paper.* www.who.int/publications/i/item/9789240054561.

Zhao, Z., Shirinpour, S., Tran, H., Wischnewski, M., & Opitz, A. (2024). Intensity- and frequency-specific effects of transcranial alternating current stimulation are explained by network dynamics. *Journal of Neural Engineering, 21*(2), 026024.

CHAPTER 12

Effects of Physical Exercise, Cognitive Training, and Multidomain Intervention on the Aging Brain

Louis Bherer and Tudor Vrinceanu

Introduction

The aging demographic is a global concern worldwide. While the increase in life expectancy is generally perceived as positive, it also comes with economic and societal concerns. Aging is an inevitable process that brings with it challenges at the individual and societal levels. Every week or so, articles are published in public media that reflect this ambivalence, some reporting about inspiring centenarians who seem to live an eternal happy life, while others ring the bell about the gigantic unaffordable societal costs of the "gray tsunami." One-sixth of the population worldwide is 60 and over in the 2020s, and the fastest-growing segment of the population is composed of those over 85 (World Health Organization [WHO], 2022). This demographic change brings challenges in managing health care, as aging is associated with physiological and psychological changes.

While chronological aging is inevitable, it does not impact everyone the same way, and literature abounds with examples of successful aging, both cognitively and physically. The heterogeneity in the profile of aging has motivated the search for protective factors that would help individuals age longer and healthier. In this context, neuroscience research thrives on unraveling the mystery of the aging brain and its potential for adaptation. Decades of research have shown that aging is a heterogeneous process that involves not only negative, but also positive, adaptations. Evidence supporting this claim, already well established over 20 years ago (Kramer et al., 2004), comes from various methodological approaches. First, prospective studies have identified lifestyle factors that are associated with positive aging patterns. Then, cross-sectional studies investigating age-related differences between younger and older adults have shown that once individual differences in terms of health determinants or lifestyle are considered, age-related differences are less clear and sometimes absent. These observations suggest that some factors can mediate the impact of aging on brain functions and that there is a level of "agency" on how we age. In other words, lifestyle choices impact the way we age. However, evidence from cross-sectional and longitudinal studies is tempered by the fact that they might also reflect selective bias and involve artifacts—that is, factors other than age—that might better explain health outcomes. Therefore, proper randomized controlled trials (RCTs) are required to draw a definitive conclusion on the impact that lifestyle factors have on cognitive and brain aging.

Decades of research using RCTs have supported that, to some extent, the brain retains some potential to adapt physically and functionally, even later in life (Brehmer et al., 2014; Intzandt et al., 2021; Nguyen et al., 2019). Evidence suggests that this wonderful potential is maintained, at least to some degree, throughout life and that lifestyle choices play a major role. The brain adapts according to some activities of daily life, and among all of them, regular engagement in physical exercise and cognitive stimulation are more prone to favor brain plasticity. Moreover, studies have investigated a myriad of ways to stimulate brain plasticity, such as aerobic training, playing games, learning a new language, practicing music, dancing, and even maintaining a healthy diet (Ballesteros et al., 2018; Cespon et al., 2018). However, covering all the amazing science that emanates from this new and innovative field of neuroscience is beyond the scope of this work. This chapter therefore discusses two approaches that have gained impressive popularity over the last decade, namely, computerized cognitive training and physical exercise training. These two domains have evolved in parallel for many years, but more recently, multidomain interventions combining both physical and cognitive components have gained global interest worldwide. However, more studies are needed to better decipher the individual potential of each approach and their potential synergistic effect in improving neurocognitive functions. The following section first briefly summarizes normal cognitive changes associated with aging, that is, neurocognitive changes that occur naturally in the course of healthy aging and are not the results of a pathological neurodegeneration process such as Alzheimer's disease or other types of dementia. Then, supporting evidence for the impact of cognitive training and physical exercise interventions on cognitive and brain functions is presented separately, followed by the studies that have investigated the effect of combining these two interventions in a multidomain approach. We conclude by highlighting the challenges in the field and proposing future directions that will help clarify the association between cognitive training, physical exercise, and cognitive plasticity.

Cognitive Aging

For the public in general, aging is associated with gradual losses of physical and cognitive functions (Aguilar-Hernandez et al., 2023; Dipietro et al., 2019; Harada et al., 2013). When it comes to brain aging, decline of memory and slowing of mental functions are the most obvious and feared inevitable changes. However, an overstated negative view is mainly driven by a confusion between normal and pathological aging. While it is true that getting older increases the risk of developing dementia, only 10.9% of adults ages 65 and older and 33.4% of those over 85 years will develop dementia (Alzheimer's Association, 2024). This is not to say that those aging without dementia will not experience negative symptoms, but changes will not lead to significant impairments or limitations in everyday life.

Moreover, the so-called normal cognitive aging is a heterogeneous process in many ways. First, all cognitive functions do not age the same way and at the same rate. Some aspects of cognition are altered very early in life, while others are relatively maintained (Harada et al., 2013). It is generally agreed that knowledge-based processes are relatively preserved (Harada et al., 2013). On the other hand, process-based functions tend to be more sensitive to the aging process (Harada et al., 2013). Aging is also accompanied by progressive cognitive slowing, as assessed with psychomotor tests such as reaction time tasks or paper and pencil tests that require fast and accurate simple responses (Verhaeghen, 2014). This cognitive slowing is pervasive and will impact most cognitive functions.

However, it has also been reported that some specific cognitive processes will show age-associated declines over and above what one would expect as being explained by mere general cognitive slowing. For instance, working memory, or the ability to maintain and consciously manipulate information, declines with advanced age at a higher rate than the decline observed in processing speed or general cognitive slowing (Fabiani et al., 2015; Nettelbeck & Burns, 2010). Specifically, age-related differences are more likely to be observed in tasks that require executive control processes such as inhibition, updating, and working memory, and even greater if the memory load (i.e., the number of items to be maintained or manipulated) is high. As we discuss below, this is likely due to the brain structures and functions supporting these cognitive processes being altered early in adult life (Harada et al., 2013). Episodic memory also tends to be sensitive to age, as older adults often show reduced recall in all episodic memory tasks (e.g., verbal or visual). The decline in episodic memory is mainly attributed to poor encoding strategies, less use of environmental support, and deficits in binding new information with existing knowledge during encoding.

Studies using structural and functional brain imaging techniques have helped gain insights into potential brain mechanisms of aging. Changes in brain volume, especially in prefrontal regions and the hippocampus have been put forth as potential accounts for the age-related cognitive changes often observed in episodic memory and executive functions (Aguilar-Hernandez et al., 2023). The brain gray matter has been reported to decrease as early as after the first 20 years of life, especially in the prefrontal cortex (Wecker et al., 2000). Although the more popular explanation for the gray matter volume change associated with aging is the death of neurons, some reports support that the neurons themselves are also decreasing in size (Harada et al., 2013). A decreased number of connections between neurons is also thought to play a significant role (Wecker et al., 2000). For example, working memory deficits have been associated with reduced or different task-related activation in frontal regions of the cerebral cortex in older adults compared with younger adults (Li et al., 2015). Aging is also associated with a degradation of the white matter tract integrity, which could play a role in the cerebral functional changes observed in older adults (Bennett & Madden, 2014; Meier-Ruge et al., 1992).

Recent studies have questioned the relationship between brain volume and functions, and more advanced techniques are now used to better understand the complexity of the interconnection between brain structures and functions (see Grady, 2012, for more on this issue). The brain vasculature is another component thought to play a crucial role in normal cognitive aging with many recent advancements. For example, a long-term gradual accumulation of damage in microcirculation components has been associated with aging (De Silva & Faraci, 2020). This is thought to affect the cerebral blood flow and impair the blood–brain barrier function (De Silva & Faraci, 2020) and, as a result, alter cognitive functioning. While those cerebral changes are expected as part of normal aging, different individuals have different trajectories depending on myriad factors, as well as their protective or damaging lifestyles.

More recently, cognitive neuroscientists have also tried to account for individual differences in cognitive performances among older adults using theoretical models like compensation and reserve (Cabeza et al., 2018). As described in detail in Chapter 9 (this volume), the concept of reserve explains why certain individuals who show signs of cerebral neuronal decline counter the behavioral symptoms (i.e., cognitive decline) through different processes of neuronal enhancement (like the creation of new neurons or repair of neuronal resources as well as the establishing of new connections). The concept of compensation has also been supported by imaging studies that show that older adults might respond to higher cognitive loads by recruiting additional neuronal resources than younger adults (Reuter-Lorenz & Cappell, 2008). Those concepts could, in part, explain the heterogeneity of the cognitive aging process. Although many of us will experience some form of physical and cognitive decline as we grow older, examples of individuals that seem to be immunized against the aging process abound. The extent to which older adults benefit from the protection from cognitive decline (as explained by reserve, maintenance, and compensation) is impacted by different outcomes, many of which are related to lifestyle choices. While education level is one of the best predictors of cognitive maintenance in late life, being cognitively and socially engaged, having a healthy diet, and exercising regularly have been shown to prevent pathological cognitive decline through brain plasticity. For example, a recent study has shown that individuals who have a healthier lifestyle also show better cognitive performance in later life, even among individuals who are at high risk of developing Alzheimer's disease, after controlling for all potential confounds, including disease biomarkers burden (Dhana et al., 2024). The researchers also found that individuals with healthier lifestyles had less disease burden following brain autopsy. They concluded that having a healthy lifestyle helps build cognitive and brain reserve, which gives patients the ability to fight age and disease-related cerebral deteriorations and preserve cognitive performance at a later age.

The notion that one could build brain reserve has been supported by many cohort and intervention imaging studies in which participants followed exercise or cognitive training programs. While the evidence is not unilateral, the association is without a doubt important. However, the need for new studies that clarify the mechanisms of action, establish dose–response, and guide prescription at an individual level is critical.

Cognitive Training

Effects on Cognitive Performance

Cognitive training can be viewed as a subtype of cognitive intervention that aims at enhancing cognitive performance and function through guided and repeated practice of tasks designed to engage certain cognitive functions. Cognitive intervention refers to a broader approach encompassing cognitive training, cognitive rehabilitation, and cognitive stimulation. Cognitive rehabilitation takes place in the context of disease-related losses of function, like after a stroke, and usually targets the recuperation of multidimensional aspects of cognition, such as memory, attention, decision making, etc. Cognitive stimulation is less oriented toward improving specific functions and usually refers to the exposure to lifestyle choices or activities that require the use of different cognitive abilities, such as learning a new language, playing music, or playing complex games. While all these approaches rely on the plasticity potential of the brain, cognitive training studies are often used to uncover the mechanisms by which cognitive and brain plasticity is maintained in older age. This is sometimes done by using laboratory-made computer-based cognitive training software or more recently commercialized packages. This medium has the advantage of individualization of task parameters while accurately recording the reaction time of the answers. By having access to this, researchers can program participant feedback, and they can modify different parameters to increase the task progression difficulty. Through computerized cognitive training, researchers can also deconstruct different cognitive processes that make up more complex cognitive abilities. A systematic review has concluded that computerized cognitive training is even more effective than traditional paper–pencil approaches (Kueider et al., 2012), and therefore it can be used to gain insight into how the brain adapts to new challenging situations.

Cognitive training itself can be divided into at least two major categories: strategy training and process-based training. Strategy training involves learning cognitive strategies on how to better use preserved cognitive functions and environmental cues to improve higher-level cognitive functions like memory and decision making. Strategy training is very effective at improving cognitive performance (in particular, memory) in individuals with cognitive impairment (Belleville et al., 2018) and is often used in rehabilitation programs. For instance, studies by Belleville and colleagues (2018) have shown that learning memory skills can help improve memory in older adults and patients with mild cognitive impairment of the amnestic type (amnestic mild cognitive impairment [MCI]). Moreover, the effect endured over 6 months and the strategies that were used were efficiently used in everyday life. Cognitive training is a valid way to promote cognition in MCI. Process-based cognitive training is generally more focused on one or a few specific functions, like working memory or attention, and it can be used to target specific basic mechanisms (e.g., inhibition). Studies from our group have been following this approach for several years now. For instance, we developed a program that involves performing two concurrent object discrimination tasks (i.e., a computerized dual-task paradigm). One could be to discriminate between numbers or objects appearing on the screen, while the second one could involve discriminating among another definitive set of objects, letters, or sounds (Bherer et al., 2005, 2006). Participants would perform both tasks independently or at the same time as fast and accurately as they can, and the program would provide individualized feedback to help improve performance.

Dual-tasking is very challenging for older adults, and this is especially true when a task involves two motor responses, one with each hand and two stimuli that involve the same input modality (visual cues for example). However, using our dual-tasking training paradigm, we observed that cognitive plasticity for executive control processes was preserved in older adults (Bherer et al., 2008), which means that both older and younger adults show the same amplitude of improvement after six sessions of training spread over 2–3 weeks. Moreover, the improvement could be generalized to new task conditions, suggesting improvement above and beyond the learning of a specific task setting. Preserved cognitive plasticity in older adults is also well demonstrated in the results of one of the largest investigations of cognitive training, the Advanced Cognitive Training for Independent and Vital Elderly (ACTIVE) study (Tennstedt & Unverzagt, 2013), in which participants performed speed of processing, attention, memory, and reasoning training. The study shows that older adults can benefit from cognitive training and that the improvement can sometimes be long-lasting, in addition to showing some level of transfer to everyday tasks, like driving. In fact, in many instances, improvement following cognitive training has also been observed in untrained tasks that served as control, suggesting that some level of transfer can be observed. However, whether the benefits of cognitive training translate to other untrained situations remains an important debated question in the field.

The so-called transfer effect has shown mixed findings, and in many cases, the transfer is most likely to be observed if the testing condition is very close in design to the training condition. Our results concurred with this, and we reported that if the response and/or the stimulus modality of the tasks changed from the training condition to the testing condition, training effects, as indexed by improved attentional dual-tasking costs, are reduced compared to the improvement observed in the training task (Lussier et al., 2012). However, the training effect does seem to generalize to some extent to untrained tasks. In support of this, a recent meta-analysis has shown that only some cognitive training programs transfer to an untrained task, and this might depend not only on the cognitive ability trained, but also on the number of trained components (Basak et al., 2020). Specifically, training programs focusing on executive functions were more likely to result in improvements in untrained tasks, but generally speaking, cognitive training programs that targeted multiple cognitive components were the best at improving performance in untrained tasks (Basak et al., 2020). Recently, a series of RCTs have been developed to study the transfer effects of working memory training in more detail (Pahor et al., 2022). The results have shown that participants who achieved higher improvement in an untrained task that relies on the same cognitive processes as the trained task are also the ones who are more likely to show improvement in untrained tasks that use completely different untrained cognitive processes. The authors have suggested that, similar to many other intervention studies in other fields (i.e., exercise, nutrition), some participants might not respond to cognitive training due to interindividual differences.

More impressively, some studies have shown that certain types of cognitive training in older adults can transfer to benefits in completely different modalities, like mobility. For example, the dual-tasking training protocol developed in our laboratory (Lussier et al., 2017) did lead to improved balance and postural control, as assessed with single- and dual-support balance, with and without cognitive load (Li et al., 2010). Similar results were presented more recently by other researchers (Marusic et al., 2022), and a systematic review and meta-analysis has reiterated the benefit of cognitive training on mobility, especially during complex walking conditions (Marusic et al., 2018). This analysis shows that computerized cognitive training for older adults could lead to functional benefits in addition to improving performance on untrained cognitive tasks.

Despite those results, some authors suggest using caution when interpreting the transfer effects of cognitive training, especially when considering the inconsistent findings in the literature, or the small effect sizes in positive studies (Lintern & Boot, 2021; Smid et al., 2020; von Bastian et al., 2024). This is often because few high-quality intervention studies are adhering to rigorous experimental designs, training programs are not reproducible, and there are various individual differences and baseline ability differences that impact the results (Traut et al., 2021). Finally, authors sometimes fail to report aspects that are likely to impact the interpretation of the results.

On the other hand, cognitive training studies that are highly contextualized, follow rigorous training programs, and respect the RCT guidelines more often tend to show positive results and higher effect sizes (Diamond & Lee, 2011; Smithers et al., 2018). A recent review study that included 13 systematic reviews and meta-analyses has reported some components that must be considered to increase the likelihood that a cognitive training program results in improvements in untrained tasks (Sanjuan et al., 2020). The authors recommend that the training program should last at least 10 weeks, with two sessions/week, of 60–90 minutes/session, be performed in a group setting, target multiple cognitive skills, use both a process-based and a strategy-based approach, and also include other components related to quality of life (e.g., stress/anxiety management, physical activity, sleep).

Recommendations on what to include for the actual content of the cognitive training programs have also been made. Briefly, the programs should be designed based on the type of population that is targeted, and they should use an individualized administration approach (see Turnbull et al., 2022, for a detailed overview of all components). However, following those guidelines does not ensure that all individuals can benefit from cognitive training. For example, a study investigating the impact of the social determinants of health on the risk of developing dementia in the ACTIVE trial has shown that greater neighborhood advantages are not only associated with a lower incidence of dementia, but also with improved effectiveness of the cognitive training program (Rebok et al., 2023). This raises an important concern about generalizability in the cognitive training literature. Specifically, future intervention studies need to ensure that the programs are culturally sensitive and take into account social class components, the health literacy level of the sample, their education level, and their language proficiency (particularly in areas with high immigration populations). One approach to address this is to include a diverse participant-partner program in the study development stage, a process that is slowly becoming more popular today. This would ensure a more efficiently individualized cognitive training program that considers social factors in addition to interindividual factors.

Results from Brain Imaging Studies

Brain mechanisms underlying cognitive training effects have been documented. Cognitive training is thought to favor brain plasticity by either delaying age-related cerebral deterioration or causing cerebral improvements. Some studies have shown that cognitive training is associated with structural and functional brain changes. For instance, a study showed functional brain changes in frontal regions after dual-tasking training in healthy individuals (Erickson et al., 2007). Dual-tasking led to reduced activity in some frontal brain regions in both older and younger adults, as well as increased activity in the left prefrontal regions in older adults. This age-specific pattern could be a sign of a compensatory mechanism since both older and younger adults show equivalent improvement in behavioral performances.

In a recent systematic review, the magnetic resonance imaging (MRI) changes found to be associated with cognitive training were both structural and functional (Intzandt et al., 2021). The structural changes more often tended to be in microstructures (decreased mean diffusivity, increased fractional anisotropy) in multiple areas of the brain. Structural changes such as increased brain volume, cortical thickness, and density and coherence of white matter tracts have also been highlighted (Belleville & Bherer, 2012). However, MRI studies report functional changes more often (Intzandt et al., 2021). Depending on the tasks used, studies report either a decrease or increase in blood-oxygen-level–dependent (BOLD) activity in frontal, parietal, and hippocampal regions (Bherer, 2015; Intzandt et al., 2021). Improved connectivity in the default mode network and increased cerebral blood flow have also been associated with cognitive training (Chapman et al., 2015). For example, Erickson and colleagues (2007) have shown that dual-tasking training results in specific patterns of brain activation changes characterized by increased activation in the left ventrolateral prefrontal cortex (VLPFC) and a decreased activation in the right VLPFC and bilateral dorsolateral prefrontal cortex (DLPFC). This suggests that cognitive training can improve efficiency as well as engage compensatory mechanisms to help older adults manage situations involving increased cognitive demand from performing multiple tasks. However, further studies are required to generalize these findings to larger groups and to investigate more diverse training protocols.

Overall, results from behavioral intervention studies and brain imaging investigations support the notion that cognitive training is a valuable option to improve attention, speed of processing, memory, and attentional control in older adults and that it can be used as a therapeutic and rehabilitation tool in clinical populations to alleviate cognitive symptoms. While transfer effects are still debated, it seems that some functional benefits can still be expected after training, such as improved balance and postural control. In addition, some brain imaging studies have documented structural and functional changes in the brain following cognitive training intervention. However, more studies are needed to further demonstrate the reliability of cognitive training, its clinical validity, and the associated neuroplasticity mechanisms.

Physical Activity and Exercise

Effects on Cognitive Performance

While cognitive training has been gaining traction in the cognitive prevention literature in the last two decades, its use has been slightly overshadowed by the physical activity and exercise training literature. Physical activity refers to the general concept of any type of body movement that results in energy expenditure (Piggin, 2020). Physical exercise training is a type of structured physical activity in which the intensity, duration, and type of activity are purposefully adjusted with the hope of improving muscular strength, cardiorespiratory functions, or flexibility. Exercise training results in a cascade of structural and biochemical changes in the body, which includes the release of signaling molecules after acute and/or chronic exercise, sometimes referred to as exerkines (Chow et al., 2022), many of which are thought to also impact brain structure and function and promote cognitive health. Alternatively, exercise is also thought to improve other health conditions (e.g., stress, sleep) or prevent chronic conditions (e.g., coronary heart diseases, metabolic syndrome, and so on) and therefore exert an indirect effect on neurocognitive aging. While many studies, including RCTs and longitudinal studies, have supported the link between exercise and improved cognitive aging, some authors have also doubted this association (Ciria et al., 2023). This is likely due to the large variability in the interventions used, and a loose definition of exercise training, but more importantly, we now understand that there is a great individual variable response to exercise training. This might explain why some studies do not find the same link between exercise and cognition, and it seems reasonable to believe that a carefully designed individualized training program that also takes into account the individual characteristics of each participant is more likely to result in improved cognitive performance.

In 2010, Sofi and colleagues performed a meta-analysis that included 15 prospective studies with more than 30,000 participants worldwide, and the results showed that engaging in vigorous exercise more than three times per week was associated with a decreased relative risk for dementia of up to 38%. Fourteen years later, a new meta-analysis (Iso-Markku et al., 2024) was performed that included 104 studies and over 300,000 participants, and the results found again that performing physical activity was associated with decreased cognitive impairment. Performing physical activity was also associated with the change in cognition over time. The authors, however, found that all the associations have a small effect size and most of the studies were of low quality. A similar pattern of results is also found in meta-analyses investigating intervention studies. For example, Colcombe and Kramer showed in 2003 that, among 18 intervention studies (run between 1966 and 2001), exercise training resulted in medium effect size improvements in executive functions and small effects in control, spatial, and processing speed. The authors also concluded that intervention programs that include a significant amount of aerobic training and last over 6 months are more likely to show larger improvements in cognition. More recent reviews that included exercise intervention studies found that, again, high-quality studies were a minority and that positive trends emerged between physical activity and cognition, but the effect sizes were small (Furtado et al., 2023; Ludyga et al., 2020). Despite the small effect sizes, the results remain important, and recent recommendations for dementia prevention have suggested limiting sedentary behavior and encouraged regular exercise (Livingston et al., 2020).

Some specific cognitive functions are more often reported to improve after exercise training, like executive functions and memory (Iso-Markku et al., 2024; Ludyga et al., 2020). However, other functions, like verbal fluency (Iso-Markku et al., 2024), processing speed (Furtado et al., 2023), and working memory (Zhidong et al., 2021), have also been found to improve following exercise training. To better understand why some training programs are more successful than others at improving cognition, reviews and meta-analyses have looked at the exercise training program components in more detail. Specifically, it looks like longer programs, as well as more intense programs, are more likely to result in cognitive improvements and, in particular, improvements in the domain of executive functions (Cabral et al., 2019; Ludyga et al., 2020). Despite this, studies have shown that even shorter programs of only 12 weeks can result in cognitive improvements. Specifically, studies from our group in which healthy older participants trained three times a week for 12 weeks with a kinesiologist closely monitoring the training have shown improvements in executive functions (inhibition, working memory, dual-tasking) and processing speed (Berryman et al., 2014; Bherer et al., 2021b; Pothier et al., 2021; Vrinceanu et al., 2022). The training programs in those studies included aerobic, resistance, and motor abilities training, either separately or in combination. The key to improving cognitive performance through such short programs might likely be the individualization of the training program to each participant and the close monitoring. In some other studies, the researchers do not follow the participants closely (e.g., participants are sent to local gyms, do not use objective training targets, or rely on self-report training journals), and as a result, it looks like those studies find positive results if the training programs are longer, 6 months or even 1 year in duration (Quigley et al., 2020).

In the past few years, the exercise training literature has made great advancements in understanding how to improve the contents of an exercise training program to maximize the improvement in cognitive performance. Our work has shown that the most efficient exercise training programs contain a combination of aerobic (continuous and interval training), resistance, and motor abilities training, are individualized based on a baseline cardiopulmonary exercise test (percent of maximal aerobic power) and one maximal repetition (rate of perceived exertion), and regularly update and increase the exercise dose (intensity and/or duration) based on progress and self-report perceived difficulty, while an expert staff monitors progression, adapts exercises, and ensures that participants follow the prescribed dose. When the training program follows those guidelines, benefits are likely to appear within 12 weeks, but the literature suggests that the longer the training program, the more likely it is to observe higher cognitive benefits. Review studies have highlighted that training programs of 6 months or 1 year are more likely to result in cognitive benefits (Quigley et al., 2020). However, it is not clear if the ideal training duration of 6 months to 1 year only reflects that there are very few carefully monitored training programs of longer than 1 year. The general conclusion is that the longer the total exercise duration (in hours) or the higher the total exercise dose, the better the chances of observing cognitive benefits (Quigley et al., 2020).

Recent studies have also identified the importance of cardiovascular fitness progression (VO_2 max change) during training as the best marker predictive of cognitive improvement. In our studies, we first identified an association between VO_2 max and improvements in executive control (Predovan et al., 2012), and more recently we have shown that VO_2 max can fully mediate the cognitive improvement following exercise training. For example, in Bherer and colleagues (2021a), we reported that in 143 participants ages 65–89 years, aerobic training predicted improvement in processing speed and attentional control, and in the case of processing speed, improvement was fully mediated by change in VO_2 max in the oldest-old group of 72-year-olds and over. We have also shown that VO_2 max mediated the difference in cognition (processing speed and executive function) between healthy participants and chronic heart failure patients or heart transplant recipients (Besnier et al., 2020). Despite those findings, some participants don't show the same physiological adaptation to exercise training. While it is still unclear why this is, recent findings suggest that exercise nonresponders might be characterized by a different phenotype that might prevent them from improving VO_2 max (Guirault et al., 2024). Since exercise nonresponders don't have the same physiological response to exercise, they might not show improvements in cognition either. However, the available literature covering this is still limited, and more studies are needed.

While aerobic training and cardiovascular improvements are crucial for cognitive improvement, it is important to mention that lighter-intensity exercise programs like yoga, tai-chi, and motor abilities training, or even dance, have also shown cognitive benefits (Gomes-Osman et al., 2018; Yang et al., 2024). It is possible that those exercises differ from classic resistance or aerobic training by having stronger impacts on secondary pathways that prevent cognitive decline (relaxation, stress management, social interactions, etc.). Another possibility is that those types of activities also involve some degree of cognitive engagement (e.g., memorizing dance patterns, involving more hand–eye coordination, or dual-tasking to a higher degree), but we discuss this in more detail in the following section of this chapter addressing the impact of multidomain interventions. Another possibility is that other types of exercise programs also result in different physiological changes that can in turn impact brain plasticity and prevent cognitive decline. A meta-analysis by Marinus and colleagues (2019) suggested that strength training alone or combined with aerobic training is more likely to lead to improved brain-derived neurotrophic factor (BDNF) than aerobic exercise alone. Taken together, this suggests that a diverse well-structured individualized training program is key to maximizing cognitive plasticity.

As new guidelines emphasize the need to properly study sex differences in research, it must be mentioned that more work must be done to address this in the exercise literature. By synthesizing the available literature, the findings are conflicting. For example, a meta-analysis conducted by Bahra and colleagues (2017) showed that the effects of physical activity training on cognitive performance differed between sexes. The study revealed that different types of physical training (aerobic, resistance, and multidomain) had greater benefits on cognitive variables in women than in men, especially for executive functions. On the other hand, a more recent *Nature* systematic review and meta-analysis showed that women benefit less from exercise and that the link between exercise dose–response and cognition differed between the sexes

(Ludyga et al., 2020). Therefore, more studies are needed, and elucidating the effects of sex on neurocognitive outcomes may help tailor targeted training programs and help reduce cognitive decline.

Results from Brain Imaging Studies

Several brain imaging studies have suggested that physical exercise induces transient and permanent changes at the structural and functional levels in the brain (Bherer et al., 2013). In a recent MRI-data-focused systematic review, exercise training has been found to increase gray matter volume in frontal and temporal regions and have a positive impact on global white matter lesion volume and atrophy (Intzandt et al., 2021). For example, seminal work from Kramer, Colcombe, and Erikson (Colcombe et al., 2006; Erickson et al., 2011; Kramer et al., 2006) has shown that aerobic training can increase hippocampus volume bilaterally, while participants in the control group show a decrease in volume.

Another study shows that exercise training over 24 months does not change white matter hyperintensities, while the control group showed up to 18.8% worsening of the white matter hyperintensities grade (Shaaban et al., 2019). In terms of functional connectivity, exercise training has been found to increase connectivity in the default mode network and central executive networks, and show either an increase or decrease in BOLD activity in the frontal, parietal, temporal, and thalamic regions (Intzandt et al., 2021). Although not as often reported, increases in cerebral blood flow and volume have also been found (Maass et al., 2015, 2016).

Yet another study has shown a link between cardiorespiratory fitness (VO_2 max) and activation in the left DLPFC during a Stroop task (Dupuy et al., 2015) using functional near-infrared spectroscopy in healthy older women. The study also observed that VO_2 max was positively associated with blood oxygenation level–dependent cerebrovascular reactivity to CO_2 in some brain regions (periventricular watershed regions and within the postcentral gyrus), which suggests that preserved vessel elasticity may be one of the key mechanisms by which physical exercise helps maintain and improve cognition in older adults (Gauthier et al., 2015).

Novel studies suggest that the development of dementia and cognitive aging are primarily dependent on specific cerebrovascular health markers both in healthy individuals and those with cardiovascular risk factors (Efimova et al., 2008; Glodzik et al., 2011). Specifically, the interplay between cerebral small vessel disease (CSVD) progression and cerebral pulsatility has been proposed as a leading mechanism. While in CSVD pathology regular exercise training is thought to exert an influence, its effectiveness remains a subject of debate in the literature. Similarly, the effect of exercise training on cerebral pulsatility is not fully understood due to the limited studies available.

Exercise-induced changes at the molecular level are also hypothesized to play a role in brain plasticity and the subsequent cognitive benefits. For example, exercise training has been shown to increase BDNF and insulin-like growth factor 1 (IGF-1; Arazi et al., 2021). In turn, BDNF has been linked to neuroplasticity and neuronal repair (Knaepen et al., 2010), and IGF-1 is thought to play a role in neurogenesis and angiogenesis (Nieto-Estevez et al., 2016). In addition, recent methodological advances in the ability to look at circulating blood proteins have opened the way to a more detailed study of the molecular mechanism linking exercise to brain plasticity by using large data and omics analyses. However, despite offering great research potential, this approach is in its infancy in the exercise and cognitive aging field, and only future studies will reveal their importance.

Multidomain Interventions Combining Exercise and Cognitive Training

Effects on Cognitive Performance

In previous sections, we saw numerous studies suggesting that exercise training and cognitive training in cognitively healthy older adults can independently help enhance cognitive performance. More recent studies have investigated whether these two approaches can be combined (multidomain training) to further synergistically enhance cognition—that is, if combining the two types of training would lead to larger improvements than would be expected from each one independently. Evidence for this can also be obtained from the exercise-only literature. For example, it has been theorized that aerobic training is likely to improve cognition through generalized biological adaptations (in particular, cardiovascular-driven) to exercise that promotes cerebral plasticity and therefore supports cognitive improvements (Netz, 2019). On the other hand, some nonaerobic low-intensity exercise training, like motor abilities training or dance, has the ability to improve cognition through distinct mechanisms (Netz, 2019). Specifically, those types of physical exercises have a certain degree of cognitive load, and the benefits of the training are likely to transfer to cognitive tests that measure those cognitive abilities that are used during training. In other words, physical exercise training also acts in part like cognitive training. This has also been experimentally proven in a study in which healthy older participants were either assigned to a cognitive-only training program, motor abilities training, or aerobic training (Vrinceanu et al., 2022). Results showed that while the cognitive training group had the highest cognitive improvement, the motor abilities training had much higher improvements in task-coordination ability than aerobic training, likely due to using those abilities as part of the training program. Therefore, to maximize the cognitive benefits, diversifying the physical exercise training component and including cognitive training components might be crucial.

Recent advancements in the field support the idea that multidomain interventions that are specifically designed to combine physical exercise and cognitive training components can lead to significant gains in cognition (Rebok, 2024b). For example, the Finnish Geriatric Intervention Study to Prevent Cognitive Impairment and Disability (FINGER) trial, a randomized controlled trial investigating the effects of a 2-year multidomain intervention (exercise training, cognitive training, and nutritional counseling) observed that cognitive functioning was improved or maintained in individuals with high cardiovascular risk factors (Cardiovascular Risk Factors, Aging, and Incidence of Dementia score) compared with a control group (no intervention; Ngandu et al., 2015). However, the design of the FINGER trial does not allow one to determine whether gains are superior in multidomain compared with single-domain interventions. To address this issue, we conducted a study combining physical exercise training biweekly and cognitive training once a week for 3 months (Desjardins-Crepeau et al., 2016).

We went further in trying to dissociate the training effects by comparing the active physical exercise training group against one doing nonaerobic stretching exercise and the active cognitive dual-tasking training component against a placebo computer condition (learning to browse the internet). Against our expectations, the results did not show superior benefits of combining both active training components relative to the computer cognitive training alone on neurocognitive tests (Desjardins-Crepeau et al., 2016). However, the combined group did perform better than the active exercise and placebo cognitive group. This is of course not completely surprising, as cognitive training that is designed to improve specific cognitive functions tends to have a greater effect than exercise simply due to the focused nature of the training (Vrinceanu et al., 2022).

It could also be the case that clinical neuropsychological tests designed to dissociate clinically significant deficits from normal cognition, used as outcomes in Desjardins-Crepeau and colleagues (2016), were not sensitive enough to detect the synergistic effect of exercise and cognitive training in healthy older adults. This idea is supported by the synergistic effect of combined intervention observed in the same trials on dual-tasking performances using an experimental paradigm. In fact, after further investigations, we observed that the group that did the combined dual-tasking training and aerobic exercise intervention did improve better in dual-tasking set cost than the other groups, which suggests the largest improvement in the working memory component of the task (Bherer et al., 2021a). These results support the notion that adding some cognitive training components to an exercise program can help maximize the cognitive benefits in seniors. This approach is further supported by a recent meta-analysis that found that adding cognitive training to an exercise training program does not impact the efficacy of the exercise training (Gavelin et al., 2021).

Evidence for the beneficial effect of multidomain interventions also comes from the literature covering clinical populations suffering from mild cognitive impairment. In fact, in a recent nationwide study, we reported that an aerobic and strength training exercise program, combined with cognitive training for 6 months, showed larger cognitive benefits compared with either one of the two independent programs or a placebo multidomain training (Montero-Odasso et al., 2022). This study was unique in comparing all potential combinations of exercise and cognitive training with placebo conditions. The study also shows that benefits could be observed, even in the presence of mild cognitive impairment.

Despite there not being a lot of studies, meta-analyses have already highlighted that multidomain interventions benefit cognition in older adults without cognitive impairment and with mild cognitive impairment (Gavelin et al., 2021; Karssemeijer et al., 2017; Sun et al., 2021). The results suggest that multidomain training is superior not only to a control group, but also exercise training alone (Zhu et al., 2016). Concerning the design of the multidomain training, there are two general approaches: sequential or simultaneous. The literature suggests that both types are superior to exercise training alone. However, simultaneous multidomain training, in which the cognitive training component is delivered at the same time as the physical exercise training component, might lead to superior cognitive benefits, although possibly not by a lot (Gavelin et al., 2021). Despite this, most studies use the sequential design mostly because it is easier to implement. This design, of course, has its limitations, as it is not clear in those studies if the effect of the multidomain training is really caused by combining the two components or if it is simply caused by performing two types of training (physical and cognitive)—and if, at the end of the day, the participants in those interventions accumulate a larger total number of hours of training. Finally, a systematic review has found some evidence that multidomain training programs could result in greater short-term cognitive benefits (Joubert & Chainay, 2018). This means that by implementing a multidomain protocol, participants might benefit from cognitive improvement faster, though very little evidence exists for this claim. If, however, this is the case, multidomain protocols would be a great solution for individuals at risk of, or living with, cognitive decline who need more aggressive cognitive rehabilitation.

Results from Brain Imaging Studies

Although limited, brain changes have also been reported in multidomain interventions. Kobe and colleagues (2016) performed a 6-month intervention combining aerobic training, cognitive stimulation, and an omega-3 supplement in individuals with mild cognitive impairment and observed increased gray matter volume in several brain regions (frontal cortex, angular cortex, precuneus, posterior cingulate cortex) in the training group, while volume decreased in controls. Another study showed that multidomain training in healthy older adults can improve the strength of the connectivity in the default mode network, as well as in the attentional networks (Pieramico et al., 2012). Finally, a systematic review investigating the impact of exercise training or cognitive training on cerebral MRI markers (Intzandt et al., 2021) found that exercise training and cognitive training have unique patterns of improvement in different cerebral MRI markers. This again supports the notion that a multidomain training intervention could improve cognition by benefiting from the pooled cerebral improvements from all different individual components of the two types of training. However, this remains to be further studied in the same design, using an intervention approach that carefully controls for other confounding factors.

Conclusion

As the world population is aging at an unprecedented rate, the quest for lowering the negative impacts of age on cognitive functions is underway. For the past few decades, researchers have tried to identify lifestyle factors and intervention programs that can maintain cognitive functions and even enhance cognitive performance in older adults. Cognitive stimulation, achieved through computerized cognitive training or a physical activity program, seems to momentarily enhance cognition and may lead to benefits in real-life situations. However, the extent to which cognitive training leads to a substantial gain in untrained tasks, the so-called transfer effect, is still a matter of debate. Nevertheless, a significant number of studies support that specific types of cognitive activities may help enhance cognition, and this is likely to translate into boosted confidence in one's cognitive performance, which in itself could lead to a transferable gain in real life. In addition, cognitive training studies offer a platform to test the extent to which cognitive plasticity is maintained in older age. That said, most studies find small effect sizes for cognitive training, and future studies are still needed to better understand the brain plasticity mechanisms involved in cognitive training.

Studies have also supported that physical activity and exercise interventions can improve cognition, and over the last two decades, advancements have been made in better understanding exercise prescription and the individual response to exercise training. These studies have shown that individualized aerobic and resistance exercise performed over several months has the potential to enhance cognition in seniors. More recent studies have investigated a wider range of physical activity, including mind–body exercise and dance, and this led to a more comprehensive investigation of the direct and indirect gains that can come from a variety of physical exercise interventions. Studies investigating the cerebral mechanisms involved in both cognitive and physical training suggest that they each have their unique benefits. Therefore, combining both cognitive training components and physical exercise training components might maximize the brain plasticity benefits.

The recent increase of interest in the combination of different types of training in multidomain interventions has shown fascinating and very promising results in the quest against age-related cognitive decline. These studies have allowed us to observe that combining exercise with cognitive stimulation is especially efficient in patients with mild cognitive impairment, but benefits in healthy seniors have also been reported.

While our understanding of the field has been growing exponentially lately, there are still some limitations and unanswered questions. For example, researchers are still looking for the ideal training plan composition for both physical and cognitive training so that they can create better prescriptions. This is a limiting factor since many components can be modified as can be observed from the very heterogeneous intervention studies available in the field. The duration of the training program is still debated, as more recent studies have shown that longer interventions are more efficient, but very few studies perform very well-controlled RCTs that are longer than 6 months or 1 year. This also raises the question of whether there is a dose–response for cognitive training or physical exercise training and, if there is one, what factors might affect it. Individual responses to physical training have also been identified, but our understanding of why some individuals react differently is still unclear. Finally, the potential impact that cognitive intervention studies might have on real-life situations, like the activities of daily living, has been somewhat studied, but it is still not clear if those effects are permanent or temporary, especially in individuals who show signs of cognitive decline and might need more aggressive interventions (Rebok, 2024a). While those are all components that will need further independent study for both physical training and cognitive training, they will also have to be further investigated in the context of multidomain training.

Moreover, recent advancements in multiomics, combined with brain imaging approaches, will likely lead to identifying new biomarkers and a better understanding of the complex mechanisms by which cognitive, exercise, and multidomain interventions promote brain plasticity, enhance cognition, and prevent cognitive decline as we age. Recent studies have identified new cerebrovascular markers as potential avenues for research in better understanding cognitive aging and dementia. In parallel, proteomic studies have started to identify potential mechanistic pathways modulated by exercise. In addition, the large amount of data that can potentially be used from e-health sources, including wearable devices that have been adopted easily by older adults (Kwan et al., 2020), will offer new approaches to studying physical activity, exercise training, and cognitive training, as well as their synergistic effect. Innovative approaches to studying multimodal training are also starting to emerge in the literature, combining multiple components, including emotion, stress management, exercise, and cognitive stimulation such as dance, dance movement therapy, and yoga. Finally, coupling this with new statistical approaches using artificial intelligence and the capacity to better manipulate and investigate large data ensures an exciting future for research in this fascinating field (Yang et al., 2024).

REFERENCES

Aguilar-Hernandez, L., Alejandre, R., Cesar Morales-Medina, J., Iannitti, T., & Flores, G. (2023). Cellular mechanisms in brain aging: Focus on physiological and pathological aging. *Journal of Chemical Neuroanatomy, 128*, 102210.

Alzheimer's Association. (2024). 2024 Alzheimer's disease facts and figures. *Alzheimer's & Dementia, 20*(5), 3708–3821.

Arazi, H., Babaei, P., Moghimi, M., & Asadi, A. (2021). Acute effects of strength and endurance exercise on serum BDNF and IGF-1 levels in older men. *BMC Geriatrics, 21*(1), 50.

Ballesteros, S., Voelcker-Rehage, C., & Bherer, L. (2018). Editorial: Cognitive and brain plasticity induced by physical exercise, cognitive training, video games, and combined interventions. *Frontiers in Human Neuroscience, 12*, 169.

Barha, C. K., Galea, L. A., Nagamatsu, L. S., Erickson, K. I., & Liu-Ambrose, T. (2017). Personalising exercise recommendations for brain health: Considerations and future directions. *British Journal of Sports Medicine, 51*(8), 636–639.

Basak, C., Qin, S., & O'Connell, M. A. (2020). Differential effects of cognitive training modules in healthy aging and mild cognitive impairment: A comprehensive meta-analysis of randomized controlled trials. *Psychology and Aging, 35*(2), 220–249.

Belleville, S., & Bherer, L. (2012). Biomarkers of cognitive training effects in aging. *Current Translational Geriatrics and Experimental Gerontology Reports, 1*(2), 104–110.

Belleville, S., Hudon, C., Bier, N., Brodeur, C., Gilbert, B., Grenier, S., et al. (2018). MEMO+: Efficacy, durability and effect of cognitive training and psychosocial intervention in individuals with mild cognitive impairment. *Journal of the American Geriatric Society, 66*(4), 655–663.

Bennett, I. J., & Madden, D. J. (2014). Disconnected aging: Cerebral white matter integrity and age-related differences in cognition. *Neuroscience, 276*, 187–205.

Berryman, N., Bherer, L., Nadeau, S., Lauziere, S., Lehr, L., Bobeuf, F., et al. (2014). Multiple roads lead to Rome: Combined high-intensity aerobic and strength training vs. gross motor activities leads to equivalent improvement in executive functions in a cohort of healthy older adults. *Age, 36*(5).

Besnier, F., Berube, B., Gagnon, C., Olmand, M., Ribeiro, P. A. B., Nigam, A., et al. (2020).

Cardiorespiratory fitness mediates cognitive performance in chronic heart failure patients and heart transplant recipients. *International Journal of Environmental Research and Public Health, 17*(22).

Bherer, L. (2015). Cognitive plasticity in older adults: Effects of cognitive training and physical exercise. *Annals of the New York Academy of Sciences, 1337,* 1–6.

Bherer, L., Erickson, K. I., & Liu-Ambrose, T. (2013). A review of the effects of physical activity and exercise on cognitive and brain functions in older adults. *Journal of Aging Research, 2013,* 657508.

Bherer, L., Gagnon, C., Langeard, A., Lussier, M., Desjardins-Crepeau, L., Berryman, N., et al. (2021a). Synergistic effects of cognitive training and physical exercise on dual-task performance in older adults. *Journal of Gerontology. Series B, Psychological Sciences and Social Sciences, 76*(8), 1533–1541.

Bherer, L., Kramer, A. F., Peterson, M. S., Colcombe, S., Erickson, K., & Becic, E. (2005). Training effects on dual-task performance: Are there age-related differences in plasticity of attentional control? *Psychology and Aging, 20*(4), 695–709.

Bherer, L., Kramer, A. F., Peterson, M. S., Colcombe, S., Erickson, K., & Becic, E. (2006). Testing the limits of cognitive plasticity in older adults: Application to attentional control. *Acta Psychologoca (Amsterdam), 123*(3), 261–278.

Bherer, L., Kramer, A. F., Peterson, M. S., Colcombe, S., Erickson, K., & Becic, E. (2008). Transfer effects in task-set cost and dual-task cost after dual-task training in older and younger adults: Further evidence for cognitive plasticity in attentional control in late adulthood. *Experimental Aging Research, 34*(3), 188–219.

Bherer, L., Langeard, A., Kaushal, N., Vrinceanu, T., Desjardins-Crepeau, L., Langlois, F., & Kramer, A. F. (2021b). Physical exercise training effect and mediation through cardiorespiratory fitness on dual-task performances differ in younger-old and older-old adults. *Journal of Gerontology. Series B, Psychological Sciences and Social Sciences, 76*(2), 219–228.

Brehmer, Y., Kalpouzos, G., Wenger, E., & Lovden, M. (2014). Plasticity of brain and cognition in older adults. *Psychological Research, 78*(6), 790–802.

Cabeza, R., Albert, M., Belleville, S., Craik, F. I. M., Duarte, A., Grady, C. L., et al. (2018). Maintenance, reserve and compensation: The cognitive neuroscience of healthy ageing. *Nature Reviews Neuroscience, 19*(11), 701–710.

Cabral, D. F., Rice, J., Morris, T. P., Rundek, T., Pascual-Leone, A., & Gomes-Osman, J. (2019). Exercise for brain health: An investigation into the underlying mechanisms guided by dose. *Neurotherapeutics, 16*(3), 580–599.

Cespon, J., Miniussi, C., & Pellicciari, M. C. (2018). Interventional programmes to improve cognition during healthy and pathological ageing: Cortical modulations and evidence for brain plasticity. *Ageing Research Reviews, 43,* 81–98.

Chapman, S. B., Aslan, S., Spence, J. S., Hart, Jr., J. J., Bartz, E. K., Didehbani, N., et al. (2015). Neural mechanisms of brain plasticity with complex cognitive training in healthy seniors. *Cerebral Cortex, 25*(2), 396–405.

Chow, L. S., Gerszten, R. E., Taylor, J. M., Pedersen, B. K., van Praag, H., Trappe, S., et al. (2022). Exerkines in health, resilience and disease. *Nature Reviews Endocrinology, 18*(5), 273–289.

Ciria, L. F., Román-Caballero, R., Vadillo, M. A., Holgado, D., Luque-Casado, A., Perakakis, P., & Sanabria, D. (2023). An umbrella review of randomized control trials on the effects of physical exercise on cognition. *Nature Human Behaviour, 7*(6), 928–941.

Colcombe, S., & Kramer, A. F. (2003). Fitness effects on the cognitive function of older adults: A meta-analytic study. *Psychological Science, 14*(2), 125–130.

Colcombe, S. J., Erickson, K. I., Scalf, P. E., Kim, J. S., Prakash, R., McAuley, E., et al.

(2006). Aerobic exercise training increases brain volume in aging humans. *Journal of Gerontology. Series A, Medicine, 61*(11), 1166–1170.

De Silva, T. M., & Faraci, F. M. (2020). Contributions of aging to cerebral small vessel disease. *Annual Review of Physiology, 82*, 275–295.

Desjardins-Crepeau, L., Berryman, N., Fraser, S. A., Vu, T. T., Kergoat, M. J., Li, K. Z., et al. (2016). Effects of combined physical and cognitive training on fitness and neuropsychological outcomes in healthy older adults. *Clinical Interventions in Aging, 11*, 1287–1299.

Dhana, K., Agarwal, P., James, B. D., Leurgans, S. E., Rajan, K. B., Aggarwal, N. T., et al. (2024). Healthy lifestyle and cognition in older adults with common neuropathologies of dementia. *JAMA Neurology, 81*(3), 233–239.

Diamond, A., & Lee, K. (2011). Interventions shown to aid executive function development in children 4 to 12 years old. *Science, 333*, 959–964.

Dipietro, L., Campbell, W. W., Buchner, D. M., Erickson, K. I., Powell, K. E., Bloodgood, B., et al. (2019). Physical activity, injurious falls, and physical function in aging: An umbrella review. *Medicine & Science in Sports & Exercise, 51*(6), 1303–1313.

Dupuy, O., Gauthier, C. J., Fraser, S. A., Desjardins-Crepeau, L., Desjardins, M., Mekary, S., et al. (2015). Higher levels of cardiovascular fitness are associated with better executive function and prefrontal oxygenation in younger and older women. *Frontiers in Human Neuroscience, 9*, 66.

Efimova, I. Y., Efimova, N. Y., Triss, S. V., & Lishmanov, Y. B. (2008). Brain perfusion and cognitive function changes in hypertensive patients. *Hypertension Research, 31*(4), 673–678.

Erickson, K. I., Colcombe, S. J., Wadhwa, R., Bherer, L., Peterson, M. S., Scalf, P. E., et al. (2007). Training-induced functional activation changes in dual-task processing: An FMRI study. *Cerebral Cortex, 17*(1), 192–204.

Erickson, K. I., Voss, M. W., Prakash, R. S., Basak, C., Szabo, A., Chaddock, L., et al. (2011). Exercise training increases size of hippocampus and improves memory. *Proceedings of the National Academy of Sciences, 108*(7), 3017–3022.

Fabiani, M., Zimmerman, B., Gratton, G., Jolicoeur, P., Lefebvre, C., & Martinez-Trujillo, J. (2015). Working memory and aging: A review. *Mechanisms of Sensory Working Memory: Attention and Perfomance XXV, 131*.

Furtado, G. E., Reis, A., Braga-Pereira, R., Caldo-Silva, A., Teques, P., Sampaio, A. R., et al. (2023). Impact of exercise interventions on sustained brain health outcomes in frail older individuals: A comprehensive review of systematic reviews. *Healthcare (Basel), 11*(24).

Gauthier, C. J., Lefort, M., Mekary, S., Desjardins-Crépeau, L., Skimminge, A., Iversen, P., et al. (2015). Hearts and minds: Linking vascular rigidity and aerobic fitness with cognitive aging. *Neurobiology and Again, 36*(1), 304–314.

Gavelin, H. M., Dong, C., Minkov, R., Bahar-Fuchs, A., Ellis, K. A., Lautenschlager, N. T., et al. (2021). Combined physical and cognitive training for older adults with and without cognitive impairment: A systematic review and network meta-analysis of randomized controlled trials. *Ageing Research Reviews, 66*, 101232.

Glodzik, L., Rusinek, H., Brys, M., Tsui, W. H., Switalski, R., Mosconi, L., et al. (2011). Framingham cardiovascular risk profile correlates with impaired hippocampal and cortical vasoreactivity to hypercapnia. *Journal of Cerebral Blood Flow & Metabolism, 31*(2), 671–679.

Gomes-Osman, J., Cabral, D. F., Morris, T. P., McInerney, K., Cahalin, L. P., Rundek, T., et al. (2018). Exercise for cognitive brain health in aging: A systematic review for an evaluation of dose. *Neurology Clinical Practice, 8*(3), 257–265.

Grady, C. (2012). The cognitive neuroscience of ageing. *Nature Reviews Neuroscience, 13*(7), 491–505.

Guirault, A., Lepretre, P. M., Trachsel, L. D., Besnier, F., Boidin, M., Lalonge, J., et al. (2024). Determinants of VO2 peak changes after aerobic training in coronary heart disease patients. *International Journal of Sports Medicine, 45*(7), 532–542.

Harada, C. N., Natelson Love, M. C., & Triebel, K. L. (2013). Normal cognitive aging. *Clinics in Geriatric Medicine, 29*(4), 737–752.

Intzandt, B., Vrinceanu, T., Huck, J., Vincent, T., Montero-Odasso, M., Gauthier, C. J., & Bherer, L. (2021). Comparing the effect of cognitive vs. exercise training on brain MRI outcomes in healthy older adults: A systematic review. *Neuroscience and Biobehavioral Reviews, 128*, 511–533.

Iso-Markku, P., Aaltonen, S., Kujala, U. M., Halme, H. L., Phipps, D., Knittle, K., et al. (2024). Physical activity and cognitive decline among older adults: A systematic review and meta-analysis. *JAMA Network Open, 7*(2), e2354285.

Joubert, C., & Chainay, H. (2018). Aging brain: The effect of combined cognitive and physical training on cognition as compared to cognitive and physical training alone—a systematic review. *Clinical Intervention in Aging, 13*, 1267–1301.

Karssemeijer, E. G. A., Aaronson, J. A., Bossers, W. J., Smits, T., Olde Rikkert, M. G. M., & Kessels, R. P. C. (2017). Positive effects of combined cognitive and physical exercise training on cognitive function in older adults with mild cognitive impairment or dementia: A meta-analysis. *Ageing Resarch Reviews, 40*, 75–83.

Knaepen, K., Goekint, M., Heyman, E. M., & Meeusen, R. (2010). Neuroplasticity—exercise-induced response of peripheral brain-derived neurotrophic factor. *Sports Medicine, 40*(9), 765–801.

Kobe, T., Witte, A. V., Schnelle, A., Lesemann, A., Fabian, S., Tesky, V. A., et al. (2016). Combined omega-3 fatty acids, aerobic exercise and cognitive stimulation prevents decline in gray matter volume of the frontal, parietal and cingulate cortex in patients with mild cognitive impairment. *Neuroimage, 131*, 226–238.

Kramer, A. F., Bherer, L., Colcombe, S. J., Dong, W., & Greenough, W. T. (2004). Environmental influences on cognitive and brain plasticity during aging. *Journal of Gerontology. Series A, Medicine, 59*(9), M940–957.

Kramer, A. F., Erickson, K. I., & Colcombe, S. J. (2006). Exercise, cognition, and the aging brain. *Journal of Applied Physiology (1985), 101*(4), 1237–1242.

Kueider, A. M., Parisi, J. M., Gross, A. L., & Rebok, G. W. (2012). Computerized cognitive training with older adults: A systematic review. *PLOS ONE, 7*(7), e40588.

Kwan, R. Y., Lee, D., Lee, P. H., Tse, M., Cheung, D. S., Thiamwong, L., & Choi, K. S. (2020). Effects of an mHealth brisk walking intervention on increasing physical activity in older people with cognitive frailty: Pilot randomized controlled trial. *JMIR mHealth and uHealth, 8*(7), e16596.

Li, H. J., Hou, X. H., Liu, H. H., Yue, C. L., Lu, G. M., & Zuo, X. N. (2015). Putting age-related task activation into large-scale brain networks: A meta-analysis of 114 fMRI studies on healthy aging. *Neuroscience & Biobehavioral Reviews, 57*, 156–174.

Li, K. Z., Roudaia, E., Lussier, M., Bherer, L., Leroux, A., & McKinley, P. A. (2010). Benefits of cognitive dual-task training on balance performance in healthy older adults. *Journals of Gerontology. Series A, Biological sciences and medical sciences, 65*(12), 1344–1352.

Lintern, G., & Boot, W. R. (2021). Cognitive training: Transfer beyond the laboratory? *Human Factors, 63*(3), 531–547.

Livingston, G., Huntley, J., Sommerlad, A., Ames, D., Ballard, C., Banerjee, S., et al. (2020). Dementia prevention, intervention, and care: 2020 report of the Lancet Commission. *Lancet, 396*, 413–446.

Ludyga, S., Gerber, M., Puhse, U., Looser, V. N., & Kamijo, K. (2020). Systematic review and meta-analysis investigating moderators of long-term effects of exercise on cognition in healthy individuals. *Nature Human Behavior, 4*(6), 603–612.

Lussier, M., Bugaiska, A., & Bherer, L. (2017). Specific transfer effects following variable priority dual-task training in older adults. *Restorative Neurology and Neuroscience, 35*(2), 237–250.

Lussier, M., Gagnon, C., & Bherer, L. (2012). An investigation of response and stimulus modality transfer effects after dual-task training in younger and older. *Frontiers in Human Neuroscience, 6*, 129.

Maass, A., Duzel, S., Brigadski, T., Goerke, M., Becke, A., Sobieray, U., et al. (2016). Relationships of peripheral IGF-1, VEGF and BDNF levels to exercise-related changes in memory, hippocampal perfusion and volumes in older adults. *Neuroimage, 131*, 142–154.

Maass, A., Duzel, S., Goerke, M., Becke, A., Sobieray, U., Neumann, K., et al. (2015). Vascular hippocampal plasticity after aerobic exercise in older adults. *Molecular Psychiatry, 20*(5), 585–593.

Marinus, N., Hansen, D., Feys, P., Meesen, R., Timmermans, A., & Spildooren, J. (2019). The Impact of different types of exercise training on peripheral blood brain-derived neurotrophic factor concentrations in older adults: A meta-analysis. *Sports Medicine, 49*(10), 1529–1546.

Marusic, U., Verghese, J., & Mahoney, J. R. (2018). Cognitive-based interventions to improve mobility: A systematic review and meta-analysis. *Journal of the American Medical Directors Association, 19*(6), 484–491.

Marusic, U., Verghese, J., & Mahoney, J. R. (2022). Does cognitive training improve mobility, enhance cognition, and promote neural activation? *Frontiers in Aging Neuroscience, 14*, 845825.

Meier-Ruge, W., Ulrich, J., Bruhlmann, M., & Meier, E. (1992). Age-related white matter atrophy in the human brain. *Annual of the New York Academy of Sciences, 673*, 260–269.

Montero-Odasso, M., Almeida, Q. J., Burhan, A. M., Camicioli, R., Li, K., Liu-Ambrose, T., et al. (2022). The SYNERGIC trial: A randomized controlled trial assessing multimodal interventions to improve cognition in mild cognitive impairment in older adults. *Alzheimer's & Dementia, 18*(S11), e061616.

Nettelbeck, T., & Burns, N. R. (2010). Processing speed, working memory and reasoning ability from childhood to old age. *Personality and Individual Differences, 48*(4), 379–384.

Netz, Y. (2019). Is there a preferred mode of exercise for cognition enhancement in older age?: A narrative review. *Frontiers in Medicine (Lausanne), 6*, 57.

Ngandu, T., Lehtisalo, J., Solomon, A., Levalahti, E., Ahtiluoto, S., Antikainen, R., et al. (2015). A 2 year multidomain intervention of diet, exercise, cognitive training, and vascular risk monitoring versus control to prevent cognitive decline in at-risk elderly people (FINGER): A randomised controlled trial. *Lancet, 385*, 2255–2263.

Nguyen, L., Murphy, K., & Andrews, G. (2019). Cognitive and neural plasticity in old age: A systematic review of evidence from executive functions cognitive training. *Ageing Research Reviews, 53*, 100912.

Nieto-Estevez, V., Defterali, C., & Vicario-Abejon, C. (2016). IGF-I: A key growth factor that regulates neurogenesis and synaptogenesis from embryonic to adult stages of the brain. *Frontiers in Neuroscience, 10*, 52.

Pahor, A., Seitz, A. R., & Jaeggi, S. M. (2022). Near transfer to an unrelated N-back task mediates the effect of N-back working memory training on matrix reasoning. *Nature Human Behavior, 6*(9), 1243–1256.

Pieramico, V., Esposito, R., Sensi, F., Cilli, F., Mantini, D., Mattei, P. A., et al. (2012).

Combination training in aging individuals modifies functional connectivity and cognition, and is potentially affected by dopamine-related genes. *PLOS ONE, 7*(8), e43901.

Piggin, J. (2020). What is physical activity?: A holistic definition for teachers, researchers and policy makers. *Frontiers in Sports and Active Living, 2*, 72.

Pothier, K., Vrinceanu, T., Intzandt, B., Bosquet, L., Karelis, A. D., Lussier, M., et al. (2021). A comparison of physical exercise and cognitive training interventions to improve determinants of functional mobility in healthy older adults. *Experimental Gerontology, 149*, 111331.

Predovan, D., Fraser, S. A., Renaud, M., & Bherer, L. (2012). The effect of three months of aerobic training on stroop performance in older adults. *Journal of Aging Research, 2012*, 269815.

Quigley, A., MacKay-Lyons, M., & Eskes, G. (2020). Effects of exercise on cognitive performance in older adults: A narrative review of the evidence, possible biological mechanisms, and recommendations for exercise prescription. *Journal of Aging Research, 2020*, 1407896.

Rebok, G. W. (2024a). Commentary on "Computerized cognitive and skills training in older people with mild cognitive impairment: using ecological momentary assessment to index treatment related changes in real-world performance of technology-dependent functional tasks." *American Journal of Geriatric Psychiatry, 32*(4), 460–462.

Rebok, G. W. (2024b). Commentary on "Multimodal exercise and cognitive training program improves cognitive function in amnestic mild cognitive impairment." *American Journal Geriatric Psychiatry, 32*(4), 475–477.

Rebok, G. W., Gellert, A., Coe, N. B., Clay, O. J., Wallace, G., Parisi, J. M., et al. (2023). Effects of cognitive training on Alzheimer's disease and related dementias: The moderating role of social determinants of health. *Journal of Aging Health, 35*(9, Suppl.), 40S–50S.

Reuter-Lorenz, P. A., & Cappell, K. A. (2008). Neurocognitive aging and the compensation hypothesis. *Current Directions in Psychological Science, 17*(3), 177–182.

Sanjuan, M., Navarro, E., & Calero, M. D. (2020). Effectiveness of cognitive interventions in older adults: A review. *European Journal of Investigation in Health, Psychology and Education, 10*(3), 876–898.

Shaaban, C. E., Aizenstein, H. J., Jorgensen, D. R., Mahbubani, R. L. M., Meckes, N. A., Erickson, K. I., et al. (2019). Physical activity and cerebral small vein integrity in older adults. *Medicine & Science in Sports & Exercise, 51*(8), 1684–1691.

Smid, C. R., Karbach, J., & Steinbeis, N. (2020). Toward a science of effective cognitive training. *Current Directions in Psychological Science, 29*(6), 531–537.

Smithers, L. G., Sawyer, A. C. P., Chittleborough, C. R., Davies, N. M., Davey Smith, G., & Lynch, J. W. (2018). A systematic review and meta-analysis of effects of early life non-cognitive skills on academic, psychosocial, cognitive and health outcomes. *Nature Human Behaviour, 2*(11), 867–880.

Sofi, F., Valecchi, D., Bacci, D., Abbate, R., Gensini, G. F., & Macchi, C. (2010). Physical activity and risk of cognitive decline: A meta-analysis of prospective studies. *European Heart Journal, 31*, 675–675.

Sun, Q., Xu, S., Guo, S., You, Y., Xia, R., & Liu, J. (2021). Effects of combined physical activity and cognitive training on cognitive function in older adults with subjective cognitive decline: A systematic review and meta-analysis of randomized controlled trials. *Evidence-Based Complementary and Alternative Medicine, 2021*(1), 8882961.

Tennstedt, S. L., & Unverzagt, F. W. (2013). The ACTIVE study: Study overview and major findings. *Journal of Aging Health, 25*(8, Suppl.), 3s–20s.

Traut, H. J., Guild, R. M., & Munakata, Y. (2021). Why does cognitive training yield inconsistent benefits?: A meta-analysis of individual differences in baseline cognitive abilities and training outcomes. *Frontiers in Psychology, 12*, 662139.

Turnbull, A., Seitz, A., Tadin, D., & Lin, F. V. (2022). Unifying framework for cognitive training interventions in brain aging. *Ageing Research Reviews, 81*, 101724.

Verhaeghen, P. (2014). *The elements of cognitive aging: Meta-analyses of age-related differences in processing speed and their consequences.* Oxford University Press.

von Bastian, C. C., Hyde, E. R. A., & Jiang, S. (2024). Tackling cognitive decline in late adulthood: Cognitive interventions. *Current Opinion in Psychology, 56*, 101780.

Vrinceanu, T., Blanchette, C. A., Intzandt, B., Lussier, M., Pothier, K., Vu, T. T. M., et al. (2022). A comparison of the effect of physical activity and cognitive training on dual-task performance in older adults. *Journals of Gerontology. Series B, Psychological Sciences and Social Sciences, 77*(6), 1069–1079.

Wecker, N. S., Kramer, J. H., Wisniewski, A., Delis, D. C., & Kaplan, E. (2000). Age effects on executive ability. *Neuropsychology, 14*(3), 409–414.

World Health Association. (2022). *Ageing and health.* www.who.int/news-room/fact-sheets/detail/ageing-and-health.

Yang, Z., Hotterbeex, P., Marent, P.-J., Cerin, E., Thomis, M., & van Uffelen, J. (2024). Physical activity, sedentary behaviour, and cognitive function among older adults: A bibliometric analysis from 2004 to 2024. *Ageing Research Reviews, 97*, 102283.

Zhidong, C., Wang, X., Yin, J., Song, D., & Chen, Z. (2021). Effects of physical exercise on working memory in older adults: A systematic and meta-analytic review. *European Review of Aging and Physical Activity, 18*(1), 18.

Zhu, X., Yin, S., Lang, M., He, R., & Li, J. (2016). The more the better?: A meta-analysis on effects of combined cognitive and physical intervention on cognition in healthy older adults. *Ageing Research Reviews, 31*, 67–79.

CHAPTER 13

Brain–Computer Interfaces and Plasticity of the Human Nervous System

Natalie Mrachacz-Kersting and Dario Farina

Introduction

A brain–computer interface (BCI) uses brain signals to control an external device without using muscles and nerves (Wolpaw, 2012). The goal for BCIs varies widely but may be divided into six broad categories: restoring, replacing, improving, enhancing, or supplementing function, and as a research tool. In any of these, using a BCI may induce plasticity of the human nervous system, even though the particular BCI is not explicitly designed to do so. Regardless of the final goal, BCIs have several fundamental components serving specific purposes, including signal acquisition (invasive or noninvasive electrodes), signal processing (feature extraction, classification, and translation), and the application (e.g., robotic actuator, virtual reality, electrical stimulator). Typically, signal acquisition using invasive electrodes or arrays is implemented for patient populations with little or no hope of recovering motor function, and here the main goal is to replace lost function. By far, the most common signal acquisition implements noninvasive techniques such as electroencephalography (EEG), functional near-infrared spectroscopy, and magnetoencephalography.

Initially, BCIs were developed to allow communication for individuals suffering from amyotrophic lateral sclerosis. However, Buch and colleagues (2008) demonstrated that BCIs may be implemented to restore motor function in stroke patients. They used magnetencephalography to record brain signals. But only 1 year later, Daly and colleagues (2009) showed that noninvasive EEG may also be implemented to detect relevant brain states correctly. Since this time, the number of investigations focused on the therapeutic use of BCIs has substantially increased (for a recent review, see Cervera et al., 2018; Mane et al., 2020; Mrachacz-Kersting et al., 2021;

Shou et al., 2023). Moreover, the application of BCIs for inducing plasticity has expanded beyond patient populations, with recent research focusing on their potential to facilitate the acquisition of new motor skills in healthy individuals (Jeunet et al., 2019; Yakovlev et al., 2020). Relearning lost motor function due to a central nervous system (CNS) insult or learning a novel motor skill in healthy individuals involves the induction of plasticity within the human nervous system (Monfils et al., 2016). Today, numerous BCIs have been tested for this purpose (Mrachacz-Kersting et al., 2021). This raises the question of how these different types of BCIs allow the induction of plasticity and what principles they follow.

Neuroplasticity: Factors Relevant to BCI Design

In their landmark 1973 experiments, Bliss and Lømo (Bliss & Lømo, 1973; Lømo, 2003, 2018) uncovered a foundational mechanism of neuroplasticity involving synaptic strength modulation, specifically through the processes of long-term potentiation (LTP) and long-term depression (LTD). This discovery has since become one of the most widely studied frameworks for understanding synaptic plasticity. Synapses that experience correlated activation of two converging inputs are strengthened, whereas those weakened by uncorrelated activity are lost, as postulated by Hebb in 1949 (Hebb, 2005). These initial studies were performed in vitro in the dentate area of the anesthetized rabbit (for a review of the discovery of LTP and LTD, see Lømo, 2018). Animal work has formed the basis for our understanding of activity-dependent alterations in synaptic strength, though there are a few studies on humans using extracted hippocampal tissue from both epileptic and tumor patients (for review, see Mansvelder et al., 2019). In both healthy and impaired humans, studies investigating plasticity at the system level have focused mainly on the primary motor cortex (M1) since it is here where direct connections with peripheral muscles originate for the control of voluntary movements. The horizontal interconnections within M1 are abundant and may be seen as the substrate for neuroplasticity (Sanes & Donoghue, 2000), which have been shown to experience significant activity-dependent plasticity (for a recent review, see Monfils et al., 2016).

A group of researchers from the University of Rostock in Germany was the first to mimic LTP and LTD noninvasively in M1 of humans (Stefan et al., 2000). Stefan and colleagues (2000) applied a single stimulation of the median nerve at three times the perceptual threshold followed, with a delay (interstimulus interval [ISI]), by a single transcranial magnetic stimulation (TMS) over that area of the motor cortex representing the abductor pollicis brevis muscle. The idea was that the peripherally generated afferent volley arrived at or just before the artificial activation of M1. When using an ISI of 25 milliseconds, 90 such pairings over a period of 30 minutes led to a significant increase in the motor evoked potential (MEP) recorded from the target muscle using electromyography. The effect outlasted the stimulation period by at least 30 minutes, was specific to the target muscle, and was dependent on the ISI, *N*-methyl-D-aspartate receptor, and calcium channel activation. Since these properties are also necessary for LTP induction in animal slice preparations, this novel paired associative stimulation (PAS) protocol was considered LTP-like. By reducing the ISI to 10 milliseconds, a depression of the MEP or LTD-like effects was observed. The PAS protocol thus requires precise timing in the millisecond range between the peripheral and central stimuli. There is emerging evidence that PAS applied at an ISI of 21.5 milliseconds and 25 milliseconds both induce LTP-like effects yet engage very different cortical circuitry.

Since its initial description, PAS has received much attention with numerous studies where the protocol was altered and adapted, such as implementing double nerve stimulation, double brain stimulation, pairing the peripheral stimulus with TMS of the cerebellum, use of different numbers of pairings, different ISIs and targeting various muscles. For a recent review, the reader is referred to the 2017 publication by Suppa and colleagues. It is now understood that while LTP- and LTD-like effects can occur in the human M1, their effectiveness is influenced by numerous factors, including participants' physical activity level (Cirillo et al., 2009). Additionally, the direction of synaptic plasticity is highly dependent on the cortical neurons' state during induction (Siebner et al., 2004), highlighting the complex interplay between neural activity states and plasticity outcomes.

Most PAS studies have focused on upper limb muscles due to their extensive and accessible representation on the motor cortex. In contrast, lower limb muscle representation is located deep within the central sulcus, necessitating higher TMS intensities to elicit a MEP. Despite these challenges, PAS protocols LTP-like effects have been successfully applied to lower limb muscles, such as the tibialis anterior (TA) and soleus, leading to significant MEP enhancements. The optimal ISI for lower limb muscles, such as 55 milliseconds for the TA, is notably longer than for upper limb muscles. This difference cannot be attributed solely to the greater distance from the brain but likely involves individual-specific factors (Mrachacz-Kersting et al., 2007; Mrachacz-Kersting & Stevenson, 2017; Roy et al., 2007). Similarly, LTD-like PAS targeting the TA shows an optimal ISI of 40 milliseconds (Mrachacz-Kersting et al., 2007; Roy et al., 2007).

PAS provides a valuable framework for studying neuroplasticity associated with motor learning. However, it requires costly equipment and specialized expertise in TMS application. A critical limitation of PAS is that the high-intensity TMS used activates a broad cortical area, which does not replicate the precise activation patterns involved in natural motor tasks. This discrepancy might explain the substantial interindividual variability in PAS outcomes, with approximately 50% of individuals not exhibiting the expected neuroplastic changes (Cirillo et al., 2017). BCIs offer a promising alternative for advancing our understanding of neuroplasticity. By utilizing brain signals generated during the performance or imagination of motor tasks, BCIs could provide more ecologically valid insights into the mechanisms underlying learning-related neuroplasticity.

An Associative BCI That Mimics PAS

BCIs for restoration of lost motor function or for learning a novel motor skill aim to induce beneficial neuroplasticity by guided neurofeedback, thereby closing the loop between the cortical activation and the contingent stimulus (Chaudhary et al., 2016;

Grosse-Wentrup et al., 2011; Mrachacz-Kersting et al., 2021). Since repeated activation of somatosensory afferents projecting to M1 has been shown to play a crucial role in motor skill learning in monkeys (Pavlides et al., 1993), it is important not only to extract the optimal brain signal associated with movement, but also to generate the corresponding afferent signal at the periphery. In addition, for a BCI that mimics PAS or LTP-like effects, the timing between the brain activation elicited through the performance or imagination of a motor task and the artificially generated peripheral feedback is of paramount importance. The core of such a system must be a fast brain switch that can accurately detect the user's motor intention within a very short latency (i.e., less than a few hundred milliseconds). This is a very challenging goal to achieve in single trials and online from EEG.

In the design of such a BCI, it is imperative that the cortex is activated. This may involve the active engagement of muscles during task performance, though often motor imagery has been implemented. Brain areas activated during the performance or imagery of a motor task are known to share similar substrates (Guillot et al., 2012; Stavrinou et al., 2007). Since activation of at least the motor cortex is preserved following stroke (Cramer et al., 2002), this type of BCI could be used to investigate motor learning in patients with complete paralysis. While research has typically focused on simple hand, arm, foot, or leg movements, more recent studies have explored complex movements (Jovanovic et al., 2020). This shift could lead to more substantial functional improvements, as both healthy subjects and animal models of stroke show that complex tasks induce significantly larger changes in structural and functional plasticity compared with simpler tasks (Pagnussat et al., 2012; Papale & Hooks, 2018; Perez et al., 2004). It is the changes in brain activation patterns in response, irrespective of the exact motor task imagined or performed, that are recognized and extracted by the algorithm within the BCI to control the required feedback.

The changes in the amplitude of the alpha (8–12 Hz) and beta (15–30 Hz) band rhythms within the sensorimotor cortex represent the initial signal of choice and are thus the most common found in the literature (Biasiucci et al., 2018; Pichiorri et al., 2015; Ramos-Murguialday et al., 2013; Rathee et al., 2019). The users have to actively achieve sufficient modulation of the amplitude of these signals. Thus, this process enables the activation of broad regions within the sensorimotor cortex, parietal cortex, insula, and lateral occipital cortex (Marchesotti et al., 2017). Such activation can potentially drive meaningful improvements in the motor control network, supporting functional recovery (Pichiorri et al., 2015). Currently, the exact sites of action and change need to be elucidated. In addition, mastering the ability to regulate sensorimotor rhythms can take healthy individuals several weeks of training, and some may not succeed in developing this skill (Ahn et al., 2013; Blankertz et al., 2010). Most importantly, the latencies for detection are in the range of seconds (Müller-Putz et al., 2010; Pfurtscheller & Solis-Escalante, 2009). It is thus questionable if they are useful regarding the precise timing required for LTP-like effects. Nevertheless, the use of such BCIs in stroke patients has shown significant functional improvements when applied over weeks of training (for recent reviews, see Cervera et al., 2018; Mane et al., 2020; Mrachacz-Kersting et al., 2021; Shou et al., 2023).

For a BCI to exhibit PAS and LTP-like properties, the cortical signal associated with the motor task must ideally be detected before motor execution. One such signal is the movement-related cortical potential (MRCP), initially proposed by Birbaumer in 1981 (Birbaumer et al., 1981). The MRCP is a slow negative potential that develops approximately 1–1.5 seconds before movement initiation. Specific temporal components of this signal are related to the planning, initiation, and performance of movement or motor imagery (Kornhuber & Deecke, 1965; Shibasaki & Hallett, 2006; Walter, 1964). The advantage of this signal is that it does not require any training by the BCI user to be evoked and specific components are closely linked to speed and force of the performed or imagined movement (Gu et al., 2009a; Gu et al., 2009b; Gu et al., 2009c; Jochumsen et al., 2013). In an initial study by our group, the MRCP was elicited in relation to a visual cue provided to the user (Mrachacz-Kersting et al., 2012). Participants were required to imagine a simple dorsiflexion of the foot across 50 trials, and this dataset was used to calculate the onset and peak negativity (PN) of the MRCP. In the subsequent 50 trials, a single electrical stimulation of the deep branch of the common peroneal nerve innervating the target muscle (tibialis anterior) was activated so that the resulting afferent volley arrived either before, at, or following the PN of the MRCP. Significant neuroplasticity was only elicited if the peripherally generated afferent signal arrived at the motor cortex during the PN. This has important implications for the design of a BCI based on the MRCP since the PN occurred –15 ± 217 milliseconds in relation to movement onset. The signal thus has to be detected before movement execution to allow sufficient time for the peripherally generated afferent signal to arrive at M1. When measured across several days, the MRCP occurs reliably with an average initial onset across subjects of –1630 ± 309 milliseconds before actual movement onset (movement onset is then the time of PN), which would allow sufficient time for detection. In later studies, we were able to show the detection in a fully online BCI with an accuracy of 73.0 ± 10.7% (and a false-positive rate of 1.3 ± 0.5 per minute), which matches those of other available BCI systems (Niazi et al., 2012; Xu et al., 2014a; Xu et al., 2014b).

An associative BCI, as described above, induces beneficial neuroplasticity in patient populations, as shown by significant improvements in clinical scales (Mrachacz-Kersting et al., 2016, 2019). It is designed to precisely mimic LTP-like mechanisms and modeled on LTP-like associative plasticity (Bliss & Lømo, 1973; Lømo, 2018; Stefan et al., 2000) and thus targets specific movement-related circuits (Mrachacz-Kersting et al., 2012, 2016, 2019; Niazi et al., 2012; Xu et al., 2014b). However, to date, the exact sites of changes have not been elucidated and warrant further investigation.

Different Approaches to Close the Loop

Feedback during BCI use is vital to close the loop between brain activity due to intention and the activation of the external device that provides the movement or the illusion of it. Hence, it may also be delivered by targeting various sensory modalities such as the visual, auditory, haptic, or proprioceptive systems. Several randomized clinical control trials aimed explicitly at functional recovery in stroke patients have used a variety of technologies, such as visual feedback with and without virtual reality (Lee et al., 2015; Pichiorri et al., 2015; Rayegani et al., 2014), robotic actuators (Ang et al., 2015, 2014; Cheng et al., 2019; Ramos-Murguialday et al., 2013), functional electrical stimulation (Biasiucci et al., 2018; Chung et al., 2015; McCrimmon et al., 2015), and single nerve stimulation (Mrachacz-Kersting et al., 2016, 2019). A novel paradigm is currently being tested in subacute stroke patients and involves applying transcranial magnetic or electrical stimulation timed with specific brain oscillation patterns (Lieb et al., 2023).

Irrespective of the type of feedback, significant improvements were seen in all the studies above, which poses the question of how one may decide which kind of feedback to supply. Indeed, there is a need to consider the effects of the state of the user's brain (idle or active), the time since the CNS insult (acute, subacute, or chronic), the level of impairment, the training status of the BCI user, and the progress of the user over time—for example, a patient who is unable to walk may initially benefit more from receiving a very synchronous nerve stimulation as feedback, while as recovery progresses, this may be changed to functional electrical stimulation or even robotic feedback. Novel studies need to be devised that can address these issues.

Conclusion

As technologies improve in the area of EEG, it is conceivable that BCI systems will be implemented outside the conventional rehabilitation setting and into the homes of patients. This may be accompanied by several limitations that need to be addressed. For example, as suggested in the introduction, regular BCI use will likely induce plastic changes within the CNS, even though the particular BCI may not be designed to do so. This may affect the signal acquired and, thus, the reliability of the features extracted for driving the external device. Indeed, we have shown for the MRCP in patients that the signal is altered significantly (Mrachacz-Kersting et al., 2019), and this likely directly impacts the performance of the classifier algorithm. Surprisingly, few studies have attempted to understand how the changes in the brain through BCI use affect the extracted brain signal and, thus, the classifier. While there is now ample evidence supporting the effectiveness of BCIs in promoting beneficial plasticity, many questions remain unanswered. These include determining the optimal dose (in frequency, intensity, and duration), identifying the best timing for BCI application and the ideal candidates, understanding the specific sites of plasticity induction, and assessing the impact of learning on BCI performance, among others. Notably, the last two points may become especially significant, as monitoring brain activation could reveal markers of plastic changes associated with functional improvements.

REFERENCES

Ahn, M., Cho, H., Ahn, S., & Jun, S. C. (2013). High theta and low alpha powers may be indicative of BCI-illiteracy in motor imagery. *PLOS ONE, 8*, e80886.

Ang, K. K., Chua, K. S. G., Phua, K. S., Wang, C., Chin, Z. Y., Kuah, C. W. K., et al. (2015). A randomized controlled trial of EEG-based motor imagery brain–computer interface robotic rehabilitation for stroke. *Clinical EEG and Neuroscience, 46*, 310–320.

Ang, K. K., Guan, C., Phua, K. S., Wang, C., Zhou, L., Tang, K. Y., et al. (2014). Brain–computer interface-based robotic end effector system for wrist and hand rehabilitation: Results of a three-armed randomized controlled trial for chronic stroke. *Frontiers in Neuroengineering, 7*, 30.

Biasiucci, A., Leeb, R., Iturrate, I., Perdikis, S., Al-Khodairy, A., Corbet, T., et al. (2018). Brain-actuated functional electrical stimulation elicits lasting arm motor recovery after stroke. *Nature Communications, 9*, 2421.

Birbaumer, N., Elbert, T., Rockstroh, B., & Lutzenberger, W. (1981). Biofeedback of event-related slow potentials of the brain. *International Journal of Psychology, 16*, 389–415.

Blankertz, B., Sannelli, C., Halder, S., Hammer, E. M., Kübler, A., Müller, K.-R., et al. (2010). Neurophysiological predictor of SMR-based BCI performance. *NeuroImage, 51*, 1303–1309.

Bliss, T. V. P., & Lømo, T. (1973). Long-lasting potentiation of synaptic transmission in the dentate area of the anaesthetized rabbit following stimulation of the perforant path. *Journal of Physiology, 232*, 331–356.

Buch, E. R., Weber, C., Cohen, L. G., Braun, C., Dimyan, M. A., Ard, T., et al. (2008). Think to move: A neuromagnetic brain-computer interface (BCI) system for chronic stroke. *Stroke, 39*, 910–917.

Cervera, M. A., Soekadar, S. R., Ushiba, J., Millán, J. del R., Liu, M., Birbaumer, N., & Garipelli, G. (2018). Brain–computer interfaces for post-stroke motor rehabilitation: A meta-analysis. *Annals of Clinical and Translational Neurology, 5*, 651–663.

Chaudhary, U., Birbaumer, N., & Ramos-Murguialday, A. (2016). Brain–computer interfaces for communication and rehabilitation. *Nature Reviews Neurology, 12*, 513–525.

Cheng, N., Phua, K. S., Lai, H. S., Tam, P. K., Tang, K. Y., Cheng, K. K., et al. (2019). Brain–computer interface-based soft robotic glove rehabilitation for stroke. *IEEE Transactions on Biomedical Engineering, 67*, 3339–3351.

Chung, E., Park, S.-I., Jang, Y.-Y., & Lee, B.-H. (2015). Effects of brain–computer interface-based functional electrical stimulation on balance and gait function in patients with stroke: Preliminary results. *Journal of Physical Therapy Science, 27*, 513.

Cirillo, J., Lavender, A. P., Ridding, M. C., & Semmler, J. G. (2009). Motor cortex plasticity induced by paired associative stimulation is enhanced in physically active individuals. *Journal of Physiology, 587*(24), 5831–5842.

Cirillo, G., Pino, G. D., Capone, F., Ranieri, F., Florio, L., Todisco, V., et al. (2017). Neurobiological after-effects of non-invasive brain stimulation. *Brain Stimulation, 10*, 1–18.

Cramer, S. C., Mark, A., Barquist, K., Nhan, H., Stegbauer, K. C., Price, R., et al. (2002). Motor cortex activation is preserved in patients with chronic hemiplegic stroke. *Annals of Neurology, 52*(5), 607–616.

Daly, J. J., Cheng, R., Rogers, J., Litinas, K., Hrovat, K., & Dohring, M. (2009). Feasibility of a new application of noninvasive Brain Computer Interface (BCI): A case study of training for recovery of volitional motor control after stroke. *Journal of Neurologic Physical Therapy, 33*, 203–211.

Grosse-Wentrup, M., Mattia, D., & Oweiss, K. (2011). Using brain–computer interfaces to induce neural plasticity and restore function. *Journal of Neural Engineering, 8*, 025004.

Gu, Y., Dremstrup, K., & Farina, D. (2009a). Single-trial discrimination of type and speed of wrist movements from EEG recordings. *Clinical Neurophysiology, 120*, 1596–1600.

Gu, Y., Farina, D., Murguialday, A. R., Dremstrup, K., Montoya, P., & Birbaumer, N. (2009b). Offline identification of imagined speed of wrist movements in paralyzed ALS patients from single-trial EEG. *Frontiers in Neuroprosthetics, 1*, 62.

Gu, Y., do Nascimento, O. F., Lucas, M.-F., & Farina, D. (2009c). Identification of task

parameters from movement-related cortical potentials. *Medical & Biological Engineering & Computing, 47*, 1257–1264.
Guillot, A., Rienzo, F. D., MacIntyre, T., Moran, A., & Collet, C. (2012). Imagining is not doing but involves specific motor commands: A review of experimental data related to motor inhibition. *Frontiers in Human Neuroscience, 6*, 247.
Hebb, D. O. (2005). *The organization of behavior.* Psychology Press.
Jeunet, C., Glize, B., McGonigal, A., Batail, J.-M., & Micoulaud-Franchi, J.-A. (2019). Using EEG-based brain computer interface and neurofeedback targeting sensorimotor rhythms to improve motor skills: Theoretical background, applications and prospects. *Neurophysiologie Clinique, 49*, 125–136.
Jochumsen, M., Niazi, I. K., Mrachacz-Kersting, N., Farina, D., & Dremstrup, K. (2013). Detection and classification of movement-related cortical potentials associated with task force and speed. *Journal of Neural Engineering, 10*, 056015.
Jovanovic, L. I., Kapadia, N., Lo, L., Zivanovic, V., Popovic, M. R., & Marquez-Chin, C. (2020). Restoration of upper limb function after chronic severe hemiplegia: A case report on the feasibility of a brain-computer interface-triggered functional electrical stimulation therapy. *American Journal of Physical Medicine and Rehabilitation*, 99(3), e35–e40.
Kornhuber, H. H., & Deecke, L. (1965). [Changes in the brain potential in voluntary movements and passive movements in man: Readiness potential and reafferent potentials]. *Pflugers Archiv fur die gesamte Physiologie des Menschen und der Tiere, 284*, 1–17.
Lee, Y.-S., Bae, S.-H., Lee, S.-H., & Kim, K.-Y. (2015). Neurofeedback training improves the dual-task Performance ability in stroke patients. *The Tohoku Journal of Experimental Medicine, 236*, 81.
Lieb, A., Zrenner, B., Zrenner, C., Kozák, G., Martus, P., Grefkes, C., & Ziemann, U. (2023). Brain-oscillation-synchronized stimulation to enhance motor recovery in early subacute stroke: A randomized controlled double-blind three-arm parallel-group exploratory trial comparing personalized, non-personalized and sham repetitive transcranial magnetic stimulation (Acronym: BOSS-STROKE). *BMC Neurology, 23*, 204.
Lømo, T. (2003). The discovery of long-term potentiation. *Philosophical Transactions of the Royal Society of London Series B Biological Sciences, 358*, 617–620.
Lømo, T. (2018). Discovering long-term potentiation (LTP)—recollections and reflections on what came after. *Acta Physiologica, 222*, e12921.
Mane, R., Chouhan, T., & Guan, C. (2020). BCI for stroke rehabilitation: Motor and beyond. *Journal of Neural Engineering, 17*, 041001.
Mansvelder, H. D., Verhoog, M. B., & Goriounova, N. A. (2019). Synaptic plasticity in human cortical circuits: Cellular mechanisms of learning and memory in the human brain? *Current Opinion in Neurobiology, 54*, 186–193.
Marchesotti, S., Martuzzi, R., Schurger, A., Blefari, M. L., del Millán, J. R., Bleuler, H., & Blanke, O. (2017). Cortical and subcortical mechanisms of brain-machine interfaces: Neural correlates of BMI-control. *Human Brain Mapping, 38*, 2971–2989.
McCrimmon, C. M., King, C. E., Wang, P. T., Cramer, S. C., Nenadic, Z., & Do, A. H. (2015). Brain-controlled functional electrical stimulation therapy for gait rehabilitation after stroke: A safety study. *Journal of Neuroengineering and Rehabilitation, 12*, 57.
Monfils, M. H., Plautz, E. J., & Kleim, J. A. (2016). In search of the motor engram: Motor map plasticity as a mechanism for encoding motor experience. *The Neuroscientist, 11*, 471–483.
Mrachacz-Kersting, N., Fong, M., Murphy, B. A., & Sinkjaer, T. (2007). Changes in excitability of the cortical projections to the human tibialis anterior after paired associative stimulation. *Journal of Neurophysiology, 97*, 1951–1958.

Mrachacz-Kersting, N., Ibanez, J., & Farina, D. (2021). Towards a mechanistic approach for the development of non-invasive brain-computer interfaces for motor rehabilitation. *Journal of Physiology, 599*(9), 2361–2374.

Mrachacz-Kersting, N., Stevenson, A. J. T., Jørgensen, H. R. M., Severinsen, K. E., Aliakbaryhosseinabadi, S., Jiang, N., & Farina, D. (2019). Brain state–dependent stimulation boosts functional recovery following stroke. *Annals of Neurology, 85*, 84–95.

Mrachacz-Kersting, N., Jiang, N., Stevenson, A. J. T., Niazi, I. K., Kostic, V., Pavlovic, A., et al. (2016). Efficient neuroplasticity induction in chronic stroke patients by an associative brain–computer interface. *Journal of Neurophysiology, 115*, 1410–1421.

Mrachacz-Kersting, N., Kristensen, S. R., Niazi, I. K., & Farina, D. (2012). Precise temporal association between cortical potentials evoked by motor imagination and afference induces cortical plasticity. *Journal of Physiology, 590*, 1669–1682.

Mrachacz-Kersting, N., & Stevenson, A. J. T. (2017). Paired associative stimulation targeting the tibialis anterior muscle using either mono or biphasic transcranial magnetic stimulation. *Frontiers in Human Neuroscience, 11*, 197.

Müller-Putz, G. R., Kaiser, V., Solis-Escalante, T., & Pfurtscheller, G. (2010). Fast set-up asynchronous brain-switch based on detection of foot motor imagery in 1-channel EEG. *Medical & Biological Engineering & Computing, 48*, 229–233.

Niazi, I. K., Mrachacz-Kersting, N., Jiang, N., Dremstrup, K., & Farina, D. (2012). Peripheral electrical stimulation triggered by self-paced detection of motor intention enhances motor evoked potentials. *IEEE Transactions on Neural Systems and Rehabilitation Engineering, 20*, 595–604.

Pagnussat, A. S., Simao, F., Anastacio, J. R., Mestriner, R. G., Michaelsen, S. M., Castro, C. C., et al. (2012). Effects of skilled and unskilled training on functional recovery and brain plasticity after focal ischemia in adult rats. *Brain Research, 1486*, 53–61.

Papale, A. E., & Hooks, B. M. (2018). Circuit changes in motor cortex during motor skill learning. *Neuroscience, 368*, 283–297.

Pavlides, C., Miyashita, E., & Asanuma, H. (1993). Projection from the sensory to the motor cortex is important in learning motor skills in the monkey. *Journal of Neurophysiology, 70*(2), 733–741.

Perez, M. A., Lungholt, B. K. S., Nyborg, K., & Nielsen, J. B. (2004). Motor skill training induces changes in the excitability of the leg cortical area in healthy humans. *Experimental Brain Research, 159*, 197–205.

Pfurtscheller, G., & Solis-Escalante, T. (2009). Could the beta rebound in the EEG be suitable to realize a "brain switch"? *Clinical Neurophysiology, 120*, 24–29.

Pichiorri, F., Morone, G., Petti, M., Toppi, J., Pisotta, I., Molinari, M., et al. (2015). Brain–computer interface boosts motor imagery practice during stroke recovery. *Annals of Neurology, 77*, 851–865.

Ramos-Murguialday, A., Broetz, D., Rea, M., Läer, L., Yilmaz, Ö., Brasil, F. L., et al. (2013). Brain–machine interface in chronic stroke rehabilitation: A controlled study. *Annals of Neurology, 74*, 100–108.

Rathee, D., Chowdhury, A., Meena, Y. K., Dutta, A., McDonough, S., & Prasad, G. (2019). Brain–machine interface driven post-stroke upper-limb functional recovery correlates with beta-band mediated cortical networks. *IEEE Transactions on Neural Systems and Rehabilitation Engineering, 27*, 1020–1031.

Rayegani, S. M., Raeissadat, S. A., Sedighipour, L., Rezazadeh, I. M., Bahrami, M. H., Eliaspour, D., & Khosrawi, S. (2014). Effect of neurofeedback and electromyographic-biofeedback therapy on improving hand function in stroke patients. *Topics in Stroke Rehabilitation, 21*, 137–151.

Roy, F. D., Norton, J. A., & Gorassini, M. A. (2007). Role of sustained excitability of the leg motor cortex after transcranial magnetic stimulation in associative plasticity. *Journal of Neurophysiology, 98*, 657–667.

Sanes, J. N., & Donoghue, J. P. (2000). Plasticity and primary motor cortex. *Annual Review of Neuroscience, 23*, 393–415.

Shibasaki, H., & Hallett, M. (2006). What is the Bereitschaftspotential? *Clinical Neurophysiology, 117*, 2341–2356.

Shou, Y., Wang, X., & Yang, G. (2023). Verum versus sham brain–computer interface on upper limb function recovery after stroke: A systematic review and meta-analysis of randomized controlled trials. *Medicine, 102*, e34148.

Siebner, H. R., Lang, N., Rizzo, V., Nitsche, M. A., Paulus, W., Lemon, R. N., & Rothwell, J. C. (2004). Preconditioning of low-frequency repetitive transcranial magnetic stimulation with transcranial direct current stimulation: Evidence for homeostatic plasticity in the human motor cortex. *Journal of Neuroscience, 24*(13), 3379–3385.

Stavrinou, M. L., Moraru, L., Cimponeriu, L., Penna, S. D., & Bezerianos, A. (2007). Evaluation of cortical connectivity during real and imagined rhythmic finger tapping. *Brain Topography, 19*(3), 137–145.

Stefan, K., Kunesch, E., Cohen, L. G., Benecke, R., & Classen, J. (2000). Induction of plasticity in the human motor cortex by paired associative stimulation. *Brain, 123*(Pt. 3), 572–584.

Suppa, A., Quartarone, A., Siebner, H., Chen, R., Lazzaro, V. D., Giudice, P. D., et al. (2017). The associative brain at work: Evidence from paired associative stimulation studies in humans. *Clinical Neurophysiology, 128*, 2140–2164.

Walter, W. G. (1964). The contingent negative variation: An electrocortical sign of significant association in the human brain. *Science, 146*, 434.

Wolpaw, J. (2012). *Brain–computer interfaces: Principles and practice.* Oxford University Press.

Xu, R., Jiang, N., Lin, C., Mrachacz-Kersting, N., Dremstrup, K., & Farina, D. (2014a). Enhanced low-latency detection of motor intention from EEG for closed-loop brain–computer interface applications. *IEEE Transactions on Biomedical Engineering, 61*, 288–296.

Xu, R., Jiang, N., Mrachacz-Kersting, N., Lin, C., Prieto, G. A., Moreno, J. C., et al. (2014b). A closed-loop brain–computer interface triggering an active ankle–foot orthosis for inducing cortical neural plasticity. *IEEE Transactions on Biomedical Engineering, 61*, 2092–2101.

Yakovlev, L., Syrov, N., Görtz, N., & Kaplan, A. (2020). BCI-controlled motor imagery training can improve performance in e-sports. In C. Stephanidis & M. Antona (Eds.), *HCI International 2020—Posters, 22nd International Conference, HCII 2020, Copenhagen, Denmark, July 19–24, 2020, Proceedings, Part I* (pp. 581–586). Springer.

CHAPTER 14

Brain Plasticity in the Age of the Internet

Martin Korte

Introduction

This chapter outlines the current results of neuroscience research on the possible effects of digital media use on the human brain, in particular with respect to neuronal plasticity and learning processes. This is of importance due to the significant amount of time that individuals spend using the internet, in particular digital media, during periods of development and learning. Given that we now theoretically have all the information of the world at our fingertips, this is changing how we store, and even value, facts and knowledge in our societies and how our brain treats this information.

Despite the several positive aspects of our digital world on the internet, which include communication with peers and use as a training tool for scholars, detrimental effects on our brains and minds have also been explored. Overall, as this book in its various chapters has shown, the human brain is a miracle of nature. It is capable of learning and adapting to constantly changing circumstances and opportunities. As defined earlier in the book, synaptic and neural plasticity is the ability of neuronal networks to continuously change their function as well as their structure. This allows us to adapt to new cultural techniques to develop and modify all kinds of skills through training. But neuronal plasticity is a double-edged sword: It can boost neuronal storage capacity and behavioral flexibility, but it can also lead to maladaptation (drug abuse, atrophy of neuronal connections). There are concerns about the negative impact of the internet and the use of generative artificial intelligence (gAI), which could lead to passive observation, rather than active learning and critical thinking. It has long been known that the absence of sensory experiences, as well as excessive one-sided training, can lead to negative changes in plasticity, resulting in the shrinking or even loss of our abilities altogether. This is even true of addiction based on processes of synaptic plasticity (Hyman et al., 2006; Tan et al., 2024), which can not only be related to drug abuse, but also to behavior (e.g., gambling disorders, or even internet addiction or strong dependence on smartphone access). It is precisely this concern that is increasingly a topic of discussion in the age of the internet in general and of smartphone use in particular.

Neurological consequences have been observed to be related to language development, learning, attention, and processing of emotional signals. This leaves us with the question of whether we still train the brains of students in the best possible way. And since learning itself, if we actively participate, lowers the risk of development of dementias like Alzheimer's disease, it also questions the way we might use processes of neuronal plasticity to keep the aging brain in shape.

The widespread use of the internet, including online gaming and internet browsing on smartphones and tablets, has transformed education globally. This trend was further accelerated during the first 2 years of the COVID-19 pandemic, when many schools and universities remained closed for prolonged periods in numerous countries. The rapid pace of this change is remarkable, with a significant surge over the past decade, but we must consider the potential costs and benefits of this transformation.

Concerns have been raised about the impact of digital media use on our brains and minds, specifically on such aspects as brain function, physical and mental health, education, social interaction, and politics. In 2019, the World Health Organization (WHO) issued strict guidelines regarding children's screen time. Additionally, California—the state that is home to Silicon Valley—announced a law (Assembly Bill 272) allowing schools to regulate the use of smartphones. These measures were prompted by research findings that linked extensive digital media use to reduced working memory capacity (Swing et al., 2010; Christakis et al., 2004; Moisala et al., 2016), psychological issues like depression, anxiety, and sleep disorders (Turkle, 2011; Hoge et al., 2017), as well as reduced text comprehension while reading from screens (Kerr & Symons, 2006). Concerning the latter, research has shown that reading complex stories or interconnected facts in a printed book results in better recall of details and connections between facts compared with reading the same text on a screen (Kerr & Symons, 2006; Mangen et al., 2019). This surprising finding is possibly related to how we associate facts with spatial and sensory cues when reading from a physical book, which seems to enhance our ability to remember (Mangen et al., 2019).

Language scientist Naomi Baron, as cited in Makin (2018), argues that reading in digital environments can also lead to superficial engagement with text. It is possible that the increased use of digital media, which often involves quickly shifting attention from one item to another, may lead to a shorter attention span and contribute to a higher prevalence of attention-deficit/hyperactivity disorder (ADHD; Swing et al., 2010). This raises the question of whether multitasking with digital media is simply correlated to ADHD or if it contributes to or even causes the increased incidence of ADHD. Two arguments support the hypothesis that excessive use of digital media is related to impairments in working memory. Simply having a smartphone in sight, even without using it, reduces working memory capacity and leads to decreased performance in cognitive tasks, as part of the working memory resources are used to ignore the phone (Ophir et al., 2009). Additionally, the more people use their smartphone for multitasking (quickly switching between mental tasks), the more easily they are distracted and perform more poorly in task-switching tests compared with users who seldom attempt to multitask (Ophir et al., 2009). These results have been disputed (see Makin, 2018). The discrepancy in results might be related to the fact that it's not digital media itself that is good or bad for our minds, but rather how we use digital media. The specific actions we take and the frequency with which we use smartphones or any other digital media are important factors to consider, a point that is often overlooked in the discussion.

Is There a Specific Neuronal Plasticity Related to the Use of Digital Media?

There is no doubt that excessive internet use affects the brain, as increased activation of specific neurons can lead to changes in neuron connectivity. Intensive learning or training can alter the wiring of neurons on both functional and structural levels (e.g., see Nudo et al., 1996; Draganski et al., 2006). Furthermore, not only neurons, but also other brain cells, such as oligodendrocytes, astrocytes, and microglia, respond to changes in neuronal activity (e.g., see Clarke & Barres, 2013; Sun et al., 2024).

The most straightforward way to explain the impact of internet and smartphone use on the human brain is to investigate whether the use of fingertips on touchscreens of smartphones and tablets leads to changes in neuronal wiring and network activity in the motor and/or the somatosensory cortex. This has been investigated by Gindrat and colleagues (2015a, 2015b). It was known before that cortical space assigned to the tactile receptors on fingertips is influenced by how often the hand is used (Elbert et al., 1995). For instance, individuals who play string instruments have a greater number of cortical neurons of the somatosensory cortex dedicated to the fingers used to play the instrument (Pantev et al., 2001). This so-called "cortical plasticity of sensory representation" has been observed in musicians and extensively studied in macaque and squirrel monkeys during repeated grasp movements (Byl et al., 1996; Nudo et al., 1996).

Touchscreen smartphones involve repeated and stereotyped finger movements. Gindrat and colleagues (2015a, 2015b) used cortical evoked potentials in response to typical touchscreen movements of the thumb, middle finger, and index finder. They compared excessive touchscreen phone users with control subjects, who only used non-touch-sensitive mobile phones. The results were noteworthy, as only touchscreen users showed an increase in cortical potentials in the thumb and index fingertips (Gindrat et al., 2015a). The study found a strong correlation between the frequency of touchscreen use and the brain response to it. Even daily variations in touchscreen use affected the size of the brain's representation of the thumb. These findings show that using touchscreens repeatedly can change how the brain processes touch sensations in the fingers, and that even short-term use can alter the brain's representation of the thumb.

Taken together, these findings demonstrate that excessive use of touchscreens has the potential to reorganize the somatosensory cortex in humans. It can then be inferred that the cortical processing abilities are continually influenced by the use of digital media. What was not investigated and should be explored in the future is whether this increase in representation of fingertips and thumb comes at the expense of other motor coordination skills. This is crucial to understand, as there could be a negative correlation between screen time and motor skills, as demonstrated by Webster and colleagues (2019), possibly due to competition in brain space for motor programs or a lack of overall physical activity.

Influences on the Developing Brain

Motor skills are just one aspect of excessive internet use. Other aspects include language, cognition, and perception of visual objects in the developing brain. Remarkably, Gomez and colleagues (2019) demonstrated that the content of digital media can affect processes of neuronal plasticity during development. To explore this, functional magnetic resonance imaging (fMRI) was used to examine brain activity from adults who had played the game *Pokémon* excessively during their adolescence.

It was previously known that object and face recognition are processed in higher visual areas of the ventral visual stream, mainly in the ventral temporal lobe (Mishkin et al., 1983). The *Pokémon* characters are a mixture of animal-like humanized figures and unique objects not typically found in human environments. The results of this study indicated that adults who have had extensive experience with *Pokémon* during childhood showed distinct distributed cortical responsiveness to *Pokémon* figures in the ventral temporal lobe, close to the areas responsible for face recognition. This was not observed in control subjects, who did not play the game. These findings—as a proof of principle—suggest that frequent use of digital media can result in a distinct and enduring mental representation of digital objects and characters, even many years after their extensive use. It is noteworthy that all *Pokémon* players showed a similar map in the ventral visual stream for *Pokémon* characters. However, it is uncertain whether these findings simply demonstrate the brain's remarkable adaptability by creating new representations for new types of objects in higher visual areas or if prolonged exposure to digital media could have negative effects on facial recognition and processing due to competition for brain resources.

In this respect, it is worth noting that studies on empathy in young adults have found a link between increased time spent with digital media and reduced ability to understand and share the feelings of others (Carrier et al., 2015; James et al., 2017). It is not clear whether this lack of empathy is due to a lack of understanding about what others are thinking (often called "theory of mind"), problems with recognizing facial expressions, or lack of exposure to peers due to spending too much online. It's important to note that some studies have found no correlation between time spent online and empathy (see reviews by Choudhury & McKinney, 2013; Lahiry et al., 2019).

Another area of interest is whether the development of language-related neuronal plasticity is affected by extensive screen time, such as watching internet videos. It is concerning that early and frequent screen use in preschoolers can significantly impact language networks, as demonstrated by advanced diffusion tensor MRI studies (Hutton et al., 2019a, 2019b). Diffusion tensor MRI is a method that provides assessments of white matter integrity in the fiber tracts of the human brain. Additionally, the authors evaluated the cognitive abilities of preschool children and tested the quality of their language processes and other higher-order cognitive skills. The extent of digital media use among preschoolers was measured with a standardized test system consisting of a 15-item screening tool for observers (ScreenQ), which aligns with the screen-based media recommendations of the American Academy of Pediatrics. The study involved analyzing the correlation between ScreenQ and the integrity of white matter tracts in the brain. Cognitive test scores, age, gender, and household income were taken into account in the analysis. The results revealed a significant correlation between excessive early childhood digital media use in preschoolers and poorer microstructural integrity of white matter tracts, particularly between Broca's and Wernicke's areas in the brain. Furthermore, these deficits in fiber tract development were found to be highly correlated with language comprehension and capacity.

The study also found that preschoolers who spend a lot of time using digital media showed lower executive functions and literacy abilities, even when their age and average household income were matched to those of control children. Additionally, their use of digital media use was linked to lower scores in behavioral measures for executive functions.

The study suggests that reading skills may be affected if fiber tracts between the language areas are not fully developed, which could impact school success. Further research could explore the correlation between screen time and school performance, as well as the comparison between traditional reading and reading on screen.

The use of electronic media may also lead to changes in reading habits, which in turn might have implications for new readers and individuals with reading disabilities. This topic has been recently explored by (Hutton et al., 2020). In their study, fMRI was used to observe children's brains as they listened to three similar stories in audio, illustrated, or animated format followed by a test of factual recall. The study compared within- and between-network functional connectivity (FC) across formats involving visual perception, visual imagery, language, default mode network (DMN), and cerebellar association. In comparison with audio, FC was reduced within the language network and increased between visual, DMN, and cerebellar networks. This suggests that using pictures and visual imagery decreased the workload on the language network. For animated stories, between-network connectivity decreased for all networks, especially in comparison with illustrated stories, indicating a preference for visual perception over network integration. These findings indicate significant differences in the functional brain network connectivity for animated and traditional story formats in preschool-age children, highlighting the benefits of illustrated storybooks in supporting language development at this age. Furthermore, digital media could influence deep reading, which may pose a threat to the development of deep reading skills in young adults (Wolf et al., 2012).

During adolescence, the brain undergoes significant development, especially in areas related to emotional and social interactions. Social media can have a strong impact on the teenage brain, as it allows them to engage with multiple peers simultaneously without direct interaction. Studies have shown that adolescents process emotions differently, and this is closely linked to their use of social media. Research has indicated changes in the volume of the amygdala, which is responsible for processing emotions, in adolescents who use social media intensely (Kanai et al., 2012; Pfeifer & Blakemore, 2012). This highlights the significant relationship between online social interactions and brain development (Meshi et al., 2015). The emotional influence, peer pressure, or sensitivity to social acceptance may make teenagers particularly vulnerable to fake or shocking information, as well as unrealistic self-expectations or difficulties in regulating emotions due to excessive use of digital media (Crone & Konijn, 2018). What is currently lacking is long-term studies to determine whether the adolescent brain is molded differently by the size of their online social network as opposed to direct personal interaction.

As a side note, there is evidence that violent games do have a profound effect on human behavior (Anderson et al., 2010). A meta-analysis of current studies demonstrates that exposure to violent video games is a highly significant risk factor for increased aggressive behavior, and is also associated with a decrease in empathy and lower levels of prosocial behavior (Anderson et al., 2010).

Cognitive Plasticity in the Age of the Internet

The studies discussed above support the notion that frequent use of digital media leads to significant changes in brain plasticity. The observed effects are remarkable and demonstrate that the brain adapts its functional and structural connections due to learning, habits, and experience (Takeuchi et al., 2014; Korte & Schmitz, 2016). This raises the question of whether extensive use of digital media may cause the brain to operate in a certain cognitive mode at the cost other of important functions, which can impact human cognition and health. The brain's ability to adapt its functional and structural connections has been shown in many human neuroimaging studies (for a review, see Engert & Bonhoeffer, 1999; Yuste & Bonhoeffer, 2001). Examples of this adaptation include studies on London taxi drivers (Maguire et al., 2000), pianists (Elbert et al., 1995), and jugglers (Draganski et al., 2004). These studies demonstrate that excessive use can stimulate the growth of new synaptic connections ("use it") while at the same time eliminating less frequently used neuronal synaptic connections ("lose it"; Hebb, 1949; Katz & Shatz, 1996) at the potential expense of others.

At the cellular level, this phenomenon has been named synaptic plasticity, as discussed in Korte and Schmitz (2016). It is widely recognized that neurons in the human cortex, hippocampus, and subcortical areas are highly adaptable. This means that changes in neuronal activity patterns (e.g., generated by intensive training) can alter synaptic function and structure. Activity-dependent synaptic plasticity affects the efficiency of synaptic transmission (functional plasticity) and changes the structure and number of synaptic connections (structural plasticity) (Martin et al., 2000; Kandel et al., 2014; Korte & Schmitz, 2016). Synaptic plasticity forms the basis for adjusting the postnatal brain to experiences and serves as the cellular mechanism for the learning and memory process. This concept was first proposed by Donald O. Hebb in 1949. He suggested that changes in neuronal activity resulting from use, training, habit, or learning are stored in assemblies of neurons, rather than in single nerve cells (Hebb, 1949). This type of plasticity occurs at the network level through the modification of synapses between neurons and is therefore referred to as activity-dependent synaptic plasticity. Hebb's postulate also introduces an important principle, suggesting that synaptic strength changes when pre- and postsynaptic neurons exhibit coincident activity (associativity), thus altering the input/output properties of neuronal assemblies. For memories to be recalled, they need to be activated together again. The response of the brain's synapses to a specific brain activity must be enhanced. For more details, refer to Magee and Grienberger (2020). This means that all regular human activity, including the use of digital media, social networks, or the internet, will leave an imprint on the brain. Whether this impact is positive, negative, or neutral depends on the activity itself and whether it comes at the expense of other activities.

In this respect, a study from Sajikumar and colleagues (2014) linking multitasking mode with cellular synaptic plasticity showed that activation of three inputs impinging on the same neuronal population in a narrow time window leads to the arbitrary strengthening of inputs, not necessarily the most important. This means the storage of relevant facts may be compromised if the input to a neuronal network in a particular brain area exceeds its processing power limit.

Note that the human brain has a limited capacity to "learn multitasking" (the ability to quickly switch between different tasks without losing time or efficiency and without increasing the error rate). For example, Rogers and Monsell (1995) found that switching between simple cognitive tasks resulted in high error rates for most individuals.

The ability to handle demanding cognitive tasks is a genetic trait, not due to plasticity-induced adaptability, according to Watson and Strayer (2010). They found that while most people experience a loss of performance when multitasking, there are individuals, called "supertaskers," who show no decline in performance. Their experiments offer strong evidence for the existence of supertaskers, but they do not provide an answer to the question about the neuronal basis for effective multitasking, which is most likely a genetic trait, rather than a result of learning and synaptic plasticity in the adult brain. Exploring this question within the context of neurobiology or neuroimaging research might help uncover the unique abilities of these supertaskers.

While no mention of supertaskers occurred before Watson and Strayer's study, several cognitive scientists before them had conducted studies to determine the neurological factors that contribute to high performers excelling beyond the average population. In a study by Jaeggi and colleagues (2007), the authors aimed to identify the neurological differences between high and low performers. They used fMRI imaging techniques to observe individuals as they engaged in a cognitively demanding task known as the *n*-back task, which is renowned for revealing individual differences in cognitive abilities such as working memory and attention. The *n*-back task involves presenting stimuli to participants, which can be auditory or visual. The participants must pay attention to a sequence of stimuli and indicate when the current stimulus matches the one from *n* steps earlier in the sequence. For instance, if the sequence of presented letters is HETH, participants should respond when they see the second H, as it was presented two letters ago. fMRI measures the changes in blood flow during the trials and serves as a proxy for neuronal activity.

Jaeggi and colleagues (2007) cross-referenced 22 brain regions of interest in the participants' brains while they performed the challenging *n*-back task. The fMRI study showed that supertaskers experience less cognitive stress when carrying out demanding tasks. Specifically, few regions in the brain of top performers are recruited during these tasks. They also identified specific regions of the brain that are important for handling demanding tasks. For instance, an increase in activation was observed in the left frontal cortex. The prefrontal cortex is involved in executive functions, such as working memory. It is not surprising that high performers use this specific part of their brain (Lara & Wallis, 2015). These results seem paradoxical, but they could be explained by the fact that high performers use the required parts of their brain (their lateral frontal areas) much more efficiently compared with middle and low performers. They do this by recruiting as little of these areas as possible (Jaeggi et al., 2007). The authors could not determine if this is a learned ability related to neuronal plasticity, a genetic disposition, or both.

Medeiros-Ward and colleagues (2015) delved deeper into this effect by using a dual *n*-back task that presented auditory and visual stimuli to supertaskers and compared their performance against that of lower-performing controls. They confirmed that multitasking of supertaskers was characterized by more efficient recruitment of the frontopolar prefrontal cortex. Furthermore, they observed recruitment of the anterior cingulate cortex (ACC) when participants engaged in the demanding dual *n*-back task. The ACC is known to mediate emotions and is involved in conflict situations, such as choosing between option A and option B. The emotional involvement may explain why supertaskers can remain calm and experience less stress when tackling demanding cognitive tasks, as they can avoid distractions and detect errors that interfere with the task at hand. Additionally, Dreher and colleagues found that damage to the frontopolar cortex, a part of the prefrontal cortex, leads to a decrease in multitasking performance. This suggests that this region is important for rapidly switching between tasks without making too many mistakes or experiencing 50% slowdown, as 98% of all normal taskers do (Dreher et al., 2008).

The research conducted by Medeiros-Ward and colleagues (2015) and Jaeggi and colleagues (2007) provides insight into the differences between typical individuals and exceptional supertaskers. It would be beneficial to explore whether regular people could develop the ability to manage the prefrontal–ACC brain network to handle not only dual tasks but also challenging ones. As workplaces become increasingly demanding, and filled with digital distractions, improving multitasking abilities would be highly advantageous for individuals in all professions.

Digital Media Impact on the Aging Brain

The effects and potential negative or positive impacts of using digital media, as well as the culture and interaction involved, might not only depend on the total time spent and the cognitive abilities engaged, but also on the age of the individual. This means that the negative effects observed in preschoolers, as have been reported by Hutton and colleagues (2019b), could be quite different from those experienced by adults (such as addiction), or from the effects on the elderly. In other words, using digital media to train the aging brain might have consequences that are quite different from the effects of screen time on preschoolers, or the constant distraction experienced by adults.

Aging is not only genetically determined but also depends on lifestyle and how the brain is used and trained (Cabeza et al., 2018). One successful attempt using digital media involved improving the attention span of elderly individuals by training response inhibition through computer games (Kuhn et al., 2017). The training was conducted on a tablet for just 2 months, and significant cognitive effects on lateral inhibition were observed compared with a control group. These findings are related to growth processes, as indicated by the increased cortical thickness of the right inferior frontal gyrus triangularis, a brain area associated with lateral inhibition. These effects, likely mediated through structural plasticity, are dependent on the time spent on the training task—the results improved in direct proportion to the training duration. In summary, it can be inferred that game-based digital training programs may promote cognitive ability in older adults, in line with other studies suggesting that attention training is mediated by increased activity in the frontal lobe (Klingberg, 2010). Other studies have supported these results by showing that computer training is a possible means for training the brain of older people (over 65 years of age), and brain-training programs can assist in promoting healthy cognitive aging (Shah et al., 2017; Pallavicini et al., 2018). However, it is also important to consider the review of Katz and colleagues (2018).

Neuronal plasticity can also be enhanced through the use of virtual reality (VR) digital tools for stroke rehabilitation. Ordinary stroke rehabilitation treatments include speech therapy, cognitive training, and physical therapy. However, many stroke survivors continue to experience functional disabilities resulting from cognitive deficits, which hinder their ability to carry out daily routines. Cognitive rehabilitation is a therapeutic approach designed to improve cognitive functioning after a brain injury, including stroke, as well as in patients with neurodegenerative disorders. Cognitive rehabilitation consists of a range of methods employed to address cognitive deficits caused by stroke. It encompasses different interventions aimed at enhancing the ability to perform cognitive tasks, achieved through the retraining of previously acquired skills and/or instructing compensatory strategies.

There are two major categories of techniques used in the cognitive rehabilitation of patients with different neurological disorders: traditional and advanced. Traditional techniques involve using cognitive strategies to retrain or improve deficits in different cognitive domains through methods such as paper-and-pencil exercises. On the other hand, advanced methods, including computer-assisted cognitive rehabilitation, use multimedia and informatics resources to enhance neurocognitive performance. In recent years, technology-based stroke rehabilitation interventions have demonstrated their potential to improve the motor and cognitive abilities, as well as the autonomy, of stroke patients. For example, studies by Hatem and colleagues (2016) and Malik and colleagues (2022) have shown promising results. The use of digital technologies in stroke neurorehabilitation has enhanced standard treatments, reducing neurological disability and improving overall daily functions.

Understanding neuronal plasticity has shown how VR can aid in the treatment of stroke patients. In most studies, VR uses computer-based simulations that enable patients to interact with multisensory environments. This allows patients to receive real-time feedback on their performance and to experience activities that closely mimic real life, albeit in a controlled environment. Using a specific digital media tool facilitates repetitive and task-specific training, actively engages patients, provides accurate and immediate feedback, and precisely measures functional improvement. Cognitive and motor rehabilitation's efficacy through virtual environments surpasses traditional real-world training. In the VR setting, patients can interact with common images featuring simulated physical properties, enabling exercises designed to stimulate key cognitive functions.

One study by Gangemi and colleagues (2023) investigated whether training sessions involving VR goggles could enhance neuroplasticity changes. The authors focused on the power band spectra of prominent electroencephalographic (EEG) rhythms (theta, alpha, and beta) in treatment and control groups before and after VR training sessions. The authors observed significant EEG-related neural improvements in the primary motor circuit of the VR-training group, indicating that the use of VR technology for cognitive recovery led to positive changes in power spectral density and time-frequency domains. The EEG data analysis indicated that VR-based training sessions resulted in a significant increase in alpha band power in the occipital areas and beta band power in the frontal areas, possibly related to improved executive functions.

The data suggest that VR-based rehabilitation can enhance clinical outcomes, even in the chronic phase of ischemic stroke, by improving neuronal plasticity processes. This finding is significant given that approximately 17 million people suffer a stroke each year, resulting in a global incidence rate of 258 in a population of 100,000. After experiencing a major stroke, patients often struggle with long-term sensory, motor, and cognitive impairments. This can include issues with attention, language, communication, visuospatial processing, learning and memory, reasoning, problem solving, and executive functions. Neurorehabilitation focuses on improving both motor and cognitive abilities to help stroke patients regain the skill they need to perform everyday activities of daily living routines and reduce the potential for psychosocial issues like depression and anxiety. It will be interesting to investigate whether digital media can be utilized in the elderly to preserve or even increase cognitive capacities, like attention, that decline after excessive digital media/multitasking at a younger age.

Mechanism of Addiction and Digital Media Usage

Synaptic plasticity plays a crucial role in shaping the postnatal development of the nervous systems and learning mechanisms. It is also associated with addiction and craving (Tan et al., 2024). In addition to classical substance-use disorders, behavioral addictions are also recognized as addictive behaviors (Brand et al., 2016). An addictive behavior is characterized by a loss of control and a compulsion to seek rewards despite serious consequences, often prioritizing short-term gratification over long-term outcomes. Conditions such as internet use disorder (IUD) and internet gaming disorder (IGD) have been included in the International Classification of Diseases, 11th Revision, by the WHO as behavioral addictions. Smartphone use disorder might be soon added to the list.

Addiction is a chronic relapsing disorder, characterized by a compulsion to seek and take substances or engage in certain behaviors, like gambling. It also involves a loss of control in limiting these behaviors or substance intake and is often associated with the emergence of negative emotions (e.g., anxiety, irritability, or dysphoria) when the substance or opportunity to engage in the behavior is not available. Neurologically, addiction is characterized by overall network changes in frontostriatal and frontocingulate circuits, which are also hallmarks of IGD and IUD (Brand et al., 2016). Adolescents might be particularly at risk (Rehbein et al., 2015). For a systematic and more detailed meta-analysis of functional and structural brain changes related to IGD, see D'Hondt and colleagues (2015) and Yao and colleagues (2017).

It is also noteworthy that some studies found a correlation between brain anatomy alterations with social networking site (SNS) addiction (He et al., 2017). Specifically, it shows that excessive interactions with social media can be correlated to gray matter alteration of brain areas involved in addictive behavior. Excessive use of social media can have a significant impact on the structure of the human brain, as reviewed by Meshi and colleagues (2015). These findings imply that neuroscience and psychology researchers should pay more attention to understanding and ultimately preventing online addiction disorders or other maladaptive behaviors related to gaming and social networking.

The effects of digital media and electronic devices on human well-being, multitasking addiction, and neuroenhancement are also noteworthy. The effects of multitasking on attention span, concentration, and working memory is a widely discussed topic (Ophir et al., 2009). It is challenging for our brains to process multiple and continuous information streams. Several experiments have investigated whether there are systematic differences in information processing styles between individuals who heavily multitask with media and those who don't (Brown et al., 2017; Uncapher et al., 2017). The results indicate that heavy media multitaskers are more susceptible to interference from irrelevant external stimuli or representations in their memory systems. This led to the surprising result that heavy media multitaskers performed worse on a task-switching ability test. This is likely because they have a reduced ability to filter out interference from irrelevant stimuli (Uncapher et al., 2017). It demonstrates that multitasking, a rapidly growing behavioral trend, is associated with a distinct approach to fundamental information processing. Uncapher and colleagues (2017) summarize the consequences of intense multimedia use as follows:

> American youth spend more time with media than any other waking activity: an average of 7.5 hours per day, every day. On average, 29% of that time is spent juggling multiple media streams simultaneously (i.e., media multitasking). This phenomenon is not limited to American youth but is paralleled across the globe. Given that a large number of media multitaskers (MMTs) are children and young adults whose brains are still developing, there is great urgency to understand the neurocognitive profiles of MMTs. (p. S62)

It is especially important to understand the information processing necessary for effective learning in the 21st-century environment. Research shows that heavy digital media multitaskers have poorer memory function, increased impulsivity, less empathy, and higher levels of anxiety (Turkle, 2011). On the neurological side, they also exhibit reduced volume in the anterior cingulate cortex. Current data indicate that switching between different tasks (multitasking) during digital media use can negatively impact academic outcomes (Uncapher et al., 2017). However, one should be careful when interpreting these results because we are not sure which way the cause-and-effect relationship goes. People with reduced prefrontal activity and shorter attention spans may be more likely to engage in media multitasking. Longitudinal studies are needed to understand this better. The overall impact of online social media on our natural social skills, including empathy and understanding other people's perspectives, is another area where we need to understand how digital media affect our thinking and perception of social cues. Out of many studies, one by Turkle (2011) should be highlighted here. Turkle conducted interviews with teenagers and adults who were heavy users of social media and other virtual environments. One of the outcomes of this study was that excessive use of social media and VR can lead to an increased risk of anxiety, a reduction in real social interactions, a lack of social skills and human empathy, and difficulties in handling solitude. Furthermore, the individuals interviewed reported symptoms related to internet and digital social media addiction.

The constant connection to hundreds or even thousands of people may be overwhelming our brains, as it drastically expands the number of people with whom we can interact closely. The evolutionary constraint might be the group size limit of approximately 150 individuals (Dunbar, 2018). This may be one of the reasons for our increase in cortical volume. For example, chimpanzees interact regularly with 50 individuals, but it may also be the limit of what our brains can achieve. Quite in contrast to this evolutionary constraint, due to social media, we are in continuous contact with a group of people that by far exceeds our neurobiological limit. What are the consequences of this cortical overtaxing? Anxiety? Attention, cognitive, and even memory deficits? Or can we adapt? So far, we have more questions than answers.

In conclusion, the brain is affected by the way we use it. It is almost obvious to expect that excessive use of digital media will alter human brains due to neuronal plasticity. It is less clear how these new technologies will impact human cognition (language skills, working memory, learning, and teaching methods) and emotional processing in a social context. One limitation is that many studies have not considered what individuals are doing online, what they are exposed to, and what types of cognitive engagement they undertake during screen time. What is clear is that digital media significantly affect human psychological well-being and cognitive performance, and this impact is influenced by the total screen time and the specific activities in which individuals are engaged in the digital environment (Reeves et al., 2020).

In the last decade, more than 250 studies have aimed to understand the effect of digital media use. Many of these relied on self-reported questionnaires, which often failed to consider the wide range of activities people engage online. However, how people use digital media and the amount of time they spend online can have different impacts on their health and behavior (Reeves et al., 2020). Researchers need a more comprehensive understanding of digital media use. In essence, they require a more precise way to measure what individuals do when they are online or using digital screens. Currently, it is often difficult to differentiate between causal effects and mere correlation. Some significant studies have already begun (Gijsen et al., 2020; Ram et al., 2019), and the Adolescent Brain Cognitive Development (ABCD) Study is also noteworthy. The ABCD Study is promoted and funded by the National Institutes of Health. It aims to investigate the impact of environmental, social, genetic, and other biological factors on brain and cognitive development. It will eventually recruit 10,000 healthy children ages 9–10 across the United States and follow them into early adulthood. The study will utilize advanced brain imaging techniques to observe brain development and brain activity during online activities and assess how these activities may influence brain maturation in specific areas. The goal is to gain insight into how online engagement may impact brain plasticity, physical and mental health, and cognitive abilities, as well as educational success. The study will also examine developmental trajectories of brain, cognitive, emotional, and academic development, and explore the influence of factors like digital media and internet use on brain development. (For more details, visit *https://abcdstudy.org.*)

It is also important to consider whether the increasing trend of all users becoming knowledge distributors themselves could pose a threat to the acquisition of solid knowledge and the need to develop original thoughts and creativity. Alternatively, could new digital technologies, such as gAI, create an opportunity to enhance teaching, learning, and information, leading us to explore new knowledge frontiers and develop more effective teaching techniques? Will the use of these technologies result in the development of completely new brain circuit arrangements, like we did when humans learned to read? Overall, while more research is needed to evaluate the potential effects of internet use on brain plasticity, it is clear that these effects will change not only how the brain develops and how we learn, but also how we socially interact.

Conclusion

This chapter outlined the current state of neuroscience research on the possible effects of digital media use on the human brain, cognition, and behavior with respect to neuronal plasticity. As shown in the chapter, this is of high importance due to the significant amount of time that individuals spend using digital media. The positive characteristics of digital media use include the capability to effortlessly communicate with peers, even over long distances, and their being used as learning tools for students and the elderly—and therefore a means of promoting neuronal plasticity. On the downside, detrimental effects on our brains and minds have also been reported in this chapter; for example, neurological consequences have been observed related to internet/gaming addiction, language development, and processing of emotional signals. However, given that much of the neuroscientific research conducted up to now relies solely on self-reported parameters to assess social media use, it is argued that neuroscientists need to include datasets with higher precision in terms of what is done on screens, for how long, and at which age.

Overall, what remains to be determined is if the increasing frequency of all users toward being knowledge distributors themselves might become a great threat to the acquisition of solid knowledge, as well as the need to develop our own thoughts and be creative. Or will these new technologies build the perfect bridge to ever more sophisticated forms of cognition and imagination, and will they enable us to explore new knowledge frontiers that we cannot even imagine at the moment? Taken together, even if much research is still needed to judge and evaluate possible effects of digital media on human well-being, neuroscience, and in particular the contribution of neuronal plasticity to these processes, can be of tremendous help in shaping a healthy relationship between our adaptable brains to digital devices.

REFERENCES

Anderson, C. A., Shibuya, A., Ihori, N., Swing, E. L., Bushman, B. J., Sakamoto, A., et al. (2010). Violent video game effects on aggression, empathy, and prosocial behavior in eastern and western countries: A meta-analytic review. *Psychological Bullettin, 136*, 151–173.

Brand, M., Young, K. S., Laier, C., Wolfling, K., & Potenza, M. N. (2016). Integrating psychological and neurobiological considerations regarding the development and maintenance of specific Internet-use disorders: An interaction of person-affect-cognition-execution (I-PACE) model. *Neuroscienec Biobehavioral Review, 71*, 252–266.

Brown, T. I., Uncapher, M. R., Chow, T. E., Eberhardt, J. L., & Wagner, A. D. (2017). Cognitive control, attention, and the other race effect in memory. *PLOS ONE, 12*, e0173579.

Byl, N. N., Merzenich, M. M., & Jenkins, W. M. (1996). A primate genesis model of focal dystonia and repetitive strain injury: I. Learning-induced dedifferentiation of the representation of the hand in the primary somatosensory cortex in adult monkeys. *Neurology, 47*, 508–520.

Cabeza, R., Albert, M., Belleville, S., Craik, F. I. M., Duarte, A., Grady, C. L., et al. (2018). Maintenance, reserve and compensation: The cognitive neuroscience of healthy ageing. *Nature Review Neuroscience, 19*, 701–710.

Carrier, L. M., Spradlin, A., Bunce, J. P., & Rosen, L. D. (2015). Virtual empathy: Positive and negative impacts of going online upon empathy in young adults. *Computers in Human Behavior, 52*, 39–48.

Choudhury, S., & McKinney, K. A. (2013). Digital media, the developing brain and the interpretive plasticity of neuroplasticity. *Transcultural Psychiatry, 50*, 192–215.

Christakis, D. A., Zimmerman, F. J., DiGiuseppe, D. L., & McCarty, C. A. (2004). Early television exposure and subsequent attentional problems in children. *Pediatrics, 113*, 708–713.

Clarke, L. E, & Barres, B. A. (2013). Emerging roles of astrocytes in neural circuit development. *Nature Revews Neuroscience, 14*, 311–321.

Crone, E. A., & Konijn, E. A. (2018). Media use and brain development during adolescence. *Nature Communications, 9*, 588.

D'Hondt, F., Billieux, J., & Maurage, P. (2015). Electrophysiological correlates of problematic Internet use: Critical review and perspectives for future research. *Neuroscience Biobehavioral Reviews, 59*, 64–82.

Draganski, B., Gaser, C., Busch, V., Schuierer, G., Bogdahn, U., & May, A. (2004). Neuroplasticity: Changes in grey matter induced by training. *Nature, 427*, 311–312.

Draganski, B., Gaser, C., Kempermann, G., Kuhn, H. G., Winkler, J., Buchel, C., & May, A. (2006). Temporal and spatial dynamics of brain structure changes during extensive learning. *Journal of Neuroscience, 26*, 6314–6317.

Dreher, J. C., Koechlin, E., Tierney, M., & Grafman, J. (2008). Damage to the fronto-polar cortex is associated with impaired multitasking. *PLOS ONE, 3*, e3227.

Dunbar, R. I. M. (2018). The anatomy of friendship. *Trends of Cognitive Science, 22*, 32–51.

Elbert, T., Pantev, C., Wienbruch, C., Rockstroh, B., & Taub, E. (1995). Increased cortical representation of the fingers of the left hand in string players. *Science, 270*, 305–307.

Engert, F., & Bonhoeffer, T. (1999). Dendritic spine changes associated with hippocampal long-term synaptic plasticity [see comments]. *Nature, 399*, 66–70.

Gangemi, A., De Luca, R., Fabio, R. A., Lauria, P., Rifici, C., Pollicino, P., et al. (2023). Effects of virtual reality cognitive training on neuroplasticity: A quasi-randomized clinical trial in patients with stroke. *Biomedicines, 11*(12), 3225.

Gijsen, V., Maddux, M., Lavertu, A., Gonzalez-Hernandez, G., Ram., N., Reeves, B., et al. (2020). The potential and the challenges of utilizing social media and other electronic communication platforms in health care. *Clinical and Translational Science, 13*, 26–30.

Gindrat, A. D., Chytiris, M., Balerna, M., Rouiller, E. M., & Ghosh, A. (2015a). L'utilisation de smartphones façonne le traitement cortical de l'information sensorielle tactile provenant de l'extrémité des doigts [Smartphone use shapes cortical tactile sensory processing from the fingertips]. *Médecine Sciences (Paris), 31*, 363–366.

Gindrat, A. D., Chytiris, M., Balerna, M., Rouiller, E. M., & Ghosh, A. (2015b). Use-dependent cortical processing from fingertips in touchscreen phone users. *Current Biology, 25*, 109–116.

Gomez, J., Barnett, M., & Grill-Spector, K. (2019). Extensive childhood experience with Pokemon suggests eccentricity drives organization of visual cortex. *Nature Human Behavior, 3*, 611–624.

Hatem, S. M., Saussez, G., Della Faille, M., Prist, V., Zhang, X., Dispa, D., & Bleyenheuft, Y. (2016). Rehabilitation of motor function after stroke: A multiple systematic review focused on techniques to stimulate upper extremity recovery. *Frontiers in Human Neuroscience, 10*, 442.

He, Q., Turel, O., & Bechara, A. (2017). Brain anatomy alterations associated with social networking site (SNS) addiction. *Scientific Reports, 7*, 45064.

Hebb, D. O. (1949). *The organization of behavior: A neuropsychological theory.* Wiley.

Hoge, E., Bickham, D., & Cantor, J. (2017). Digital media, anxiety, and depression in children. *Pediatrics, 140*, S76–S80.

Hutton, J. S., Dudley, J., Horowitz-Kraus, T., DeWitt, T., & Holland, S. K. (2019a). Associations between home literacy environment, brain white matter integrity and cognitive abilities in preschool-age children. *Acta Paediatrica, 109*, 1376–1386.

Hutton, J. S., Dudley, J., Horowitz-Kraus, T., DeWitt, T., & Holland, S. K. (2019b). Associations between screen-based media use and brain white matter integrity in preschool-aged children. *JAMA Pediatrics, 1174*(1), e193869.

Hutton, J. S., Dudley, J., Horowitz-Kraus, T., DeWitt, T., & Holland, S. K. (2020). Differences in functional brain network connectivity during stories presented in audio, illustrated, and animated format in preschool-age children. *Brain Imaginging and Behavior, 14*, 130–141.

Hyman, S. E., Malenka, R. C., & Nestler., E. J. (2006). Neural mechanisms of addiction: The role of reward-related learning and memory. *Annual Review of Neuroscience, 29*, 565–598.

Jaeggi, S. M., Buschkuehl, M., Etienne, A., Ozdoba, C., Perrig, W. J., & Nirkko, A. C. (2007). On how high performers keep cool brains in situations of cognitive overload. *Cognitive Affective and Behavioral Neuroscience, 7*(2), 75–89.

James, C., Davis, K., Charmaraman, L., Konrath, S., Slovak, P., Weinstein, E., & Yarosh, L.

(2017). Digital life and youth well-being, social connectedness, empathy, and narcissism. *Pediatrics, 140*(Suppl.), S71–S75.

Kanai, R., Bahrami, B., Roylance, R., & Rees, G. (2012). Online social network size is reflected in human brain structure. *Proceedings of the Royal Society B: Biological Sciences, 279*, 1327–1334.

Kandel, E. R, Dudai, Y., & Mayford, M. R. (2014). The molecular and systems biology of memory. *Cell, 157*, 163–186.

Katz, B., Shah, P., & Meyer, D. (2018). How to play 20 questions with nature and lose: Reflections on 100 years of brain-training research. *Proceedings of the National Academy of Sciences, 115*, 9897–9904.

Katz, L. C., & Shatz, C. J. (1996). Synaptic activity and the construction of cortical circuits. *Science, 274*, 1133–1138.

Kerr, M., & Symons, S. (2006). Computerized presentation of text: Effects on children's reading of informational material. *Reading and Writing, 19*, 1–19.

Klingberg, T. (2010). Training and plasticity of working memory. *Trends in Cognitive Science, 14*, 317–324.

Korte, M., & Schmitz, D. (2016). Cellular and system biology of memory: Timing, molecules, and beyond. *Physiological Reviews, 96*, 647–693.

Kuhn, S., Lorenz, R. C, Weichenberger, M., Becker, M., Haesner, M., O'Sullivan, J., et al. (2017). Taking control! Structural and behavioural plasticity in response to game-based inhibition training in older adults. *Neuroimage, 156*, 199–206.

Lahiry, S., Choudhury, S., Chatterjee, S., & Hazra, A. (2019). Impact of social media on academic performance and interpersonal relation: A cross-sectional study among students at a tertiary medical center in East India. *Journal of Education and Health Promotion, 8*, 73.

Lara, A. H., & Wallis, J. D. (2015). The role of prefrontal cortex in working memory: A mini review. *Frontiers in Systems Neuroscience, 9*, Article 173.

Magee, J. C., & Grienberger, C. (2020). Synaptic plasticity forms and functions. *Annual Review Neuroscience, 8*, 43–95.

Maguire, E. A., Gadian, D. G., Johnsrude, I. S., Good, C. D., Ashburner, J., Frackowiak, R. S., & Frith, C. D. (2000). Navigation-related structural change in the hippocampi of taxi drivers [see comments]. *Proceedings of the National Academy of Sciences, 97*, 4398–4403.

Makin, S. (2018). Searching for digital technology's effects on well-being. *Nature, 563*, S138–S140.

Malik, A. N., Tariq, H., Afridi, A., & Rathore, F. A. (2022). Technological advancements in stroke rehabilitation. *Journal of the Pakinstan Medical Association, 72*, 1672–1674.

Mangen, A., Olivier, G., & Velay J. L. (2019). Comparing comprehension of a long text read in print book and on kindle: Where in the text and when in the story. *Frontiers in Psychology, 10*, 38.

Martin, S. J., Grimwood, P. D., & Morris, R. G. (2000). Synaptic plasticity and memory: An evaluation of the hypothesis. *Annual Review Neuroscience, 23*, 649–711.

Medeiros-Ward, N., Watson, J. M., & Strayer, D. L. (2015). On supertaskers and the neural basis of efficient multitasking. *Psychonomic Bulletin and Review, 22*(3), 876–883.

Meshi, D., Tamir, D. I., & Heekeren, H. R. (2015) The emerging neuroscience of social media. *Trends of Cognitive Science, 19*, 771–782.

Mishkin, M., Ungerleider, L. G., & Macko, K. A. (1983). Object vision and spatial vision: Two cortical pathways. *Trends of Neurosciences, 6*, 414–417.

Moisala, M., Salmela, V., Hietajarvi, L., Salo, E., Carlson, S., Salonen, O., et al. (2016).

Media multitasking is associated with distractibility and increased prefrontal activity in adolescents and young adults. *NeuroImage, 134*, 113–121.

Nudo, R. J., Milliken, G. W., Jenkins, W. M., & Merzenich, M. M. (1996). Use-dependent alterations of movement representations in primary motor cortex of adult squirrel monkeys. *Journal of Neuroscience, 16*, 785–807.

Ophir, E., Nass, C., & Wagner, A. D. (2009). Cognitive control in media multitaskers. *Proceedings of the National Academy of Sciences, 106*, 15583–15587.

Pallavicini, F., Ferrari, A., & Mantovani, F. (2018). Video games for well-being: A systematic review on the application of computer games for cognitive and emotional training in the adult population. *Frontiers in Psychology, 9*, 2127.

Pantev, C., Engelien, A., Candia, V., & Elbert, T. (2001). Representational cortex in musicians. Plastic alterations in response to musical practice. *Annals of the New York Academy of Sciences, 930*, 300–314.

Pfeifer, J. H., & Blakemore, S. J. (2012). Adolescent social cognitive and affective neuroscience: Past, present, and future. *Social Cognitive and Affective Neuroscience, 7*, 1–10.

Ram, N., Yang, X., Cho, M-J., Brinberg, M., Muirhead, F., Reeves, B., & Robinson, T. N. (2019). Screenomics: A new approach for observing and studying individuals' digital lives. *Journal of Adolescent Research, 35*, 16–50.

Reeves, B., Robinson, T., & Ram, N. (2020). Time for the human screenome project. *Nature, 577*, 314–317.

Rehbein, F., Kliem, S., Baier, D., Mossle, T., & Petry, N. M. (2015). Prevalence of Internet gaming disorder in German adolescents: Diagnostic contribution of the nine DSM-5 criteria in a state-wide representative sample. *Addiction, 110*, 842–851.

Rogers, R. D., & Monsell, S. (1995). Costs of a predictible switch between simple cognitive tasks. *Journal of Experimental Psychology: General, 124*(2), 207.

Sajikumar, S., Morris, R. G., & Korte, M. (2014). Competition between recently potentiated synaptic inputs reveals a winner-take-all phase of synaptic tagging and capture. *Proceedings of the National Academy of Sciences, 111*, 12217–12221.

Shah, T. M., Weinborn, M., Verdile, G., Sohrabi, H. R., & Martins, R. N. (2017). Enhancing cognitive functioning in healthly older adults: A systematic review of the clinical significance of commercially available computerized cognitive training in preventing cognitive decline. *Neuropsychology Review, 27*, 62–80.

Sun, W., Liu, Z., Jiang, X., Chen, M. B., Dong, H., Liu, J., et al. (2024). Spatial transcriptomics reveal neuron-astrocyte synergy in long-term memory. *Nature, 627*, 374–381

Swing, E. L., Gentile, D. A., Anderson, C. A., & Walsh, D. A. (2010). Television and video game exposure and the development of attention problems. *Pediatrics, 126*, 214–221.

Takeuchi, T., Duszkiewicz, A. J., & Morris, R. G. (2014). The synaptic plasticity and memory hypothesis: Encoding, storage and persistence. *Philosophical Transactions of the Royal Society of London. Series B, Biological Sciences, 369*, 20130288.

Tan, B., Browne, C. J., Nobauer, T., Vaziri, A., Friedman, J. M., & Nestler, E. J. (2024). Drugs of abuse hijack a mesolimbic pathway that processes homeostatic need. *Science, 384*, eadk6742.

Turkle, S. (2011). *Alone together: Why we expect more from technology and less from each other.* Basic Books.

Uncapher, M. R., Lin, L., Rosen, L. D., Kirkorian, H. L., Baron, N. S., Bailey, K., et al. (2017). Media multitasking and cognitive, psychological, neural, and learning differences. *Pediatrics, 140*(Suppl.), S62–S66.

Watson, J. M., & Strayer, D. L. (2010). Supertaskers: Profiles in extraordinary multitasking ability. *Psychonomic Bulletin and Review, 17*(4), 479–485.

Webster, E. K., Martin, C. K., & Staiano, A. E. (2019). Fundamental motor skills, screen-time, and physical activity in preschoolers. *Journal of Sport and Health Science, 8*, 114–121.

Wolf, M., Ullman-Shade, C., & Gottwald, S. (2012). The emerging, evolving reading brain in a digital culture: Implications for new readers, children with reading difficulties, and children without schools. *Journal of Cognitive Education and Psychology, 11*(3), 230–240.

Yao, Y. W., Liu, L., Ma, S. S., Shi, X. H., Zhou, N., Zhang, J. T., & Potenza, M. N. (2017). Functional and structural neural alterations in Internet gaming disorder: A systematic review and meta-analysis. *Neuroscience & Biobehavioral Reviews, 83*, 313–324.

Yuste, R., & Bonhoeffer, T. (2001). Morphological changes in dendritic spines associated with long-term synaptic plasticity. *Annual Review of Neuroscience, 24*, 1071–1089.

CHAPTER 15

Concluding Thoughts on Neuroplasticity

Jordan Grafman and Paolo Nichelli

This volume contains chapters identifying the major forms of neuroplasticity that can be studied and promoted in healthy human volunteers and patients after brain damage. Besides the various electroencephalographic and functional imaging methods used in humans, the neurophysiological processes that underlie plasticity continue to be studied in animals at the level of synaptic physiology and ultrastructure after repeated stimulation.

There is evidence that neuronal differentiation and synaptic remodeling occur well into adulthood in animals and perhaps in humans. For example, neurogenesis in adulthood appears to occur in both the hippocampus and selected regions within the cerebral cortex. It is unclear what functional role new neurons play in previously existing networks. Perhaps they contribute to the enrichment of neural connectivity in brain regions most active during learning, such as the hippocampus. Neurogenesis and synaptic remodeling would be ideal mechanisms to assist brain regions partially damaged by brain injury and other lesions to recover their functions. However, because recovery of function after brain injury is rarely, if ever, complete, their contributions to recovery of function may be restricted by cortical space constraints on the emergence of new neurons and damage to the pathways by which neural precursors access damaged areas. On a larger scale, from a phylogenetic standpoint, the rapid development of technology, which allows new ways to promote access to human knowledge (e.g., the internet and artificial intelligence), is likely to induce changes in cortical specialization and brain functional connectivity.

Fundamental questions about how plasticity induces functional cooperation between brain regions can be asked. Why does the ability to shift functions between sites decline over development and aging? This may be the result of the necessity to stabilize connectivity between maturing brain areas dedicated to distinctive functional computations. The increasing degree and stability of this connectivity suggests that the networks themselves are committed to a particular functional representation. If functional substitution was permitted beyond the early stages of the formation of these networks, then continuous and substantial reorganization of distributed networks would be required for their efficient operation. Therefore, it is likely that the increasing connectivity required for learning is directly related to the increasing functional commitment of brain areas throughout life. A second question about plasticity emerges from the observation of cross-modal activation of the primary visual cortex in the early blind. Traditional notions about deafferentation lead one to expect atrophy and/or "denervation hypersensitivity" of a maladaptive kind in the visual areas of the blind. Instead, evidence suggests that the modality-independent processing capabilities of the visual cortex (e.g., discrimination of width, angles, and feature conjunctions) can be used to process spatial information from more than one sensory source. This is a remarkable departure from the idea that cortical functions are assigned to areas entirely based on input routing, rather than processing architecture.

Clinical approaches to enhancing recovery of cognitive function in patients recovering from traumatic brain injury have historically been implemented in an atheoretical way. Early approaches relied simply on massed repetitive practice in various domains of function (e.g., memory, attention). More recent efforts at rehabilitation have begun to use treatments motivated by cognitive neuroscientific models of neuroplasticity. Despite this increasing sophistication, there have been too few clinical trials that included large numbers of subjects or adequate controls, and most rehabilitation studies have compared programs of stimulation with supposedly neutral interactions or to no intervention at all, rather than investigating the validity of specific interventions on specific outcomes. Furthermore, the therapeutic strategies used in these studies were not always developed with systems and cognitive neuroscience findings in mind, much less motivated by computational models of plasticity. Although some recent counterexamples exist, the rehabilitation field has often lagged behind other specialties in clinical neuroscience in adapting basic science findings to the clinic. Importantly, the patient must be motivated and engaged in research-derived efforts to improve their functioning. So, in tandem with procedures that are designed to improve and utilize neuroplastic mechanisms to accomplish functional goals, the application of rewards and reinforcement to motivating the patient to participate in neuroplasticity trials is critical to the success of the intervention.

Fortunately, many conceptual frameworks for neuroplasticity exist that could lead to optimal rehabilitation methods. We suggest that proven methods for inducing changes in the cortical topography at the network level and rerouting or unmasking latent input and output to the affected network should guide the development of new rehabilitation techniques for patients with brain injury. Testing of paradigms designed to cause and manipulate neuroplasticity in healthy volunteers and patients will help investigators find the key conditions for neuroplastic change. Such paradigms may also lead to "challenge" studies using pharmacological and other agents to enhance or prevent neuroplastic changes. Indeed, the future looks promising as we probe the limits of functional neuroplasticity in adult humans with brain injury while answering fundamental questions about the stable and dynamic topography of information processing.

Despite the promises of modern cognitive neuroscience techniques and theories, translational aspects of laboratory-based studies are critical since their implementation in a therapeutic environment may have limitations, and it is fair to wonder about their usefulness once a person returns home. This latter challenge will be critical along with determining whether the tradeoffs between the encouragement of positive changes in one function potentially compromises another function. As noted above, an important aspect of plasticity is rewarding patient engagement to optimize the utility and persistence of effort during training. Finally, given that learning and training programs often don't generalize, the targeting of the neuroplastic training will be critical if such training is to have notable effects, in general, on everyday life and responsibilities. Otherwise, the training toward a meaningful outcome for the patient must be considered. The rapidity of modern artificial intelligence methods will also aid neuroplasticity by providing, at a minimum, compensatory software to aid the patient in accomplishing their goals, taking into account learning rates, optimal learning strategies, and contextually relevant actions.

We hope that the chapters in this volume allow you, the reader, to have a broad, up-to-date introduction to many of the approaches used to facilitate plasticity in the brain, and we hope that you are stimulated to consider these approaches in your own research and practice.

Index

Note: *f* or *t* following a page number indicates a figure or table

B

C

D

E

F

G

H

I

Q

R

S

T

V